A Guide to Patient Recruitment

Today's Best Practices and Proven Strategies

Diana L. Anderson, Ph.D.

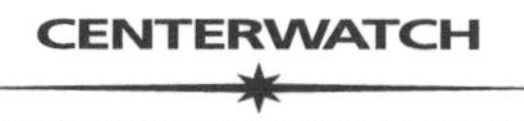

CenterWatch, Inc.
22 Thomson Place, 36T1
Boston, MA 02210
Phone: 617.856.5900
Fax: 617.856.5901
www.centerwatch.com

ISBN 1-930624-11-5

CenterWatch Book Editor: Whitney Allen
CenterWatch Publisher: Ken Getz
Design and Production: Liz Abbate
Printing: Innovative Printing Group, Inc.

Foreword

Patient recruitment in its true sense seems almost mystical. For example, why does one investigator site enroll consistently better than another, how do we measure the outcomes of recruitment initiatives, what works, what doesn't and why? These questions must and should be answered as pharmaceutical research becomes increasingly complex. There is an expected two- to three-fold increase in the number of chemical entities that will be discovered by 2005, and genomics will revolutionize the discovery process, making more candidate compounds available for evaluation than we could have dreamed of ten or even five years ago. These facts make it clear that we will need far more volunteers for clinical studies and that the field of patient recruitment, still in its infancy, must evolve to help take these discoveries forward.

A Guide to Patient Recruitment: The Best Practices and Proven Strategies is an effort to begin to build a body of knowledge based on outcome data in the area of recruiting and retaining subjects in clinical trials. Leading experts in the field have generously shared their knowledge for this book. I believe it is fair to say that this information previously has not been captured elsewhere. Each chapter covers information that will help guide the reader. This text will serve as a manual in planning, developing and implementing strategies for successful recruitment based on actual metrics.

In addition, I am hopeful this information will serve to convince sponsors of the importance of evaluating the potential of well planned patient recruitment strategies and understanding how the increasing amounts spent in this area are being utilized.

—Diana L. Anderson

Table of Contents

TABLE OF CONTENTS (continued)

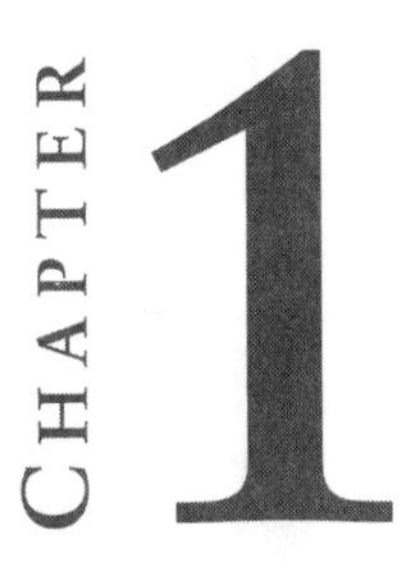

Professionalizing The Process of Patient Recruitment: A History and Overview of Today's Issues

Diana L. Anderson, Ph.D.; Rheumatology Research International

INTRODUCTION

Well-planned initiatives aimed at accelerating patient enrollment in clinical trials are key to the clinical development process. The need for active recruitment efforts stems from the fact that new clinical research starts for pharmaceuticals are rising, and commercial investigational new drug (IND) submissions have been growing steadily over the past few years.[1] (Table One) Additionally, the number of subjects per NDA currently averages 3,900 and is growing by 7% annually. European averages are about the same.[2] But the most promising investigational compounds cannot move forward unless there are enough subjects available for testing. As technological advances lead to pipelines rich with new chemical entities (NCE), sponsors will face the growing challenge of identifying patients who will enroll and complete the resulting clinical trials, which currently number in the range of 50,000 to 60,000 annually.[3] And as sponsors continue outsourcing study conduct activities, investigative sites are assuming more responsibility for enrollment.

Data from 400 clinical trials suggest that patient enrollment represents 22.3%, nearly one-quarter of the entire clinical development

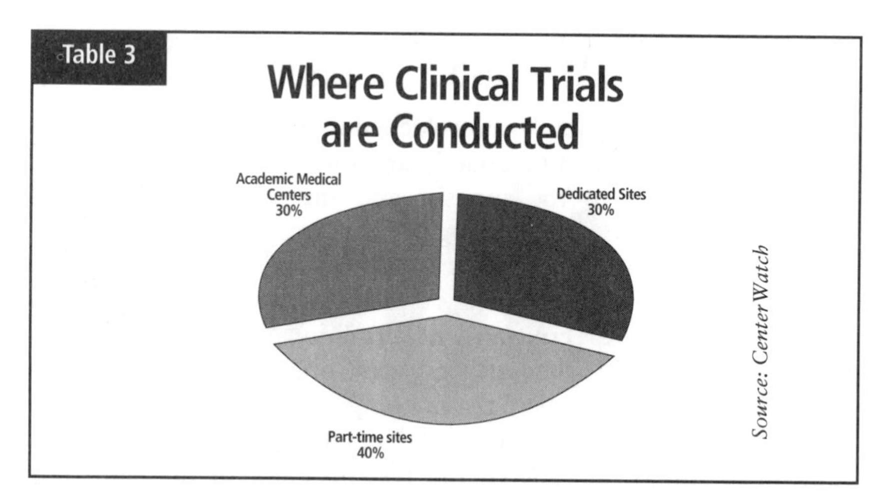

by staff dedicated for this purpose.[5] Since then, a diversity of techniques has emerged including use of proprietary patient databases, centralized call centers, centralized recruitment campaigns and web-based recruiting.

RECRUITMENT TODAY

In less than a decade, there have been remarkable changes in approaches to patient recruitment. At major SMOs, larger independent sites and patient recruitment companies, rudimentary recruiting methods have given way to the development of professional, well-organized strategies led by staff dedicated to recruitment efforts. At the same time, today's sponsors generally understand the need for additional funds to support patient recruitment initiatives outside of the medical practice. In fact, they are now investing significant resources in patient recruiting. This is an important shift in mindset because evidence suggests that approximately two-thirds of enrolling patients are self-referred.[6] That is, they have responded to external recruitment efforts, as opposed to having been referred by their physicians, who may be investigators for studies of interest.

The study conduct market is highly fragmented, and the vast majority of sites are neither SMO-affiliated, nor large enough to justify a study recruiter. In fact, according to CenterWatch, a U.S. based publishing and information service for the clinical trials industry, part-time sites account for approximately 40% of all study conduct dollars. (Table Three) So, the reality is that even today, many sites do not conduct enough clinical trials to justify development of sophisticated patient recruitment systems at the site level.

One way to address this issue is through the use of professional recruitment groups, fairly new players on the clinical trials scene.* These companies can structure entire recruitment campaigns, including the design and placement of advertising, detailed follow-up and fine-tuning the strategy as the project unfolds. Also, professional recruitment companies typically have databases of patients to access for direct mail activity.

The use of patient databases as a source of potential study subjects is a strategy under scrutiny. Simply possessing a large database does not necessarily translate into an understanding of clinical trials, nor an ability to identify appropriate patients for a therapeutic-specific recruitment program. For example, how would a professional recruiting organization identify a group of potential patients in its database who might qualify for an osteoarthritis study? What about for a rheumatoid arthritis study? Is the company's database designed to differentiate between these two forms of arthritis?

The point is that large numbers of general responders do not guarantee appropriate candidates. For example, identifying 30,000 people in a database who claim to have arthritis does not mean that there will be enough candidates to fulfill a study commitment to enroll 150 patients in a Phase III rheumatoid arthritis study being conducted at ten sites. To be a useful recruiting tool for difficult-to-enroll studies, a database should be refined to the point that it can select relatively pre-qualified potential patients, given specific parameters. Also, it should not be the sole source of potential patients. Good patient recruitment firms know that use of the database is only part of larger, more diversified strategies that are therapeutic-specific.

It is worth mentioning that issues surrounding patient database ownership are being discussed frequently. There are legitimate concerns, as well as legal ones, about the confidentiality of the information contained within them, and who will have access to it. John Isidor, an attorney, and CEO of Schulman Associates, a central IRB, says, "Contracts need to be created to determine to whom a database belongs." He also suggests that when potential subjects are being pre-screened for studies, they should be advised as to what may be done with the confidential information that is provided during the pre-screen. When Web sites are internal patient databases to satisfy enrollment targets. If enrollment from this patient population database does not fulfill enrollment projections, sites often turn to print, radio or television advertising. With this approach comes the creation of materials designed to advertise the study.

Prior to publishing or airing recruitment advertisements, the site or recruitment vendor must submit the material to the study's selected IRB for review. Until the late 1990s, IRBs generally reviewed this collateral at no charge, but this practice changed by the end of the decade. Starting at that time, a number of large independent and academic IRBs began charging fees to review this material if submitted after the initial package, containing the investigator brochure and protocol. John Isidor, of Schulman Associates, explains that the need to charge reflects the tremendous increase in the number of advertising materials submitted for review, and the requisite increase in time needed to conduct these reviews. "We started to get a voluminous amount of recruitment materials submitted after the initial package. Some were easy to review, but many were time-consuming because they made specific reference to inclusion/exclusion criteria and other items that required revisiting the protocol to determine their accuracy." At the time of this writing, Schulman Associates does not charge an additional fee to review patient recruitment materials if they are submitted as part of the initial regulatory package.

Table 5 **Sample Fees to Review One Patient Recruitment Advertisement Submitted After the Initial Review**

$100 per piece X 50 investigators=$5000

Doing some forward thinking can translate into significant savings in IRB fees. For example, the fee that an IRB charges to review one advertising piece submitted after the initial regulatory package may exceed $100 per investigator per piece.[7] Therefore, if an SMO develops two advertisements, and that SMO has three investigators participating in a study, IRB fees to review the two advertisements may be more than $600, i.e., (two pieces X $100 per piece) X (three investigators). The fees can add up quickly if a central IRB is reviewing materials for a fifty-site study using fifty investigators. (Table Five) Those same marketing materials would have been reviewed at no additional charge had they been submitted with the initial package. In negotiating the patient recruitment budget, recruitment groups need to make sponsors aware of this change in IRB fee structure, since sponsors foot the bill.

PATIENT RECRUITMENT ETHICS

In May 1999, *The New York Times* ran two investigational articles highlighting questionable patient recruitment practices. The first story, "Drug Trials Hide Conflict for Doctors" was the result of a ten-month investigation. During this time period, *The New York Times* obtained thousands of confidential contacts between health care professionals and pharmaceutical sponsors, that suggests conflicts of interest, whereby researchers received cash for influencing patients to join clinical studies. The article also referred to documented cases of investigators receiving additional bonuses for being top recruiters or reaching enrollment targets ahead of schedule. According to the article, physicians who do not participate in a trial can receive finder's fees for making referrals to participating doctors.[8]

The second article, "A Doctor's Drug Studies Turn Into Fraud" describes the case of a California physician who was so dazzled by the large sums and accolades he earned for being a top enroller that he and his staff recruited patients with a zeal that can only be described as a most extreme example of fraud. Not only were there examples of coercion, but some patients' lives were endangered when the doctor refused to allow patients suffering adverse events to withdraw from trials. The doctor was sentenced to fifteen months in federal prison.[9]

These articles stirred up a controversy that resulted in two separate inquiries conducted by the Office of Inspector General (OIG) of the Department of Health and Human Services. Specifically, the first directive was to look at recruitment practices and research sponsored by the drug industry, and the second was to determine whether there is adequate oversight in place to detect possible fraud by clinical investigators. The first inquiry examined use of private doctors in research, and whether this creates conflicts of interest between the doctor's obligations to the patient and responsibilities to the drug company sponsoring the trial. OIG examined use of financial incentives to encourage doctors to accelerate patient recruitment, including payments made for each patient enrolled, and bonuses used to encourage trials in a particular therapeutic area are possibly more motivated to enter a trial than those who learn about studies in a passive manner, such as noticing a flyer in a doctor's waiting room or spotting an advertisement in the local newspaper." (Table Thirteen) He adds that Internet users are better educated, have higher household incomes and may have a higher likelihood of completing a study.

Table 13 **Therapeutic Areas Most Frequently Viewed On the CenterWatch Web Site**

Therapeutic Area	% of Trial Views
Oncology	20.5%
Gastroenterology	10.5%
Neurology	8.5%
Cardiology/Vascular	8.0%
Endocrinology	7.0%

Source: CenterWatch

One of the most important indicators of Internet efficacy is the number of Internet users seeking trial information who ultimately enter a trial as a result of that initial effort. Only about 8 to 10% of fifty million Americans suffering from chronic conditions have ever participated in a clinical trial. This is in direct contrast to visitors to CenterWatch's Web site, 23% of whom have been clinical subjects.[16] In 1998, CenterWatch conducted a survey of nearly 1400 individuals. Results showed that 63% of those visiting the CenterWatch Web site are interested in participating in clinical trials, and 38% of all patients viewing CenterWatch trial postings report contacting a research center. About half of clinical trials postings on the Internet are for phase III trials.[17] For further information on use of the Internet for patient recruitment, see Chapter Nine.

THE RELATIONSHIP BETWEEN PATIENT RECRUITMENT AND RETENTION

Patient recruitment is the precursor to patient retention. Felix Khin-Maung-Gyi, Pharm.D., CEO of an independent IRB comments that retention of patients in clinical trials is the result of various factors, all directly linked to the human interaction between the site and the potential patient. It starts from the very beginning with advertising that is to be simple, direct and non-coercive. Assuming the patient qualifies for the study, and wishes to enroll, the next step is the informed consent document. This form should provide sufficient and understandable information without being so lengthy and highly technical that the potential patient is too intimidated to sign it. Also, it should be well-presented by staff who are caring. If a patient does not understand the study, he is more likely to be disappointed and drop out.

Following enrollment and randomization, the patient has periodic contact with the site. Barring adverse reactions, this is where good interpersonal relations have a particular impact on retention. Clinical coordinators are often overstressed, and typically juggle the competing priorities of multiple studies. If the patient senses that the coordinator or other site professionals are rushing through a patient visit, or are indifferent, the patient may feel uncomfortable, and not want to return. Contrast this scenario with a positive experience, particularly if the patient is doing well on the study drug. That patient will be more inclined and motivated to remain in the study.

DataEdge, LLC, a data service for the pharmaceutical industry, reports that there are no data at this time to document how many enrolled patients stay in studies, but drop out rates correlate to specific therapeutic areas.[18] Patients in antibiotic studies, for example, tend to drop out because they start feeling better. However, in studies where the investigational drug is tantamount to disease treatment, such as cancer or HIV, the retention rate is higher.

To boost retention, sites can perform small gestures that yield big results, such as mailing reminder cards for upcoming appointments, or simply calling the day before the scheduled appointment.

GEOGRAPHIC NUANCES

As a global industry, pharmaceutical companies place studies in various countries, often simultaneously. Recruiting techniques must vary country to country, recognizing and respecting different regulations, and sensibilities. A case in point is the tale of an American-based SMO holding focus groups in Canada to gauge reactions to various magazine advertisements designed to recruit for a study for an investigational arthritis medication. This research turned up numerous findings, namely that recruitment advertisements in Canada should target Canadians. Referrals to U.S.-based investiga-

[7] Data from Rheumatology Research International presentation, "Ethical and IRB Issues in Patient Recruitment: Practical Suggestions and Guidelines." 1999.

[8] "Drug Trials Hide Conflicts for Doctors." *The New York Times*. Kurt Eichenwald and Gina Kolata. May 16, 1999.

[9] "A Doctor's Drug Studies Turn Into Fraud." *The New York Times*. Kurt Eichenwald and Gina Kolata. May 17, 1999.

[10] "U.S. Officials are Examining Clinical Trials." *The New York Times*. Kurt Eichenwald. July 14, 1999.

[11] *Recruiting Human Subjects: Pressure in Industry-Sponsored Clinical Research*. Office of Inspector General, OEI-01-97-00195. p. 2. June 2000.

[12] *Ibid.*, p. 4-5.

[13] *Institutional Review Boards, A Time for Reform*. Department of Health and Human Services, Office of Inspector General. OEI-01-97-00193. June 1998. p. 6.

[14] *Ibid.*, p. 3.

[15] *www.nielsen/netratings.com*, June 2000.

[16] "Surf's Up." *Applied Clinical Trials*. Kenneth Getz and Ann Kennon. May 1998. pp. 58-61.

[17] *Ibid.*, p. 59.

[18] Mark Hovde, President of DataEdge LLC.

AUTHOR BIOGRAPHY

Diana L. Anderson, Ph.D., is the President and Chief Executive Officer of Rheumatology Research International. RRI provides contract research, site management services, communications and custom publishing exclusively in the field of rheumatology. In her role as CEO, Dr. Anderson has lead RRI to become the only comprehensive provider of rheumatology services.

Dr. Anderson previously served as Chief of Operations for Metroplex Clinical Research Center (currently Radiant Research, Dallas), a large multi-specialty investigator site. She has also held positions in marketing and administration in hospital based settings.

She has been and continues to be a leader and innovator in the area of patient recruitment in clinical trials and has spoken and published extensively both nationally and internationally in the area of patient recruitment. In addition, she is the author of the book "50 Ways to Cope with Arthritis," in its second printing.

Her vision for the ongoing growth and professionalism of the field of patient recruitment has recently been focused on the goal of developing a body of knowledge specific to patient recruitment. This text, "A Guide to Patient Recruitment: Today's Best Practices and Proven Strategies," is the beginning of that vision.

Dr. Anderson has contributed to many professional organizations in the areas of rheumatology and clinical research. She is currently a Board member of Rheumatology Research International and the Association of Clinical Research Professionals. She has also served on the Boards of the American College of Rheumatology, Association of Rheumatology Health Professionals and the National Arthritis Association.

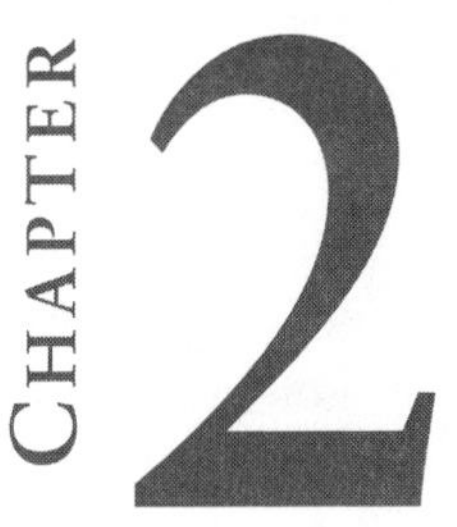

Benchmarking the Process of Patient Recruitment: Practices and Behaviors in the Current Recruitment Climate

Kenneth A. Getz, CenterWatch

Every year, several million people participate in clinical trials to support new drug applications (NDAs) submitted to the Food and Drug Administration. This level of participation represents less than 10% of the more than sixty million people who have severe, life-threatening and chronic illnesses in the United States.[1] It would seem relatively easy to find and retain highly motivated study participants from this population for NDA submissions. But that is hardly the case.

At present, the majority (nearly 80%) of clinical trials conducted in the United States must extend enrollment by at least one month beyond the study completion period.[2] This results in significant direct costs for the study sponsor. Extended enrollment periods can also cause delays in new product introductions—a substantially higher cost that is due to missed market opportunity. Nearly two-thirds of investigative sites feel that the challenges of patient recruitment and retention are becoming more difficult.[3]

The goal of this chapter is to present data that capture the current climate for patient recruitment. Several key issues are posed to frame data that are based on primary and secondary sources recently published in major trade and peer-reviewed journals.

NUMBERS OF PATIENTS WHO VOLUNTEER AND ENROLL IN CLINICAL TRIALS ANNUALLY

An estimated 45,000 to 60,000 phase I to III protocols are conducted annually in the United States. An average of sixteen patients is required to complete a protocol, across all therapeutic areas and phases I to III. In total, between 750,000 to 900,000 study subjects will complete clinical trials for new drug applications (NDAs)—many of which will be submitted to the Food and Drug Administration.[4]

The largest numbers of subjects are needed for phase III programs. Seven out of ten study subjects—also called evaluable patients—need to be recruited to support phase III programs for an NDA submission. Slightly less than one in five will be recruited for phase II programs. And 10% of total evaluable patients per NDA will be part of phase I studies.[5]

However, most estimates of total study subjects in annual clinical trials fail to capture the much higher numbers of patients that must be drawn into clinical trials in order to yield the required number of subject completions. For example, for every patient who completes

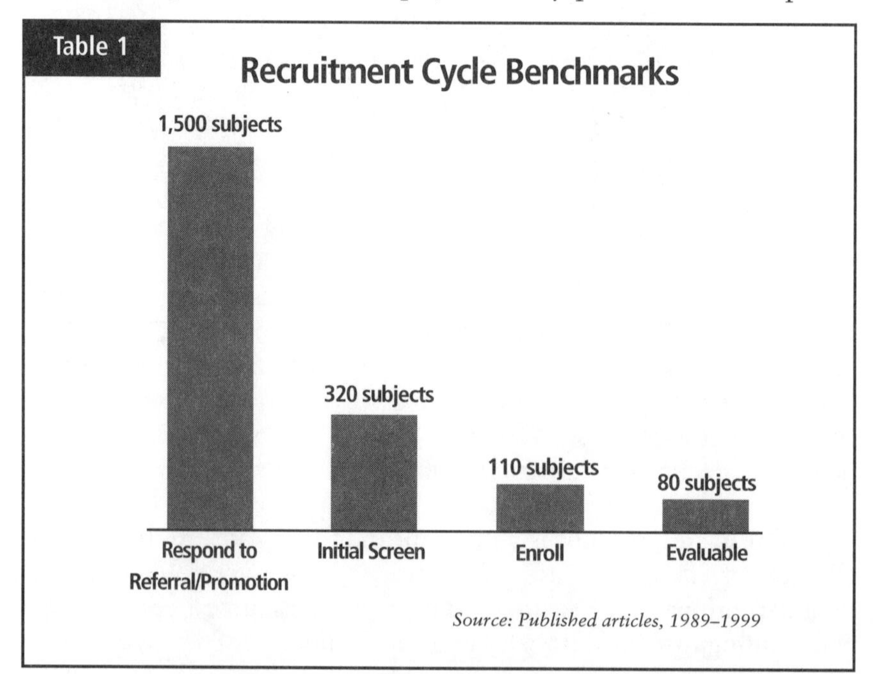

Source: Published articles, 1989–1999

a phase I to III clinical trial, three other patients will have an initial screening but will fail to be randomized or then drop out after randomization (see Table One).

These conversion rates are an aggregation of data from published articles and more than twenty case studies between 1989 and 2000.[6] And, these rates are conservative. Several recent studies suggest that fewer patients are responding to recruitment promotions and fewer still are now completing clinical trials. Using the benchmark conversion rates in Table One, an estimated 2.8 million to 3.6 million people participate in industry-sponsored clinical trials annually. In other words, each year, several million individuals make a conscious decision, and make the effort, to take part in an initial screening with study staff to determine eligibility.

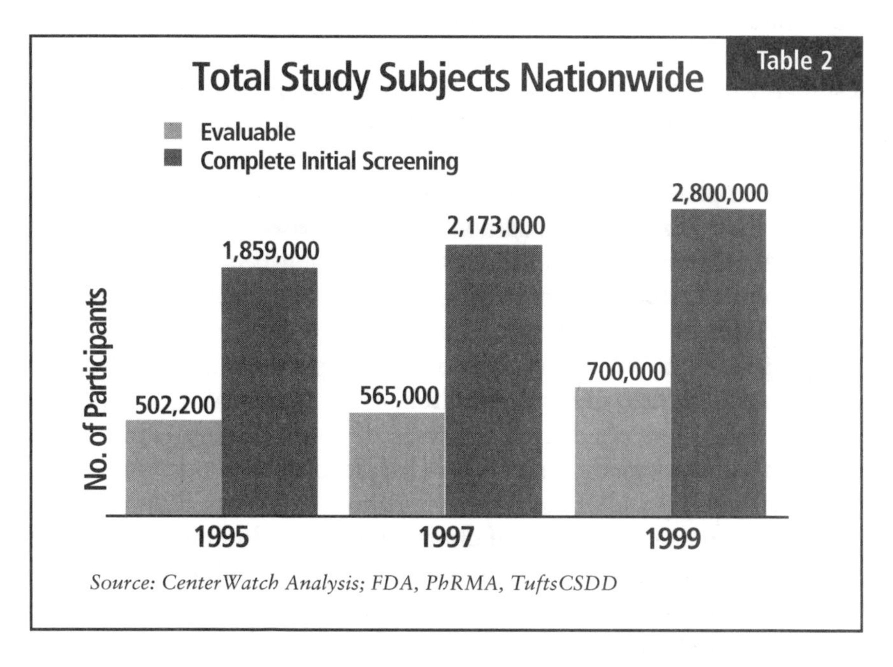

Source: CenterWatch Analysis; FDA, PhRMA, TuftsCSDD

These figures represent more than 14,000,000 people who were involved—albeit briefly—in clinical trials in 2000 (See Table Two).[7] This includes those individuals who contacted an investigative site as a result of a professional referral or who responded to a patient recruitment promotion or advertisement. This may reflect some duplication as certain individuals may be contacting investigative sites several times each year to learn about volunteer opportunities. Still, the figures illustrate the challenges of attempting to generate

underwent clinical observation over a forty-year period. Although the course of the disease was well-known and effective antibiotic therapy was available, no treatment was offered for thirty-three years.[16]

Tuskegee is only one barrier creating a more difficult recruitment climate among the Black community. Many minorities perceive that they are receiving health care attention that is sub par. Although an underlying premise of clinical research is that medical advances will benefit all members of the American public, many minority populations do not feel that they share equally in these benefits.[17]

Due to the lack of available data, it has long been believed that the typical study subject is male. Recently gathered data suggest otherwise. It now appears that the gender mix of study volunteers has been distributed equally since 1966.[18] In a recent October 2000 report published by *Controlled Clinical Trials*, the authors reviewed 100,000 clinical trials published in reputable journals including the *Lancet*, NEJM, JAMA and the *Annals of Internal Medicine* between 1966 and 1998. The authors found that 55% of clinical trials involved both men and women, 12% involved men only, and 11% involved women only. Approximately 21% of the published clinical trials did not specify gender. The authors also noted a higher incidence of male participants involved in cardiovascular studies, a disease that has been long mistakenly believed to affect men disproportionately. And, among cancer trials, women are two-and-a-half times more likely to have been enrolled than are men.

Whereas gender mix in clinical trials appears to be relatively balanced, there is no question that protocol designs have historically addressed disease as it manifests in adult males. During the past decade, public pressures have fueled stricter government requirements for gender-specific studies in both NIH and industry sponsored research projects. Pharmaceutical and biotechnology companies have also sought ways to increase the market potential for new and existing drugs by gathering clinical data to make specific claims about drug safety and effectiveness among women. As a result, clinical trials are increasingly being designed to assess gender-specific medical treatment safety and efficacy.

Another key characteristic of study subjects is that they are uniquely motivated to find and access new medical treatments. And, there is a great deal of data to support this characteristic. Of the three million people who participate in clinical trials in the United States, an estimated 40% receive their primary care from a staff-model HMO or managed care provider. More than 70% of the U.S. population receives its primary care through a managed care network.[19] Still, study volunteers are expressing a high motivation level as they are stepping outside their health care network, often without the permission of their primary care physician or nurse.

There has been a dramatic shift in study participant self-referral behavior. In a survey conducted among several hundred patients in 1995, only one-third of patients said that they self-referred into a clinical trial. Their physician or nurse referred them to a clinical trial nearly two-thirds of the time. In 1999, 58% of patients said they self-refer into a clinical trial and less than 40% said that their physician or nurse had referred them.[20]

Clinical research coordinators, clinical investigators and study staff strongly agree that today's patients are more informed about their medical conditions and their treatment options. Driven in large part by health care reform during the past decade, patients are less trusting of a single medical opinion. And patients and their advocates want to take more responsibility for their treatment decisions. However, motivation to seek out information about treatment options has not extended rapidly into the clinical research arena. With the exception of those patients with the most severe and life-threatening illnesses, most people do not readily consider clinical research a treatment option. And their providers of primary and specialized health services—again with the exception of severe, life-threatening illnesses—typically do not suggest or recommend clinical trial participation.

In a survey conducted in 2000 among 1,000 people, 77% said they have never spoken with their physician or nurse about participating in clinical trials.[21] Only one in five patients (22%) have. These findings suggest a major opportunity for the NIH and industry to educate patients, the general public and health professionals on the value and the risks and benefits of clinical research participation.

HOW POTENTIAL STUDY PARTICIPANTS IDENTIFY CLINICAL TRIAL OPPORTUNITIES

Investigative sites have traditionally turned to the following approaches in order to identify potential study subjects: Chart review, walk-ins, professional referrals, phone screens, study notices and bulletins and direct mail to patients and physician practices. During the past decade, investigative sites have also dramatically increased their use of the mass media to reach prospective volunteers, newspaper ads, radio advertising, television and more recently, the Internet. These strategies are covered in depth throughout this book.

Interestingly, recruitment approaches vary by investigative site type. And, the recruitment approaches used by investigative sites have a direct impact on the type of volunteer enrolled in clinical trials (see Table Three). Traditional investigative sites (i.e., major medical centers and part-time sites) rely more heavily on their own patients or on physician referral. More than 70% of major medical centers, for example, say that their study subjects come from internal sources, including physician faculty and affiliated physician networks.

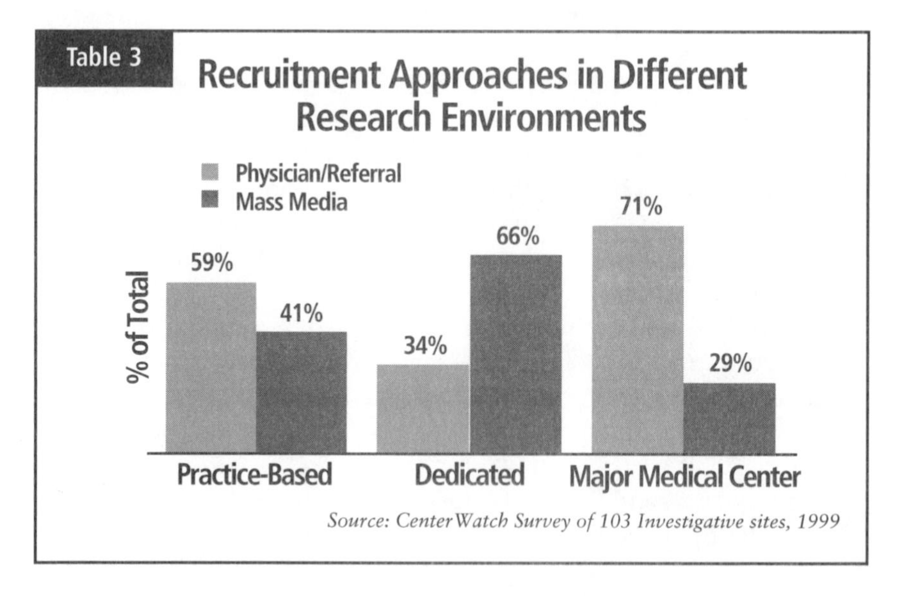

Source: CenterWatch Survey of 103 Investigative sites, 1999

Part-time sites, investigative sites that derive revenue from both clinical practice and clinical trials, report a mix of approaches that favor the patient community that they directly serve. These traditional study conduct providers tend to attract a larger percentage of patients from actual use settings where patients are seen and treated by their primary care or specialty care providers.

Dedicated investigative sites, including many that are site management organizations, are research centers sites that derive almost 100%

of their revenue from clinical trial activities—relying heavily on mass media advertising and promotion to find study subjects. Certain dedicated sites maintain a full-time staff of principal investigators and study coordinators. In these instances, study volunteers are often seen only during a clinical trial and not in an actual use setting.

Ultimately, the variability in patient recruitment approaches across investigative site environments raises issues about where sponsors and CROs should place their clinical trials and the amount of dollars that should be budgeted for patient recruitment approaches. This variability in recruitment behavior across investigative site types extends beyond the United States. The use of mass media for patient recruitment is growing in parts of Europe as well.[22]

Today, patients still prefer to gather their general health and medical information from their physician or nurse. In a survey of 1,000 people in the United States:

- 38% of respondents said they turn to their doctor or nurse for health information;
- One out of four (26%) respondents browse the Internet for this information;
- Approximately one in five (19%) refer to the newspaper or other mass media for health-related information; and
- Less than 5% turn to a friend for health information.[23]

In the same survey, the vast majority of people (85%) felt that it is very important that their doctor or nurse get involved/or refer them to a clinical research program. Yet, as mentioned earlier, only 22% of the general public reports that their doctor or nurse ever mentions clinical trials as a treatment consideration.

The above statistics touch on sources for general health information. Another recent survey looked specifically at where patients learn about clinical trials.[24] This data is skewed toward individuals who completed a clinical trial within the past year:

- Almost half of study subjects (46%) said that a physician or nurse actually referred them to the trial;
- One third (35%) of study volunteers said they learned about a trial through mass media venues--newspapers, TV, radio, magazines and press releases;

- Less than one in ten study subjects reported that they first learned of a clinical trial through the Internet; and
- Approximately 2% of study subjects reported that they learned of a clinical trial through cold calls that originated from a research center.

When an individual learns about a clinical trial, they are most likely to call the research center by telephone, with 70% choosing to do so. One in five (19%) prefer to show up at a research center in person. At present, 10% prefer to contact a center by e-mail.[25]

MOTIVATORS OF CLINICAL TRIAL PARTICIPATION

Based on a survey of more than 1,000 study volunteers who had completed phase II and III clinical trials within the past year, the largest percentage (60%) of study subjects get involved to find a more effective treatment.[26] Approximately one in four study volunteers get involved for altruistic reasons—they hope to advance science. Only 11% of study subjects say they become involved primarily to earn extra money. And less than one in ten (6%) volunteer to participate in order to receive better medical care and for help covering the cost of therapy (Table Four). These findings are consistent with the results of similar surveys conducted in the early 1990s.

Interestingly, a high percentage—61%—of the general public say that they would likely get involved in a clinical trial. In this survey of 1,000 U.S. residents, 96% said that they do perceive value in clinical research. However, in a recent Harris Interactive poll of several

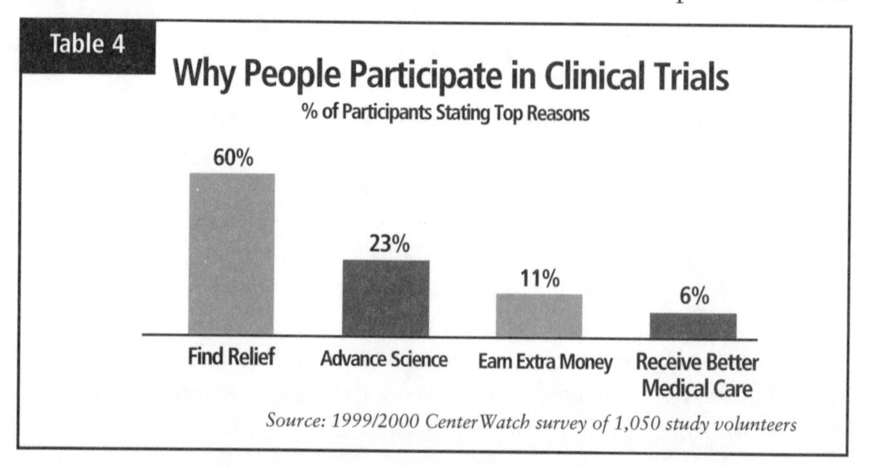

thousand Americans, of patients who are aware of a suitable clinical trial, most, 71%, choose not to participate.[27]

There are similar results with Internet-based listings of clinical trials. At present, only an estimated 34% of individuals follow up with investigative sites when they find an appropriate clinical trial listing on the CenterWatch web site. In a recent survey, the top reason why people choose not to participate has to do with study design (Table Five). The most frequently mentioned concern, by nearly half of 1,050 respondents, is fear of receiving a placebo instead of the active drug.

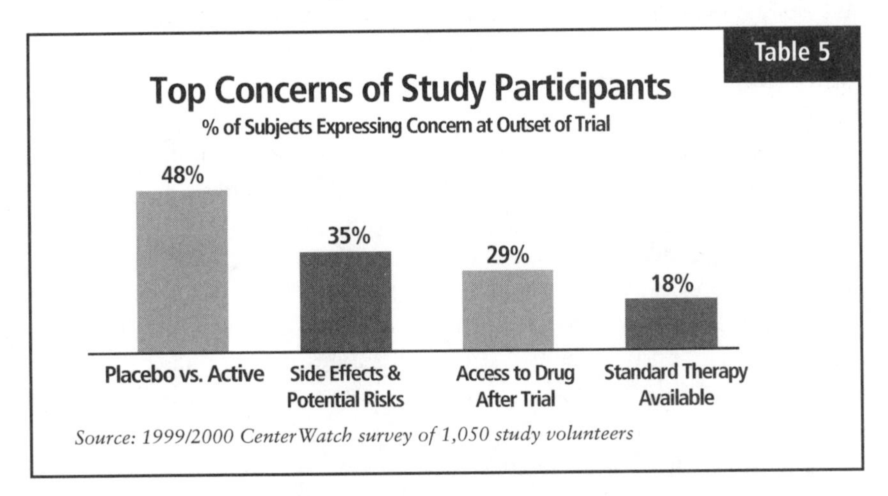

Source: 1999/2000 CenterWatch survey of 1,050 study volunteers

INDUSTRY SPENDING TO FACILITATE PATIENT RECRUITMENT

It is estimated that combined, sponsors, CROs and sites spent $375 million in 2000 on patient recruitment activities. This represents less than 5% of total clinical development spending.[28]

Based on surveys of several hundred investigative sites, an estimated $215 million is directly allocated by the investigative sites for the purposes of patient recruitment.[29] This figure does not include the costs of routine personnel and overhead. This figure represents spending for marketing programs—typically local promotional programs including flyers, outreach initiatives, mailings and limited mass media activities. Investigative sites report that they spend approximately 6% of every study grant on patient recruitment promotion.[30]

While it is true that sponsors are paying larger than average grants-per-study to investigative sites, increased grant spending is not the result of rising costs-per-patient. Cost-per-patient has risen less than 5% annually from approximately $4,500 in fees-per-patient in 1990 to $6,500 in 1999. When adjusted for inflation, the cost-per-patient has been essentially flat. This suggests that investigative sites are conducting a growing number of procedures per patient for less average funding per procedure.[31]

The amount paid to investigative sites, when adjusted for inflation, is hardly rising, meaning that at the same time that recruitment is becoming more difficult, sites are doing more with less. Study costs are rising because more procedures are being performed on each study volunteer. This factor is contributing to increased difficulty in study subject compliance and retention.

Pharmaceutical and CRO companies spend an additional $175 to $200 million directly on mass media patient recruitment promotions for phase I to III programs.[32] Much of this spending is allocated to advertising agencies to cover large regional and national campaigns to support patient recruitment programs. A portion of sponsor and CRO spending may also be going to investigative sites as remedial support. As a result, sponsors and CRO spending on patient recruitment may include some duplication of investigative site spending.

The vast majority (93%) of investigative sites report that they rely on their study coordinator(s) for most patient recruitment responsibilities. Yet study coordinators, busy running most daily research study activities, are typically not trained to manage large marketing and promotional programs. Less than one in three (28%) investigative sites report that they depend on administrative support to direct patient recruitment initiatives.[33] Only 13% of investigative sites report having a dedicated patient recruitment specialist. This is an interesting and concerning fact given that investigative sites and sponsors strongly agree that patient enrollment rates are the single largest determinant of repeat business.

SUMMARY

The data presented in this chapter provide a snapshot of the current climate for patient recruitment. In closing, it is important to note that there are numerous forces, countering one another, that have the potential to dramatically change the nature of patient recruitment.

For example, clinical projects are more ambitious today than ever before. Several seminal studies have been recently published that document the rising number of clinical studies per new drug application (NDA), the growth in the number of procedures performed per protocol and the increasing numbers of study subjects required per NDA.

Drug pipelines are also growing at a faster rate given the impact of new drug discovery technologies including high throughput screening, combinatorial chemistry, and pharmacogenomics. In 1993, there were an estimated 4,000 projects in the drug development pipeline. In 2000, that number has almost doubled.[34] The number of new drugs entering this pipeline is projected to grow by 12% annually during the next five years. This is almost twice the growth rate of new drugs entering the pipeline during the past five years.

There is significant pressure on pharmaceutical companies to increase their development productivity and to improve the performance of drugs once they enter the market. Industry observers expect sponsor companies to invest far more heavily in the coming years to improve the patient recruitment process during clinical development in order to gather more data about investigational treatments and to prime the market, to engage more physician prescribers, prior to product launch. The patient recruitment process has historically been the largest single cause of delays in clinical development.

A number of factors cause recruitment difficulties. For example, protocols may be too stringent, resulting in eligibility requirements that exclude too many. Protocols may be too demanding. And as a result, patient volunteers are asked to contribute more than is reasonable to subject themselves to unpleasant and invasive procedures. There may be too many trials competing for the same patients. Or, clinical trials may be competing with medical therapies that, although not ideal, are effective enough to diminish interest in accessing a therapy that is only available through clinical trial participation. Lastly, potential study subjects may associate a high level of risk with participating in clinical trials. To date, NIH and industry have not effectively educated the general public about the importance of clinical research. Doing so would benefit all parties involved in the clinical trial process—patients, health professionals and clinical research professionals.

Several process and technology changes are addressing some of the difficulties described above. As a result, we may eventually see a decline in the number of evaluable patients per NDA; a decrease in the number of procedures per clinical trial; and a decline in the number of studies per NDA.

Over time, electronic data management technologies may make it easier to target specific patient populations. Electronic data management technologies may also arm study sponsors and staff with real-time abilities to monitor and improve clinical trial performance. The Internet may become a more viable distribution channel to reach potential study subjects. And, this approach may offer cost advantages over other mass media approaches.

Pharmacogenomic research and studies for special populations (e.g., pediatrics, minorities and gender-specific) may drive smaller clinical trials in which far more targeted and select patients will be recruited. Sponsor companies are also committing resources and attention to developing protocols and project plans that are more targeted to real world patient populations. These approaches may result in more inclusive eligibility criteria.

Investigative sites are forming larger and broader networks that include a variety of health providers, including tertiary care and community-based physicians, private-payor and managed care settings, and multi-specialty and population-specialty environments.

These are but a few of the changes in clinical development practices that may have profound effects on the patient recruitment process in the coming decade. Understanding of the process today combined with the application of exciting solutions to address process improvement areas, will no doubt facilitate the use of more effective strategies and practices in the new frontiers of patient recruitment.

REFERENCES

[1] US Census Bureau, Statistical Abstract of the United States, August 2000.

Lightfoot, Gary. "Where Will the Patients Come From?" *CenterWatch Newsletter*, 1996. Volume 3 Issue 4. Pages 8-9.

[2] Getz, K. "Meeting and Extending Enrollment Deadlines." *PAREXEL Pharmaceutical R&D Statistical Sourcebook 2000*. Page 104.

[3] Zisson, S. "Losing Ground in the Battle Against Development Delays." *CenterWatch Newsletter*, 1998. Volume 5 Issue 12. Pages 1, 3-6.

[4] CenterWatch Editors. "Grant Market to Exceed $4 Billion in 2000." *CenterWatch Newsletter*, 2000. Volume 7 Issue 11. Pages 1, 6-10.

[5] *Ibid.*

[6] *Ibid.*

Lovato et al. "Recruitment for Controlled Clinical Trials Literature Summary." *Controlled Clinical Trials*, 1997. Volume 18. Pages 328-357.

Silagy, C.A. et al. "Comparison of Recruitment Strategies for Large Scale Clinical Trials in the Elderly." *Journal of Clinical Epidemiology*, 1991. Volume 44. Pages 1105-1114.

Spilker, B. and Cramer J. "Patient Recruitment in Clinical Trials." *Raven Press*, 1992. Pages 39-59.

Swinehart, J.M. "Patient Recruitment and Enrollment in Clinical Trials: A Discussion of Specific Methods and Disease States." *Journal of Clinical Research and Pharmacoepidemiology*, 1991. Volume 5. Pages 35-47.

Yusuf, S. et al. "Selection of Patients for Randomized Controlled Trials: Implications of Wide or Narrow Eligibility Criteria." *Statistics in Medicine*, 1990. Volume 9. Pages 73-83.

[7] CenterWatch Editors. "Grant Market to Exceed $4 Billion in 2000." *CenterWatch Newsletter*, 2000. Volume 7 Issue 11. Pages 1, 6-10.

[8] *Ibid.*

[9] Llewellyn-Thomas, H.A. et al. "Patients' Willingness to Enter Clinical Trials: Measuring the Association with Perceived Benefit and Preference for Decision Participation." *Social Science & Medicine*, 1991. Volume 32. Pages 35-42.

Lovato et al. "Recruitment for Controlled Clinical Trials Literature Summary." *Controlled Clinical Trials*, 1997. Volume 18. Pages 328-357.

Spilker, B. and Cramer J. "Patient Recruitment in Clinical Trials." *Raven Press*, 1992. Pages 159-179.

[10] Comis, R. "Harris Poll Data on Public and Patient Views of the National Cancer Clinical Trials." Presented at the Institute of Medicine's Clinical Research Roundtable, Washington DC, September 25, 2000.

[11] CenterWatch Editors. "A Word from Clinical Trials Volunteers." *CenterWatch Newsletter*, 1999. Volume 6 Issue 6. Pages 1, 9-13.

Comis, R. "Harris Poll Data on Public and Patient Views of the National Cancer Clinical Trials." Presented at the Institute of Medicine's Clinical Research Roundtable, Washington DC, September 25, 2000.

Getz, K. "Study Volunteer Behaviors and Attitudes in Industry-Sponsored Clinical Trials." Presented at the Institute of Medicine's Clinical Research Roundtable, Washington DC, September 25, 2000.

[12] US Census Bureau, Statistical Abstract of the United States, August 2000.

[13] Lovato et al. "Recruitment for Controlled Clinical Trials Literature Summary." *Controlled Clinical Trials*, 1997. Volume 18. Pages 328-357.

[14] CenterWatch Editors. "Reaching Out to Minority Investigators." *CenterWatch Newsletter*, 1997. Volume 4 Issue 1. Pages 1, 7-9.

Henderson, L. "Reaching Out to Minority Subjects." *CenterWatch Newsletter*, 2000. Volume 7 Issue 3. Pages 1, 10-14.

Lauerman, J. "Building Bridges to the Minority Community." *CenterWatch Newsletter*, 1996. Volume 3 Issue 2. Pages 1, 4-7.

[15] *Ibid.*

[16] Dunn et al. "Protecting Study Volunteers in Research." *CenterWatch Publications*, 2000. Pages 8-11.

[17] CenterWatch Editors. "Reaching Out to Minority Investigators." *CenterWatch Newsletter*, 1997. Volume 4 Issue 1. Pages 1, 7-9.

Henderson, L. "Reaching Out to Minority Subjects." *CenterWatch Newsletter*, 2000. Volume 7 Issue 3. Pages 1, 10-14.

[18] Meinert, C. "Study Finds Women Not Under-Represented in US Clinical Trials." *Controlled Clinical Trials*, October 2000.

[19] Getz, K. "Study Volunteer Behaviors and Attitudes in Industry-Sponsored Clinical Trials." Presented at the Institute of Medicine's Clinical Research Roundtable, Washington DC, September 25, 2000.

[20] CenterWatch Editors. "A Word from Clinical Trials Volunteers." *CenterWatch Newsletter*, 1999. Volume 6 Issue 6. Pages 1, 9-13.

Getz, K. "Study Volunteer Behaviors and Attitudes in Industry-Sponsored Clinical Trials." Presented at the Institute of Medicine's Clinical Research Roundtable, Washington DC, September 25, 2000.

[21] Woolley, M. "Research!America Poll Data on Attitudes Toward Medical Research." Presented at the Institute of Medicine's Clinical Research Roundtable, Washington DC, September 25, 2000.

[22] Allen, W. "No Advertising for Patients in Europe? Not True!" *CenterWatch Newsletter*, 1999. Volume 6 Issue 12. Pages 4-5.

[23] Woolley, M. "Research!America Poll Data on Attitudes Toward Medical Research." Presented at the Institute of Medicine's Clinical Research Roundtable, Washington DC, September 25, 2000.

[24] Getz, K. "Study Volunteer Behaviors and Attitudes in Industry-Sponsored Clinical Trials." Presented at the Institute of Medicine's Clinical Research Roundtable, Washington DC, September 25, 2000.

[25] *Ibid.*

[26] *Ibid.*

[27] Woolley, M. "Research!America Poll Data on Attitudes Toward Medical Research." Presented at the Institute of Medicine's Clinical Research Roundtable, Washington DC, September 25, 2000.

[28] Getz, K. "Study Volunteer Behaviors and Attitudes in Industry-Sponsored Clinical Trials." Presented at the Institute of Medicine's Clinical Research Roundtable, Washington DC, September 25, 2000.

[29] Henderson et al. "Sites Prosper...But Financial Health Threatened." *CenterWatch Newsletter*, 2000. Volume 7 Issue 1. Pages 1, 10-14.

[30] *Ibid.*

[31] *Ibid.*

CenterWatch Editors. "Grant Market to Exceed $4 Billion in 2000." *CenterWatch Newsletter*, 2000. Volume 7 Issue 11. Pages 1, 6-10.

[32] Getz, K. "Study Volunteer Behaviors and Attitudes in Industry-Sponsored Clinical Trials." Presented at the Institute of Medicine's Clinical Research Roundtable, Washington DC, September 25, 2000.

[33] Henderson et al. "Sites Prosper...But Financial Health Threatened."

CenterWatch Newsletter, 2000. Volume 7 Issue 1. Pages 1, 10-14.

[34] CenterWatch Editors. "Grant Market to Exceed $4 Billion in 2000." *CenterWatch Newsletter*, 2000. Volume 7 Issue 11. Pages 1, 6-10.

AUTHOR BIOGRAPHY

Kenneth A. Getz is the President and Publisher of CenterWatch, a Boston-based company that focuses on the clinical trials industry. CenterWatch is a subsidiary of the Medical Economics Company. CenterWatch provides a variety of information services used by pharmaceutical and biotechnology companies, CROs and investigative sites involved in managing and conducting clinical research. CenterWatch publications include the CenterWatch newsletter, the *CWWeekly* fax news bulletin and *JobWatch*, a monthly listing of career and educational opportunities for clinical research professionals. CenterWatch also publishes a variety of services for consumers including *New Medical Therapies* reports on promising new medical treatments in development as well as its well-known CenterWatch Clinical Trials Listing Service™, at *centerwatch.com*, on the Internet.

Prior to CenterWatch, Mr. Getz worked for over seven years in management consulting, first with Arthur D. Little and then with Corporate Decisions (a spin-off of Bain & Company) where he assisted pharmaceutical and biotechnology companies develop and implement business strategies to improve clinical development performance.

Mr. Getz is a well-known speaker at industry conferences and has published over 100 articles and chapters in a variety of journals and books including *Scrip Magazine, Applied Clinical Trials, The Drug Information Journal, Pharmaceutical Executive, The Medical and HealthCare MarketPlace*, and *Clinical Research and Regulatory Affairs*. Mr. Getz serves on a variety of boards and committees including the Institute of Medicine's Clinical Research Roundtable, the Drug Information Association's Steering Committee for the North Americas, and the Association for Clinical Research Professional's Future Trends Committee.

Mr. Getz holds an MBA from the J.L. Kellogg Graduate School of Management at Northwestern University and bachelor's and master's degrees, Phi Beta Kappa, from Brandeis University.

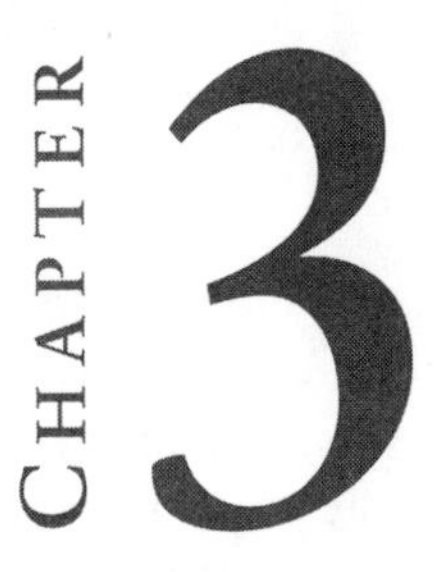

Ethical and Confidentiality Based Issues in Subject Recruitment Today

Felix A. Khin-Maung-Gyi, Pharm.D., M.B.A. and
Matthew D. Whalen, Ph.D.; Chesapeake Research Review, Inc.

This chapter is not meant to be an exhaustive treatise of ethics and/or regulations of biomedical and behavioral research. The intention of this chapter is simply to raise awareness of issues relating to ethics in the course of drug development research (particularly in the United States as of the beginning of the 21st Century) and specifically to recruitment of subjects into clinical trials. The reader is directed to other authoritative texts for more elaborate discussions on the history and principles of ethics, evolution of the regulations governing clinical research and informed consent concerns.[1-5]

INTRODUCTION

Societal awareness of issues in clinical research is often promoted as a result of crises, challenges or major events, whether domestically or internationally. Often, the development of applications of ethics is spurred on by these same events, either to assist in resolving the crisis or challenge or to strengthen national and international regulation.[6-11]

From the Nuremberg Code[12] to the Declaration of Helsinki[13], to The Belmont Report[14], to the guidelines from the Council for

International Organizations of Medical Sciences (CIOMS)[15], what has come to be known as bioethics in biomedical research has been defined through principles.

Fundamental to the Nuremberg Code is the requirement of informed consent from potential subjects and the adequate evaluation of both the risks entailed as well as the science, in order to justify inclusion of human subjects, prior to their participation in research. In addition to consideration of clinical and scientific matters, the Declaration of Helsinki addresses the need for the research to be reviewed by an independent body. The Belmont Report, resulting from a National Commission's efforts, outlines basic principles of respect for individuals and articulates the need for the population who bearing the risk(s) of participating in research also enjoy the benefits of the findings.

It is primarily those sentinel documents that regulate authorizing the Institutional Review Board (IRB) as the governing entity overseeing the protection of the rights and welfare of human subjects participating in research. (21 Code of Federal Regulations, Part 56). Similarly, regulations governing the scope and content of informed consent (21 Code of Federal Regulations Part 50) were also generated based on these documents and principles within. (Noteworthy is the fact that while the regulations cited above relate to FDA regulated products, there exist similar regulations for all federally funded research involving human subjects.)

Ethical Review Boards (ERBs) and Institutional Review Boards (IRBs), collectively referred to here as IRBs, in compliance with governing regulations, apply those regulations and principles in making determinations related to protecting the rights and welfare of human subjects participating in a range of research activities.

In addition to sound clinical and scientific design of proposed research, key principles that have served as touchstones for all individuals involved in research include, for example, autonomy and permission. These principles emphasize freedom of individual choice and appropriate acknowledgment by an individual to participate in clinical research. They are the core of both being informed and giving consent. Complementing these principles are those of voluntary participation (that is, the subject does so without coercion; or, more practically in today's healthcare environment, with minimal coercion).

Individual awareness, on the other hand, of the availability of a research study, specific to the individual's therapeutic needs, are met through access to information directly or indirectly and actively or passively as provided by the researcher or their staff. Direct-to-consumer advertising, notices of ongoing research studies posted in clinics and referral (by lay personnel and professional staff) are examples. Such recruitment efforts for pharmaceutical company sponsored studies recently have become more concerted, better coordinated and funded, in an attempt to enhance timely and efficient enrollment of subjects into clinical research studies.

Both HHS's Office of Human Subject Protections (OHRP, formerly the Office of Protection from Research Risks, OPRR) and the FDA interprets[16] the use of such efforts to be the beginning of the informed consent process as well as study subject selection. As such, although specific and clear regulatory guidance remains nebulous at best, all forms of recruitment, direct advertisement in particular, is required to receive IRB review and approval prior to implementation and use.

Recent reports[17, 18] issued by the U.S. Office of the Inspector General (OIG) found that the system charged with protecting the rights and welfare of subjects is deficient in consistently applying ethical review and oversight of recruitment activities. The reports criticized the lack of regulatory will and direction in empowering IRBs to act with authority and consistency. The reports suggest that the lack of adequate oversight has resulted in improper subject identification, selection and inclusion into clinical studies with harm to some.

On point, a bioethicist recently wrote:

> Clearly and unequivocally [in U.S. federal regulations] protecting prospective subjects and research participants from coercion and undue influence is the responsibility of the institutional review board (IRB). Until very recently, in general, the public has trusted that the IRB system, coupled with the integrity of the physician-investigator, has been sufficient to meet the task...But the pressures to recruit and retain subjects are evolving in ways that increase the prospect for coercion at the same time that serious questions are being raised about the ability of the IRB system to do its job...[However,] what no regulatory reform can assure is that IRBs develop and manifest moral courage.[19, 20]

Simply and concisely, this provides a thumbnail sketch of what a bioethical perspective looks like when brought to bear on subject recruitment practices. Paralleling the OIG's findings and recommendations, the constituent of the clinical research process (or team member) most identified with safeguarding human subjects is the IRB. Regulations and standards of accepted practice in the United States have presumed that an IRB must have "moral courage" in order to deliberate appropriately what is and is not in the best interest of subjects when it comes to recruitment. Notice, also, that this "moral courage" cannot be defined regulatorily, legally, ethically, clinically or scientifically define-able. Rather, it is a phenomenon of the discussion and deliberation process that occurs among scientists and non-scientists making up the IRB.[19, 20]

What operates both behind and beyond moral courage is ethics. All ethics are based on principles. Bioethics are simply those principles utilized for medical and healthcare purposes, including those of research. Applied ethics are the practical implementation of those principles. By tradition, bioethics is necessarily "applied ethics," since the development of bioethics is intimately tied to the history of the development of both the glory and the infamy of clinical research. The tradition of bioethics, domestically and internationally, includes principles found in documents developed to focus specifically on clinical research, such as the Nuremberg Code, the Helsinki Agreement, the Belmont Report (in the U.S., and a basis for the Code of Federal Regulations), and the CIOMS documents.

The volume and complexity of clinical research being conducted, fueled by rapidly advancing technology, continues to increase in response to market and public pressures. Equally significant is the public attention being drawn to clinical research by the popular press. As a result, clinical investigators, their study staff, sponsors of the research, as well as IRBs, are challenged to find "moral courage" in the conduct of clinical research. One means for doing so is to incorporate honest and comprehensive debate and application of current and alternative strategies for subject recruitment in the context of ethics.

The challenge for all participants is the juggling or balancing of appreciation of regulations, law, well-constructed clinical science, and financial and economic pressures along with the practical necessities of conducting trials as well. The challenge is even greater because regulations, laws and ethical principles function similarly, and multi-dimensionally.

- they provide baselines, or the minimum requirements;
- they are highly subject to interpretation and application; and,
- they rely on interpretive bodies to determine precedents and rationale for decisions—many of which are subject to change over time even when considering the exact same issues.

While charged with protecting the rights and welfare of human subjects, the IRB itself is not a patient advocacy body (i.e., advocate for a specific therapeutic area such as cancer); nor is it a judiciary entity; nor a scientific peer review committee in a strict definition; nor an instrument of public policy; nor a regulatory affairs department; nor an ethics committee. Yet, it must take into account these various and variant concerns and apply all those doctrines when debating subject protection issues for any given research project.

If an IRB were an advocacy body, it would demand, for example, that drugs with pharmacological activity for a range of cancers be tested for the only group the IRB advocates. If the IRB were a judicial entity, it would recommend promulgation of new laws. If the IRB were a scientific and clinical committee, it would be responsible for designing (or worse, re-designing) proposed research. Current U.S. regulations specifically prohibit the IRB from making a decision to approve a project based on "...(considering) possible long-range effects of applying knowledge gained in research (for example, the possible effects of research on public policy) as among those risks that fall within the purview of its responsibility." (21 CFR 56.111(2)) If the IRB were a regulatory affairs department, it might demand that information submitted for governmental regulatory consideration include certain documents. If the IRB were strictly an ethics committee, simply in the name of "fairness," the sponsor of the research may be asked to bear the costs of all procedures and activities related to research.

One can begin to appreciate that if an IRB were to take a firm position on any one of these areas, research would be paralyzed, or at best slowed to the point of being counter-productive for individual recipients of the research and society in general. Hence, for better or for worse, the challenge of juggling and balancing is one quite familiar for IRBs.[20]

potential subjects bad? Shouldn't patients be told of research that might be of benefit to them? How is advertising of research any different than any other type of advertising? If a patient were referred to another physician for participation in a research, wouldn't the physicians have the patient's best interest in mind before suggesting enrollment in a study?

Different phases of drug development research and different biomedical and behavioral research processes have different ethical issues. Recruiting subjects, therefore, confronts ethical issues associated both with study start-up and with different phases. The principle that appears to be violated when potential subjects enter studies based on mis-information, intentional or inadvertent, is coercion.

Coercion

From the vantage of an IRB, the IRB is the group charged with reviewing and approving any information that a potential subject reads relating to a specific clinical trial as part of recruitment. That information includes the whole media of recruitment (including graphics, music, text, layout, format and so on). After all, the material and campaign are also the beginning of the informed consent process: the first opportunity the potential subject has to begin to become informed about a trial.

Hence, being informed, or misled, is a process beginning with that information.

This reality places significant restraints on the creativity of public relations, media and advertising professionals. Recognizing that the goal of such professionals is to convince the buyer to agree to the message. What IRBs, as well as sponsors and site personnel must separate is information from misinformation. Suspending disbelief is useful in assuming that the intention is not to: mislead; suggest that participating in research is better in some shape or form; imply that the research is "new and improved" compared to standard therapies; or overly promise financial or other therapeutic incentives for participation.

As the clinical research enterprise becomes more competitive and, with the assistance of mass media, the realities and perception of fraud increases, it is ethically incumbent upon those participating in research to examine what other types of fraud can exist beyond that of illegal handling of revenues or misappropriation of pharmaceuticals. In brief: the information and messages of recruitment campaigns can be coercive, not simply influential. A more critical perception, or issue, is that those behind the message are participants in fraud.

A more obvious aspect of coercion involves inducements to participate or continue in the study. Inappropriate inducements may be offered to the subject, investigator and investigator's staff, colleagues who refer patients to participate or to the potential subject's friends or family. While the potential harm to subjects being coerced to remain in the study for reasons solely due to receiving monetary or other inducements is readily evident, less obvious is the involvement of health care professionals. There exists a prevailing concern that incentives to physicians to refer patients or to investigators to accelerate enrollment are a conflict of interest, not to mention potential violations of local laws, regulations and medical codes of conduct.[21,22]

Each IRB makes its own judgments in the area of payment to/for subjects participating in clinical research trials. Their basis for decisions is the principles of distributive justice (from the Belmont Report and other documents on research ethics) and avoidance of unacceptable inducements for subject participation (e.g., lack of coercion). While the U.S. regulations are silent on this issue the "Canadian Tri-Council Policy Statement in Ethical Conduct for Research Involving Humans" provides some guidance for IRBs from the perspective of a proportionate approach in reviewing the incentives and conflicts of interest. The document suggests that the IRB evaluate the nature of the conflict of interest and make a subjective determination of relative magnitude. So, if the IRB perceives the conflict to be relatively small, the investigator is asked to disclose this conflict. The investigator, however, would be asked to abandon involvement if the conflict is determined by the IRB to be significant.

An IRB does consider other factors in its deliberations about whether a proposed payment for a clinical trial subject is reasonable. The factors may vary depending on the project being considered, and not all are applicable in every instance. The deliberation of such factors is, again, driven by reference to ethical principles, as well as practical understanding of the clinical research process and regulatory requirements and guidelines.

These factors include the purpose of the payment (e.g., acknowledging the altruistic participation of the subject, thanking a person; reimbursement for an expense; compensation for time or lost wages; or compensation for a subject's efforts or pain because of research procedures). They also include the level of risk compared to benefit; as well as factors related to the autonomy of the subject (e.g., age, dependent relationship with study staff, the person's economic status, among others).

Other factors include the nature of the payment (cash, cash-equivalent, an object of value; as well as the impact of the payment as it may be related to privacy or confidentiality, such as the necessity of reporting earnings to the IRS or other federal, state and local authorities).

Access to healthcare itself is an inducement to participate in research. This is especially true in economically disadvantaged countries and communities, and in circumstances of disease states for which there are no, or not enough, viable alternatives. To avoid real or perceived conflicts and issues of coercion, IRB deliberation has to include not only the matter of payment to subjects but also other inducements to participate.

Equitability is yet another factor of concern, raising questions such as: what is the range of variation of compensation among sites in a multi-site study; how wide is the range; what accounts for the range; is there a potential bias for/against inclusion of certain subjects; and how do community attitudes and local conditions impact the types and amounts of compensation offered in one area versus another?

As an aside, if a physician practice simply wishes to announce participation in clinical research, as a broad announcement, such promotion does not require IRB review and approval. Information associated with a specific study, however, does require IRB review and approval. Hence, the IRB's purview with respect to screening potential subjects includes review of everything from scripts used by call center interviewers to simple flyers tacked onto walls of clinics.

Screening Subjects & Confidentiality

Identification of eligible subjects, in addition to the recruitment processes mentioned above, may include review of existing databases correlating inclusion and exclusion criteria to patient medical histories and demographics. Historically, only the patient's physician and caregiver evaluated patients in physician practices. The mounting economic pressures on physicians and clinical researchers to remain competitive have resulted in exploration of the use of patient profiles in an attempt to accelerate enrollment.

More efficient screening of potential subjects is a crucial element of recruitment and retention efforts. Hence, systematic attention has been focused on this facet of the clinical research process; so much so that a burgeoning sub-industry has grown up around the screening process. Dampening enthusiasm, however, is lack of regulatory guidance and, as a result, a potentially conservative posture among IRBs (that is, when the regulations are silent, IRBs exist to manage risk following what makes reasonable ethical sense). Moreover, with heightened awareness about the privacy of medical records, associating subject records, including the case report form, is not an extreme legal extension.

Faced with the twin threats of regulatory and legal sanction, the clinical research enterprise has been somewhat hampered in its efforts to recruit more efficiently. The ethical dimension of the matter, however, has less to do with individual freedom and more to do with informed consent and permission.[1] Simply stated, patient records should not be reviewed for research-related activities without prior permission from the patient or legally authorized representative. Similarly, following obtaining consent from the patient, mechanisms should exist to enable the patient to withdraw consent at any time without jeopardizing any of the benefits to which the patient is otherwise entitled. The ability to identify those who: have given consent and the subsequent removal of their names should they rescind the consent, or, request that they not be contacted for research-related activities, should be inherent to any process where database screening is considered.

Two final points regarding confidentiality:

- With or without technology, there is no such thing as complete confidentiality; and to convey otherwise is disingenuine, if not immoral.

- Working with technology transforms the issue of confidentiality and privacy to one of security in no small measure. As a result, even the methods of technology come under the purview of ethical review.

SUMMARY

The fact that IRBs are over burdened to meet today's burgeoning demands of the drug/device/biologics development and clinical research enterprise is well known and accepted. While regulatory is assigned to the IRB, it would be counterproductive to place the burden of oversight regarding the protection of the rights and welfare of human subjects solely on one part of the clinical research enterprise.

Not only from an ethical perspective but also from that of practicality, trust is the underpinning of the clinical research enterprise:

- patients' trust in care providers and caregivers;
- trust of volunteers founded in the assumption that researchers will adhere to the highest principles of clinical and scientific care in conducting the research;
- researchers' trust that the sponsor of the research will utilize the information collected from subjects in good faith in an appropriate manner, applying the highest standards;
- sponsors' trust that the researchers have the core competencies necessary to collect clean data in a timely manner; and,
- regulatory agencies' trust that all participants in the research process will abide by all applicable regulations.

Table One (following) illustrates the relationship between all those involved/affected by the research process. Violation of trust by any of the participants in the scheme results in tremendously negative results. Many times it is easy to place the blame of wrong doings on another party. However, it is incumbent on each of us not to violate that trust ultimately given to us by the subject.

At a basic level, compassion is understood mainly in terms of empathy—our ability to enter into and, to some extent share others' suffering.... This causes one who is compassionate to dedicate themselves entirely to helping others overcome both their suffering and the causes of their suffering.

-The Dalai Lama, from Ethics for the New Millennium

In terms of reviewing, deliberating, and approving subject recruitment approaches, this mission seems particularly pertinent in the new millennium and in the global marketplace of clinical research. The reader is advised to further reference the Office of Inspector General's report on Sample Guidelines for Practice.[17]

FROM A VANTAGE OF THE IRB: A PERSONAL AFTERWORD

Instead of looking at what the IRB is not and trying to derive what it is, as one of my first IRB mentors, and the Chair of our independent IRB now, is fond of summarizing the mission of the IRB as: "To preside, provide and guide."

Both ethics and IRBs have evolved significantly over the last ten years. Or, rather, the interpretation of both has changed. The role of the IRB and the evocation of ethics throughout the clinical research enterprise has become more pervasive.

In times of such change, it is important, in my opinion, to recall our heritage as well as to prepare for more and different responsibilities. That is, to maintain the intention of originating principles, regulations and guidelines, while adapting to changed circumstances, among the most significant of which are public opinion and social need.

Because I also have had the good fortune to gain experience at the Sponsor, CRO and site levels, I have come to appreciate the importance of all participants in the research process understanding the challenges each other faces, including recruitment.

From the biomedical research industry's perspective, one of the greatest challenges is finding appropriate subjects, as well as to assure that representation of a variety of people affected by specific diseases becomes part of the recruitment effort.

The burden of doing so may fall particularly to investigational sites and to organizations utilized to recruit subjects.

APPENDIX I

Practical Guidelines

The following are suggestions that may provide a practical approach to recruitment issues:

Recruiting Subjects: Advertisements, Flyers, Letters

A very simple, short "notice" format is appropriate. It should contain: that you are conducting a research study and a brief objective of the study; what drug/device/biologics is involved (and/or therapeutic area involved); general description of subjects to be enrolled; and a contact person. Subsequent direct screening during enrollment of subjects will give subjects the opportunity to get additional information and to ask any questions to clarify information in the short notice.

For more elaborate recruitment notices, the following may assist in order to meet the spirit and letter of federal government regulations:

- This is a research study in which you/your organization, by name, is participating.
- What exactly is being studied that impacts the individual subject.
- The duration of the study and what is expected of the individual subject. For example, the number of visits to your facility in the course of the study, and what the subject must do, such as keep a diary or use a drug or device.
- The benefits that the subject will receive only as directly related to the study: for example, free study-related drug/device/biologics, free study-related tests (and what kinds), free study-related examinations (and what kinds).
- Monetary compensation—separate from benefits—that the enrolled subject may expect to receive, including travel expense reimbursement.
- A statement that includes, "If you or someone you know is

interested in participating, please contact...," and indicate an individual and his/her phone number.

- The name of a specific person who may be the Principal Investigator, the Research Coordinator or a designated staff member of your organization or practice.

- Use of "research" or "investigational" as descriptors rather than words like "new" (or any similar term suggesting 'improved' or 'better' or 'different therefore having more advantage').

- If the recruitment material includes graphics: Look carefully at any illustrations in the literature to assure they are appropriate to the subject population being studied (in terms of gender, ethnicity, age, for examples) and that the illustrations are inclusive of the diversity of the population upon which are being drawing for recruitment. This is particularly true for human representations.

- Note also that typefaces used and size need to be carefully considered so that they do not constitute misleading enticements; as might the overemphasized use of the word "free."

- Avoid language that focuses on your site, your organization or your reputation as opposed to what subjects need to know—words like: "the largest," "most experienced" and "leading expert"—or words and phrases that suggest the same thing.

- Specifically regarding indications of benefits, suggestion of coercion is a critical concern.

Recruiting Subjects: Using Audio and Visual Media

All the suggestions made that apply to print materials also apply to audio and visual presentations, especially those relating to graphics. In audio and visual presentations, the same sensitivity can be shown in selecting appropriate voices, actors or dynamic images.

Making such selections means balancing what might appeal to the populations particularly targeted for the study with the regulatory guidelines relating to inclusion of minority and women populations. Additional appreciation needs to be considered if special populations are being recruited (such as children, physically or mentally challenged, institutionalized individuals, among others).

Another dimension of audio and visual presentations are the stagings and settings. Dramatic images, or sounds, that suggest a level of competency, trust or credibility that is not accurate to the study or study site being advertised can be coercive. For example:

- A video presentation using settings or scenes which display large complexes of buildings or equipment to suggest an excellence of facilities that in fact will not be used;
- A sound-/look-alike actor with resemblance to a trusted authority in a specific community, or in society, used in a manner that is not highly obviously humorous;
- A web site with graphics and interactivity highly appealing to a particular population that also emphasizes financial compensation and/or suggests that being a 'professional subject' is a viable means of making a living.

The fundamental approach is to keep the advertising piece clear, simple and accurate. Neither the FDA nor the IRB is looking for award-winning creativity, which might be construed to be coercive.

Inclusion, Access & Confidentiality of Human Subjects

Database

The screening process for enrollment of subjects subsequent to their recruitment gives the study coordinator another opportunity to get additional information from the prospective subjects in order to develop a database assuring that all appropriate populations have access to participation.

In developing site databases of any kind, including adoption of already-created practice systems, it is critical to build in confidentiality protection for each subject or applicant. Requirements of the sponsor organization may or may not be sufficient from regulatory, legal or ethical perspectives, since the sponsor does not necessarily have either complete access to the systems or the right to protect them.

One way to anticipate potential issues concerning inclusion, access, and confidentiality is to plan the study anticipating that the following questions can be answered with "YES" (that is, ways in which something might have been done better) after the study is over:

- Could you tell that the study population described in the protocol fairly reflects the eligible population in clinical practice by: (a) age; (b) gender; (c) ethnicity?

- If you used multiple sites, is the above still true?

- Could you access this type of information in a way that provides general results only or in a coded fashion, preventing correlation of this information with the name of the subject?

- Were there conditions of the study excluding certain populations: for example, the number of visits to your facility in the course of the study (issue of subjects' access to transportation); and what the subject must do, such as keep a diary or use a drug or device (issue of subjects' literacy or innumeracy capability)?

- Were financial benefits realized appropriately—that is, involving balancing short-term discomforts, indignities, risks with longer-term gains and risks for the use of the subject's body?

- Were the subjects enrolling in the study primarily for the financial benefits they gained? (Issue here, appreciating that 'how much is too much' is circumstantial: the benefit to the subjects are financial to such a degree that discomforts, indignities or risks they might otherwise not assume are temporarily ignored by subjects at the risk of physical and/or emotional harm).

REFERENCES

[1] Engelhardt HT. *The Foundation of Bioethics*. New York, NY: Oxford University Press; 1996.

[2] Beauchamp TL, Childress J. *Principles of Biomedical Ethics*. New

York, NY; Oxford University Press; 1996.

[3] Levine RJ. *Ethics and Regulation of Clinical Research*. New Haven, CT: Yale University Press; 1988.

[4] Grisso T, Applebaum PS. *Assessing Competence to Consent to Treatment*. New York, NY; Oxford University Press; 1998.

[5] Hartnett T, editor. *The Complete Guide to Informed Consent in Clinical Trials*. PharmSource Information Services, 2000.

[6] Epstein KC, Sloat B. *Drug Trials: Do People Know the Truth about Experiments? In the Name of Healing*. Cleveland, OH: The Plain Dealer; December 15, 1996.

[7] Sloat B, Epstein KC. *Drug Trials: Do People Know the Truth about Experiments? Using Our Kids as Guinea Pigs*. Cleveland, OH: The Plain Dealer; December 16, 1996.

[8] Epstein KC, Sloat B. *Drug Trials: Do People Know the Truth about Experiments? Foreign Tests Don't Meet U.S. Criteria*. Cleveland, OH: The Plain Dealer; December 17, 1996.

[9] Sloat B, Epstein KC. *Drug Trials: Do People Know the Truth about Experiments? Overseers Operate in the Dark*. Cleveland, OH: The Plain Dealer; December 18, 1996.

[10] Weiss R, Nelson D. *U.S. Halts Cancer Tests in Oklahoma*. Washington, DC: The Washington Post; July 11, 2000.

[11] Weiss R, Nelson D. *FDA Faults Penn Animal Tests that Led to Fatal Human Trial; Genetic Research Killed Teenager*. Washington, DC: The Washington Post; July 12, 2000.

[12] The Nuremberg Code. JAMA. 1996;276:1691.

[13] World Medical Association Declaration of Helsinki: Recommendations Guiding Medical Doctors in Biomedical Research Involving Human Subjects. Adopted by the 18th World Medical Assembly, Helsinki, Finland, June 1964 and amended by the 29th World Medical Assembly, Tokyo, Japan, October 1975, 35th World Medical Assembly, Venice, Italy, October 1983, 41st World Medical

Assembly, Hong Kong, September 1989, and the 48th General Assembly, Somerset West, Republic of South Africa, October 1996.

[14] National Commission for the Protection of Human Subjects. The Belmont Report. Washington, DC: US Government Printing Office; 1979.

[15] Council for the International Organizations of Medical Sciences. International Ethical Guidelines for Biomedical Research Involving Human Subjects. Geneva, Switzerland: CIOMS; 1993.

[16] FDA Information Sheets. *Guidance for Institutional Review Boards and Clinical Investigators*. Rockville, MD: 1998.

[17] Office of Inspector General. *Recruiting Human Subjects: Pressures in Industry-Sponsored Clinical Research*. www.dhs.gov/progorg/oei. June 2000.

[18] Office of Inspector General. *Recruiting Human Subjects: Sample Guidelines for Practice*. www.dhs.gov/progorg/oei. June 2000.

[19] DeRenzo EG. *Coercion in the Recruitment and Retention of Human Research Subjects, Pharmaceutical Industry Payments to Physician-Investigators, and the Moral Courage of the IRB*. IRB, A Review of Human Subjects Research. March-April 2000; 22(2):1-5.

[20] Chesapeake Research Review, Inc. *On Being an IRB*. IRB, A Review of Human Subjects Research. September–December, 1995; 17(5,6):12-16.

AUTHOR BIOGRAPHIES

Dr. Felix Khin-Maung-Gyi, for more than fifteen years, has provided consultation and professional development as well as managed research units and projects. Dr. Gyi has worked internationally. Roles have included: clinical scientist and project and program leader in both private and academic sectors. He has also restructured and managed an academic medical center IRB.

In addition to research project management and coordination, other areas of his expertise include human subject protection, pharmacovigilance, and inter-sector partnerships among industry, government, academia and non-profits.

Recent professional appointments include: IRB Forum Chair and Task Force Member, Principal Investigator Certification, Association of Clinical Research Professionals (ACRP); and Member, Council for Certification of IRB/IEC Professionals of Applied Research Ethics National Association (ARENA). He is also on the Editorial Board of Clinical Trials Advisor.

Previously, Dr. Gyi has worked for pharmaceutical (both domestic and international), medical, professional services, and healthcare organizations. Throughout his professional career, Dr. Gyi has also served on university faculty, including, until recently, at an academic medical center.

Dr. Gyi received the Doctor of Pharmacy degree from Duquesne University; and the M.B.A. (Executive Program) from Loyola (MD) College. He has completed Clinical Pharmacy residencies in both pediatric and adult medicine and done post-graduate studies in drug development, regulations and medical research. His undergraduate work in Pharmacy included a concentration in Microbiology.

Dr. Matt Whalen has over twenty years experience in advising on managing organization and work unit change, including start-up through mature organizations. Since 1987, Dr. Whalen has maintained a practice in executive and senior management coaching representing leadership in each of the five sectors of the workplace.

Dr. Whalen has also been called "an expert on workplace trends," quoted in media ranging from **Executive Update** and **New Woman** to **Money, USA Today**, and **Reader's Digest**. Authors of two mass market books (one on global business development, the other on organization and individual change) have acknowledged him as a primary resource. He is serving in a similar capacity for a forthcoming book on Research Ethics.

Immediately prior to co-founding Chesapeake Research Review, Inc., Dr. Whalen served as a Vice President of the Washington, DC region of an international management consulting firm. Clients included both **Forbes** and **Inc.** 500 companies, federal agencies, and trade associations. Earlier, he ran the office of a national consulting firm, directing a company-wide task force reorganizing services and functions.

Active in economic development as well, Dr. Whalen coordinated two industry/government partnerships, winning a Presidential Citation.

Throughout his professional career, he has also served on university faculty at institutions including Temple University, Trinity College and University of Maryland in areas ranging from Business and Public Policy to American Cultural Studies.

His Ph.D. focus was science, technology and society (University of Maryland, College Park). Post-graduate work included Mediation (University of Vermont) and Organization Development (Georgetown University).

Table 1 of Chapter 3

Network of Formal Relationships of the Clinical Research Enterprise

The Expanded 'Flow' of Information

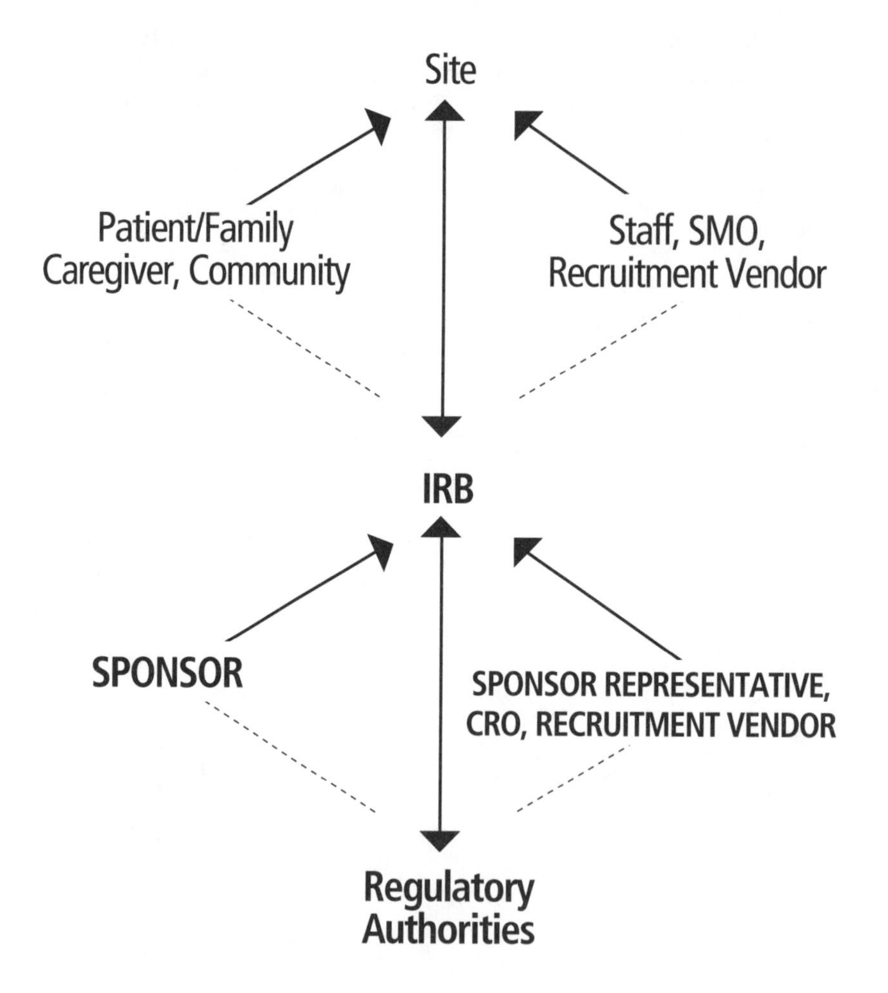

Definition: Formal relationships include a range of agreements from employment arrangements, informed consent form permissions, and investigator compliance documents (like the 1572), to negotiated contracts.

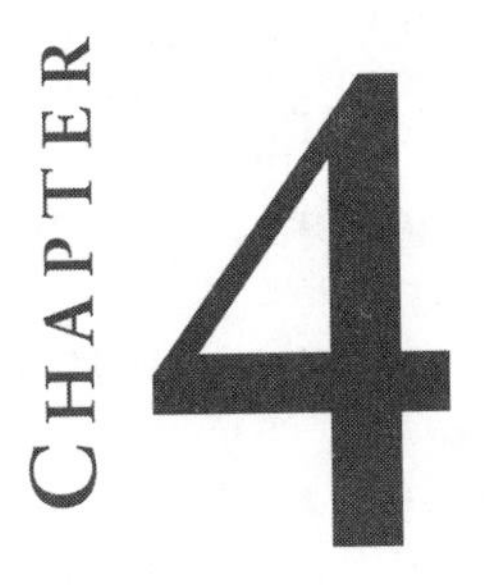

Budgeting and Contracting in Patient Recruitment

Bonnie A. Brescia, BBK Healthcare, Inc.

In the field of patient recruitment for clinical trials, considerations of budgeting and contracting are becoming increasingly essential to success. This chapter challenges clinicians, administrators, sponsors and others involved in clinical trials to think more strategically in deciding when, where, how and why to budget and contract for patient recruitment.

Until recently, patient recruitment was exclusive to the physician investigator's role in a clinical trial. Patients for clinical trials were largely drawn from the physician's practice, and the sponsor paid for that access as part of the physician's total compensation. A separate budget for centralized patient recruitment was rare.

As the number of clinical trials increased and competition grew among companies testing similar compounds and procedures, recruiting patients from physician practices was not enough. It became necessary to find new methods for attracting participants. Individual study sites began spending money on promotional campaigns with widely varying degrees of success. For every success there were more failures, and the duplication among sites of effort was inefficient and wasteful.

Management within sponsor organizations soon began analyzing the return on investment for patient recruitment efforts, challenging the marketplace to reevaluate the concept of decentralized versus centralized campaigns and budgets. The first organizations to attempt centralized programs were clinical research organizations (CROs). However, CROs lacked expertise in direct-to-consumer promotions, and soon it was necessary to find others that could analyze the process and develop a marketing communications strategy for patient recruitment as a distinct effort. Many early, centralized recruitment budgets were often inflated, even exorbitant. More recently, the pooling of patient recruitment expertise distributed throughout the clinical trial community, sponsors, sites, CROs, SMOs and communications agencies, has resulted in a more strategic approach to budgeting for patient recruitment.

Today it remains ever more critical to accelerate and improve patient recruitment for clinical trials. Every day that a study is delayed can be measured not only in costs to continue running the study, but also in lost revenue from the potential product. Developing and managing a budget is essential to protect product potential. There is no substitute for being first to market with a new or improved product, and that must be factored into the budgeting process for successful completion of the clinical trial. It is important to remember that without patients, there would be no data; considering patient needs should therefore be a priority as the budget is developed.

This need for achieving recruitment success in an efficient, cost-effective and process-oriented manner has led to the growth of strategic contracting as a budget management tool. Performance-based contracting between sponsors, sites, CROs and communications specialists is an effective method for distributing the risks involved in the increasingly competitive field of clinical trial recruitment.

In an ideal world, it would be possible to predict and control for all the variables that contribute to a successful patient recruitment campaign. The minimum budget necessary to guarantee results could be determined in advance of study launch. However, the controls available in research studies rarely apply in the open marketplace. A protocol conducted in January of one year would require a sig nificantly different recruitment approach if conducted in June of the following year. Two protocols investigating the merits of the same compound in two different populations also would require distinct strategies to ensure success. Therefore, every protocol will demand its own budgeting strategy. What follows is a process to assist project leaders in understanding the variables that affect the recruitment budget, which when evaluated, lead to a comprehensive patient recruitment budget.

BEFORE BUDGETING

Before sitting down to write a budget, there are many questions and factors to consider. This section provides an overview of key questions to ask about the trial, introduces a method for estimating numbers of patients needed at each recruitment stage to fulfill the final randomized requirement, discusses the factors essential to determining budget size and scope, considers the question of using a centralized or a decentralized budget and explores the options of competitive recruitment for sites. A review of these issues will pave the way to drafting a strategically sound budget.

ANSWERING KEY QUESTIONS

Before creating a patient recruitment budget, develop a protocol recruitment profile by answering several key questions. Keep this profile as a reference throughout the recruitment planning, budgeting and contracting process. Answer these questions now and refer to them while reading the next few sections.

- How many randomized participants are needed?
- How many patients must be screened to enroll the target number?
- How many sites are planned?
- Where will they be located geographically?
- How much of the recruitment effort, if any, can the sites handle?
- Is this study pivotal (e.g., providing data for NDA?) or is it an earlier phase?
- How important is the product/compound to the company's business strategy?
- Does the company have recent recruitment experience in this therapeutic category?
- What is the timeframe for beginning and completing the study?

- How onerous are the inclusion/exclusion criteria?
- What is the incidence of the disease/condition?
- Are there competitive treatments already available?
- Are all sites under a central IRB or individual IRBs?

DETERMINING A RECRUITMENT FUNNEL

In order to recruit the target number of enrolled patients for a study, a much greater number of potential participants must be reached through promotional efforts. This larger pool of candidates will be winnowed down as their eligibility and appropriateness for the study is further scrutinized, creating a "funnel" effect. Before developing a patient recruitment budget, it is important to make assumptions about the recruitment funnel for each study. These assumptions provide initial performance metrics against which a program can be measured. They also form the basis for many decisions that will affect program design and allocation of resources. Essentially, this model projects the number of individuals who must respond to a promotional program in order to generate a target number of patients who will pass through the various screens and ultimately be randomized into a study.

The first step in using the recruitment funnel method is to determine how many individuals an investigator is likely to see for a medical evaluation in order to enroll (randomize) one patient into the study. It should be noted that not every individual referred to a site for medical evaluation will make and keep an appointment. Next comes the determination of how many people must pass a preliminary screening for key demographic and basic medical history in order to

Table 1 The Recruitment Funnel Concept

Stage of Enrollment	Numbers needed to enroll/randomize one individual	Numbers extraploated to enroll/randomize 750 individuals
Inquiries	24	21,000
Referred to sites	8	7,000
Made and kept appts.	6	4,500
Medically eligible	2	1,500
Enrolled/randomized	1	750

be appropriate for an in-person medical evaluation. Last is the determination of how many people are needed to call the study site or central toll-free number in order to generate the desired number of individuals who will pass the preliminary screening. See Table One for an example of the recruitment funnel concept.

Understanding how many people must be reached to effectively enroll the target number of patients has a significant effect on the budget. The protocol promotional profile offers insight into the need for reaching greater or lesser numbers of individuals in order to reach required screening and enrollment ratios. For example, in a diabetic neuropathy study, ten patients might need to be screened in order to enroll one patient. However, the promotional campaign may need to reach 1,000 people in order to generate the ten qualified callers that will result in one enrolled patient. In this scenario, the ratio of callers to enrollees may be so great that the investigative site may be understaffed to generate or respond to this volume of inquiries. Thus, the budget would be expanded to allow for additional personnel or the use of a centralized response center to field patient inquiries.

Use of the recruitment funnel can also serve as an early feasibility assessment of employing marketing communications tactics to achieve recruitment goals. If it becomes apparent from this type of analysis that a significant percentage of the potential patient pool (i.e., more than 5%) must respond to marketing communications, then it may be necessary to consider more significant strategic recommendations in addition. For example, other strategic tactics could include reducing number of patients, broadening scope of recruitable patients or increasing number of study sites.

CONSIDERING BUDGET FACTORS

Evaluating the factors in a budget help determine its size and scope. No matter how large or small your trial, certain factors don't change. A certain level of strategy, research and development costs are required. Other factors are variable and depend on the number and location of markets, number of sites and patients and more.

Timing

The timing of when a budget is developed affects which elements can be included or must be eliminated because the timelines for their implementation fall outside the recruitment window. The earlier in the clinical trial process that the patient recruitment budget is considered, the more likely it is that recruitment will be accomplished in a timely and cost-effective manner. There are several stages when a patient recruitment budget is typically considered.

At Protocol Development

The earliest moment to consider the budget is concurrently with development of the trial protocol. Decisions about patient definition and selection, investment of time and other factors affect recruitment efforts. For example, rather than planning a trial with 100 sites in 100 different media markets, consider grouping the 100 sites in twenty media markets. Not only will this save in marketing costs, but in other expenditures as well. For example, travel costs for investigator meetings and site monitoring also may be reduced. Planning the budget at this point provides the most control over options and choices.

At Study Launch

This is a second common point at which budgets are developed. When patient recruitment is pinpointed as a problem at this stage, some options may be reduced. For example, sites are likely to be already contracted, thus, changes in number and location of sites or modifications to the protocol to improve patient-friendliness may be too cumbersome to implement. But there is still an opportunity to bring a proposal to management and perhaps prevent some of the lost time and revenue that occurs in rescue mode.

Rescue Mode

Once the study has started and patient recruitment is recognized as a problem, the costs in time and effort for a supplemental recruitment program are at a premium. Advertising costs may be locked in at an expensive time of year. Some outreach options such as public relations may be unavailable because, although they are effective and cost-efficient, they require long lead times to implement and bear fruit. Marketing may be limited to less-than-optimum materials already developed and approved by IRBs, or new materials may need to be developed and approved dependent on the constraints of the IRBs. When options are limited, costs go up.

Difficulty of Protocol

Once the protocol is written, it can be used to estimate the recruitment cost per patient. There are factors in each protocol that make it easier or harder to recruit patients. Protocol factors that often increase recruitment difficulty include a placebo arm, satisfactory existing treatments in the therapeutic category being studied, one or more invasive procedures, limited prevalence/incidence of the disease and resultant difficulty of subject identification. Factors that might make recruitment easier include likelihood of medical insurance coverage, no satisfactory existing treatments in the category, wide demographic population being studied, long lead time to study start date and use of a central IRB.

Number of Patients/Number of Sites

Both of these factors increase costs incrementally. The more patients that are needed, the more money is required to recruit. Likewise, the more sites in the study, the more resources that must be allocated to cover the media markets and the costs of creating and producing materials. Each site has start-up costs and each requires monitoring. Decisions must be made about whether to distribute promotion across more sites or limit the number of sites and provide more funds for promotion.

Location of Sites

Deciding on the location of sites will affect the budget. Locating multiple sites in one media market is a cost-saving strategy. Placing them in densely populated areas is another strategy to increase the number of potential participants reached with fewer dollars. Analyzing past and potential site performance is important to determine which sites would be most effective to include. Does the site have a dedicated recruitment specialist or marketing manager? If so, it's more likely they will know how to use promotional funds effectively.

Management Priorities

How important is the drug being studied to the sponsor's overall business strategy? The answer will affect budgeting decisions. If the drug already has a revenue stream and the study will help to extend or expand that revenue stream, management will probably be more willing to spend money on recruitment to shorten the overall length of study duration. The same may hold true for promising new compounds with the first-to-market position at stake. Project leaders should not assume that because patient recruitment has not been budgeted as a separate effort in the past, that management would not support a sizeable recruitment budget today.

CHOOSING A CENTRALIZED OR DECENTRALIZED BUDGET MODEL

One of the first considerations in setting a patient recruitment budget is to determine whether to use a decentralized or centralized budget or a combination of both. In the days when sponsors contracted solely with physicians, recruitment budgets were managed by investigators and associated site staff. Under this decentralized model, clinicians managed the entire process of patient interaction, from initial recruitment, through the course of the study to collecting, analyzing and reporting data. Patient recruitment components, such as patient screening, special events and advertising, were line items in the investigator's budget. Pharmaceutical companies chose investigators based on their reputations, ability to recruit patients and proposed budgets. Over time, clinical trials became more competitive. Sites had to become more sophisticated and reach outside their own practices to recruit patients. Their costs went up and duplication of efforts became common as each site created its own versions of study and promotional materials.

Budget centralization was introduced to address these issues. In this model, the sponsor originated strategy and media materials and then communicated the message and disseminated the materials to investigators and sites. For direct-to-consumer campaigns, call centers were added into the budget to centralize patient screening and processing because the volume of respondents became too high for individuals at sites to handle.

Once the rule, decentralized budgets may soon become the exception. However, there are some instances that may make decentralization the optimum choice. When the number of participants in a trial is small, distributing recruitment funds to individual sites may be more efficient. If the study needs eighty-five patients from seven sites, providing each site with a budget of $10,000 to execute local promotion would be less expensive than engaging a communications firm to develop a single campaign. It is reasonable to assume that sites will be able to deliver some percentage of the target number of patients from their existing practice or databases. This higher-than-average allocation of promotional funds is likely to fill in the gap.

Allocating funds on a per site basis is also an advantage when a local effort is the most effective way to reach potential patients, e.g., a screening event, or when leveraging existing relationships is essential, e.g., using physician referral to find patients. Decentralized budgets, which leave promotional responsibilities with the study sites, can also reduce the workload for sponsor staff as compared to centralized budgets, which sponsor staff must manage.

Centralizing the budget is often the most effective model for patient recruitment. Especially for large trials and Phase IIb or later trials, the benefits of centralization are many. Centralization offers economies of scale, requiring the performance of work only once and preventing duplication of efforts. Centralization also results in more effective tracking. When call centers are used to collect information as a central source, sponsors are not dependent on numerous sites to submit reports relating to recruitment promotional data. Project managers can determine early on whether sufficient resources are being deployed to generate sufficient number of potential study participants to meet enrollment. A weekly analysis of recruitment performance enables course corrections to reallocate budgets to the most effective strategies or sites.

Control over the budget also gives sponsors greater control over promotional content. When investigators manage the budget, there may not be a mechanism for sponsor review and approval of promotional materials. In an era when regulatory energies are being focused on investigator ethics in recruitment, sponsor-initiated, IRB-approved campaigns may provide greater control over regulatory compliance.

Sometimes, a combination of centralized and decentralized budgeting works well. For example, a trial might be launched through a centralized TV or radio campaign and then followed up with sites running print ads as needed to complete enrollment. The choice of centralized, decentralized or combination budgeting for recruitment is a strategic decision that will affect the study's outcome as measured in time to completion and total cost to completion. This decision also will affect the contracts executed with outsource suppliers.

DECIDING TO RECRUIT COMPETITIVELY OR NOT

Deciding how to motivate sites to recruit also affects the patient recruitment budget. With competitive recruitment, sites are rewarded financially for the number of patients they enroll. Media support is equalized across markets to provide a level playing field. Sites compete to recruit the most patients. An alternative approach is to budget fixed amounts unevenly among the sites depending on expected recruitment performance. In this model, higher performing sites are supported with higher budget amounts, ensuring higher recruitment rates. In both approaches, the funds to both support the promotional effort and reward the sites are allocated in the marketing and media portion of the budget. The promotional budget in either case may be the same, but there is a difference in how it is spent.

Knowledge of site performance is key to making the decision to choose a competitive recruitment or alternative model. If there is no history of site performance, then competitive recruitment might be a good choice. In competitive recruitment, the first sites to enroll the most patients are rewarded. Should there be knowledge and experience of some sites as proven high performers, allocating funds by known performance levels may make more sense. In this case, it is not as important to enroll patients first as to enroll patients at a consistently higher rate than other sites.

In the competitive recruitment approach, sites are challenged to recruit a minimum number of patients at a certain fee per patient evaluated, with the opportunity to increase earnings for recruitment over the quota. For example, if 500 patients are needed from fifty sites, sponsors budget and contract for ten patients per site, but offer compensation for up to thirty patients recruited. Thus, the sites that are good at recruiting generate more revenue from their research effort. Less effective sites receive less or may be dropped from the study. However, there are operating costs to administer a study even for a non-performing site. Spending more promotional dollars on fewer sites may result in a lower overall study budget. Again, the decisions made about recruitment have the potential to affect many line items in the study's operational budget that are not directly related to recruitment.

With this model, sponsors must be careful to provide equal promotional support to all sites. Support should be equalized by effort, not dollars. This means that sites in more expensive media markets may receive more money to reach the same target audience that a less expensive market may need fewer funds to find. While it may seem obvious that radio advertising in New York City is more expensive than in Tulsa, Oklahoma, few decentralized recruitment budgets account for these wide variations in media costs market to market.

Equalizing these costs across markets is done by assigning a target rating point or number of impressions for promotion in each market. Rating points represent the percentage of the marketplace that is exposed to an advertising message. Impressions are the number of people who are exposed to the message. Rather than budgeting a flat amount per site or per market, it is wise to consider budgeting for a number of impressions generated or percentage of the marketplace to be reached. See Table Two for an example of equalized support across different media markets.

Comparision of Media Costs, Target Market Women 25-54 — Table 2

Market (Rank)	Total Gross TV Costs/ 50 TRPs*	Total Gross Radio Costs/ 50 TRPs	Sunday Newspaper Gross Costs, 7"x7" SAU**	Total by Market
New York (#1)	$22,775	$30,100	$14,762***	$67,637
Los Angeles (#2)	$24,200	$37,900	$16,065	$78,165
Seattle (#12)	$8,550	$11,150	$6,173	$25,873
Birmingham (#39)	$2,363	$3,250	$4,865	$10,478
Tulsa (#59)	$2,000	$2,150	$2,436	$6,586

Source:
Gross TV Media Market Guide, Spring 2000 Q3 Projections
Newspaper Sunday open rates; SRDS June 2000
**TRP: Target rating points*
***SAU: Standard adjusting unit*
****New York Daily News size is based on non-SAU 4cx7" (28")*

In the alternative model, no effort is made to support sites equally. In fact, more promotional funds to support recruitment efforts are allocated to the sites that are already known to be the best recruiters. Based on site performance levels, sites can be divided into several tiers. At the lowest tier are the sites that may or may not reach their quota. They receive a set amount of promotional support. For sites that, with the addition of extra funds can reach beyond their recruitment quota, more is budgeted. Top performers receive the greatest budget support. The extra effort ensures that the best performers recruit the most patients. Many project managers set initial budgets for the first ten patients enrolled. If a site demonstrates strength in recruitment, the project manager can pull from a contingency fund to further support that site in recruiting additional participants. This approach can be deployed within a centralized or decentralized budgeting model.

As in many other budgeting decisions, the approach to allocating promotional dollars by site (or market) can affect the overall outcome of other aspects of the study. Despite efforts to equalize resources, many project managers have found that competitive recruitment creates tensions within the clinical trial community. Despite the initial inequities in the tiered support model, participating sites in these programs appreciate that some effort has been made to match study promotions with their capacity to manage the results of an outreach campaign.

DRAFTING A BUDGET

Having made pre-budgeting decisions, the process of drafting a budget is easier and more efficient. Using the knowledge gained, it is time to draft a budget. Although most organizations crave a budget standard for recruitment, there is no industry-wide accepted practice for patient recruitment budgeting. In the field, wide variations in budget allocations are seen.

At BBK Patient Recruitment, budgeting is approached from one of two perspectives. In one approach, the budget is built from the ground up depending on the assessment of the protocol and its recruitment challenges. In the other approach, a fixed budget is provided that is then allocated to provide the greatest return on investment. In a "from-the-ground-up" budget, each protocol is evaluated to determine its relative difficulty of enrollment. When a direct-to-consumer promotional campaign is required to meet enrollment goals, an average of $1,200 per enrolled (randomized) patient is applied as a baseline for budgeting. For example, if 750 individuals must be recruited to an influenza study that has been assessed as having an average difficulty, $900,000 would be calculated as a planning measure. For a study that requires multiple endoscopies and has extensive exclusion criteria, it might be determined that the protocol has twice the difficulty of the influenza study. In this case, the planning budget would be based on an assumption of $2,400 per enrolled (randomized) patient.

Some of BBK's clients prefer to budget for recruitment using standards that have been set for other direct response advertising programs they've conducted. In these cases, the number of inquiries required is the critical factor in setting the budget. Target costs per inquiry can range from $50 to $250 depending on the percent of people in the marketplace who are eligible to respond to promotion based on having the condition under investigation. In this scenario, if 10,000 individuals are needed to call the toll-free phone number and the population is relatively easy to target, such as type 2 diabetics, then the budget might be set at $75 per inquiry, or $750,000 for the program as a whole.

Often project managers have a fixed amount of money that can be invested in patient recruitment, regardless of evidence that suggests a bigger budget may be necessary to complete recruitment. In this situation, it is important to evaluate all of the potential program elements on a return-on-investment basis. It may be more prudent to allocate all of a $200,000 budget to a single promotional activity if that activity has the potential to generate 50 percent of the inquiries or randomized patients required.

This section outlines the common components of a patient recruitment budget and provides a budget worksheet that can be used as a planning tool in drafting a project budget.

BUDGET COMPONENTS

Depending on the size of the budget, not all components come into play, but all should be considered. Each component is followed by a list of representative expenses contained within it.

Research and Planning: Focus groups, database searches, purchase of existing reports on therapeutic category and sufferers, consulting services (such as for protocol design) and population tracking and demographics.

Creative Development: Creation of a graphic identity system or study logo, preparation of materials including letterhead, brochures, print and broadcast advertisements, direct mailers, posters, flyers, Web sites, etc. (Hints: Budget for creative development separately from production. Send all materials for regulatory and IRB approval at one time. Incur production costs on a phased, or as-needed basis. Save money by not producing all materials until their deployment is warranted. Save time by not returning for supplemental regulatory/IRB approval in mid-stream.)

Production: Production of approved pieces from creative development; includes printing, copying and collating, production of radio or television commercials, talent fees, photography and/or illustration rights, web programming, etc.

Marketing and Media
Media Placement: Ad space in newspapers, on the Web or in outdoor media; ad time on the radio, TV or cable; list rental; postage for direct mail programs.

Publicity: Development of press kits, press releases and public service announcements. Separate charges will be incurred for distributing materials via mail or wire services. Professional fees for conducting media follow-up, coordinating news coverage, and coaching study spokespersons.

Community Outreach: Participation in existing gatherings and events (e.g., health fairs, senior center meetings, church groups).

Internet Outreach: Creation of a Web site, postings on electronic bulletin boards, listings on other sites.

Special Events: Organization of study-specific events coordinated by the sponsor or sites.

IRB Approvals: Costs for approval differ depending on the IRB. Some IRBs will charge per item, some per campaign and others will negotiate volume discounts for review of the same materials on behalf of a multitude of sites.

Project Management and Reporting: Personnel (whether in-house or outsourced), technology licenses for project management software.

Call Center Operations:
(Hint: Separate the fixed from the variable costs in the budget. In the fixed line item, include start-up costs and minimum monthly charges. In the variable budget, put all items that are tied to number and disposition of calls.)
Fixed Costs: Start-up fees, operator training, computer programming of screener, database design, standard report package.

Variable Costs: Inbound operator costs (most often charged on a per-minute basis which will vary depending on the complexity of screening and level of personnel required), outbound calls, customized reporting, distribution and fulfillment of requests for information, customized services to support sites with patient scheduling, follow-up, appointment reminders.

Site Support Services: Personnel liaison with sites, site training, hiring or subcontracting staff, coaching, newsletters, web sites, teleconferencing, patient scheduling, mailing, onsite staff, software.

Site Incentives: Recognition gifts as allowed by sponsor or site management, thank yous, newsletters, plaques.

Patient Incentives: Compensation, parking stipends, books, gift certificates, newsletters, cards and communications.

Miscellaneous Expenses: Out-of-pocket expenses, shipping and delivery, travel costs, teleconferencing, supplies, overhead charges.

OTHER BUDGETARY CONSIDERATIONS

Hiring a Call Center

When a Call Center is Mandatory
When a patient recruitment media campaign includes broadcast advertising and public relations, there is a potential to generate a large number of calls (fifty or more) per day. If it is a national campaign or covers more than ten media markets, this level of calls could persist for several days or weeks at a time. On their own, study sites would be unable to handle the volume. Calls would back up, potential patients would not receive callbacks and patients would be lost. To ensure candidates are responded to immediately and processed efficiently, a call center is essential. When spending $1 million on a media campaign to inspire callers, it is worth another $270,000 to ensure those callers are processed efficiently otherwise the effort could be wasted.

Choosing a Dedicated or Shared Environment
Professional call centers can be contracted to be dedicated only to

one client or to answer calls for many clients. It is of course more costly to contract a dedicated call center, and it is rarely justified unless a company has multiple (over a dozen) studies in recruitment phase at the same time. Far more common are shared environment call centers, where operators take calls for many clients and studies. This way costs are shared, and there is no charge for down time when operators are not answering calls for a particular study.

Patient Recruitment Budget Worksheet

The worksheet includes examples of budgets for comprehensive and moderate recruitment programs. Referring to the sections above, use the columns on the right side of the worksheet to draft a new budget or to organize a current program budget.

Patient Recruitment Budget Worksheet

Budget Component	Large Budget ($1.5M)		Moderate Budget ($250,000)		Sample Budget	
	%	$	%	$	%	$
Research & Planning	4	60,000	10	25,000		
Creative Development	4	60,000	15	37,500		
Production	12	120,000	15	37,500		
Marketing & Media (media placement, publicity, community outreach, Internet outreach, special events)	40	600,000	40	100,000		
IRB approvals	2	30,000	2	5,000		
Project Management & reporting	7	105,000	10	25,000		
Call Center Operations	18	270,000	0	0		
Site Support Services	6	90,000	8	20,000		
Site Incentives	2	30,000	0	0		
Patient Incentives	5	75,000	0	0		
Site Administration						
Miscellaneous Expenses						
Total		$1.5M		$250,000		

AFTER BUDGETING

There are several considerations that follow the drafting of a budget. There will always be changes and unexpected circumstances that should be allowed for in a contingency budget. Many studies require ongoing maintenance in the form of efforts to retain patients, which may necessitate additional funding outside of the recruitment budget. In addition, once all of these budgets are complete, it is essential to gain the confidence and approval of management to go forward. The following section explores these areas.

Planning a Contingency Budget

No matter how thorough the initial planning, inevitably there will be changes during the course of the recruitment period that cannot be anticipated. Contingency budgets provide project managers with the resources to respond to changing conditions. However, not all organizations view contingency budgets in the same way. Some see planning a contingency budget as part of the process. Others perceive it as a sign of incompetence. Still others prefer to budget more money than is necessary in the main budget and then plan to spend only two-thirds of it. When planning the budget, it is important to know the nature of the organization involved. Generally, a contingency budget should be planned below the line of the main budget. Factors that require contingency might include the following:

Miscalculations: Not enough candidates are calling in, more are needed; or the target number of patients is calling, but qualification rates are lower than expected.

Not all IRB Materials Approved on Schedule: Approval may have to be sought in phases, with a percentage of sites receiving approval up front and the rest later. In this case, the recruitment efforts will be executed piecemeal, resulting in higher labor and production charges. Another effect of delayed approval could be delayed media placement. Since advertising rates change seasonally, a delay in project execution that moves a media placement buy from February to April could result in as much as a twenty percent increase in costs as 2nd and 3rd quarter rates are more expensive than 1st quarter. Fourth quarter rates are the most expensive of all.

Sites Added or Withdrawn: Adding sites increases costs in many areas, including patient recruitment; withdrawing sites may mean shifting budget amounts and burden to remaining sites.

Changes in Protocol: These changes often affect the messaging, media and outreach efforts, e.g., if the age is changed from 18-70 to 12-70, the strategy must be adapted to reach a younger audience.

Considering Retention Costs

If a trial runs 26 weeks or longer, it is worth considering a budget for retaining patients in the study. For multiyear trials, a retention budget is mandatory. This should be a budget separate from patient recruitment and contingency recruitment costs.

To keep patients involved and motivated, it is important to budget for ongoing communication with them, just as for investigators and site coordinators. It is helpful to solicit feedback from participants to determine the nature of communications or support they value most. Usually, they want more information about the study and how to best manage their disease state. Educational information makes participants feel valued. Carrying the study's logo or graphic identity on to the development of retention materials is a logical means of continuing the connection between study, participants and site staff.

Consider the call center a resource for retention as well, investing in training for follow up calls, continued appointment scheduling and confirmation, surveys and polls. The call center can be a key tool in maintaining positive contact with patients.

As for patient recruitment estimating, there are no accepted industry standards for budgeting for patient retention. At BBK Patient Recruitment, costs per patient are estimated at $100 (U.S.) per patient per retention year as a starting point in the planning stage. If the study is particularly complicated and requires more frequent interaction with patients, then a higher budget may be in order.

Selling the Budget to Management

Even the most carefully thought out budget does not guarantee management support for new approaches to recruitment. It is necessary to understand the politics and dynamics of the management style of the organization granting approval. Knowledge of the company's previous experience, confidence level and commitment to a product or study is important in planning the strategy for achieving approval of the budget.

Outsourcing Supervisors: There is a growing trend in the pharmaceutical industry to identify internal individuals and departments as responsible for serving as resources and sometimes gatekeepers in the budgeting process. Based in the clinical, financial or communications areas of a company, they provide knowledge of outsourced resources, evaluation of outside suppliers, guidance through the competitive bidding process, negotiation procedures and more. Teaming with these experts and gaining their endorsement can be of great assistance in selling the budget to management.

One-shot vs. Phased Approvals: Depending on the nature of the company, there are different strategies for seeking approval. If confidence in a budget is high, and the management has had positive experiences in budgeting patient recruitment, then one-shot, or comprehensive, budget approval may be possible. When confidence is lower, and the company may have had little or unsatisfactory experience with centralized patient recruitment, a phased approach might be best. Suggesting a $300,000 demonstration project on a $1.5 million budget could encourage gradual buy-in. Successful completion can be presented as proof–of-concept and full approval requested. Once again, it is important to understand the politics and preferred management style of the company.

Performance Projections: It is an easy and worthwhile exercise to anticipate management challenges to a patient recruitment budget.

Performance Projections — Table 3

Source	Inquiries	Refer Ratio	Referrals to Sites	Enrolled
Networking	2,000	2:1	1,000	425
Publicity	8,000	4:1	2,000	830
Direct mail	3,000	3:1	1,000	425
Advertising	10,000	5:1	2,000	830
Total	23,000	4:1	6,000	2,510

Table 4 **Return on Investment**

Source	Inquiries	Cost/ Inquiry	Referrals to Sites	Cost/ Referral	Enrolled	Cost/ Enrolled
Networking	2,000	$128	1,000	$256	425	$602
Publicity	8,000	$60	2,000	$240	830	$578
Direct mail	3,000	$106	1,000	$318	425	$748
Advertising	10,000	$91	2,000	$455	830	$1,096
Subtotal	23,000	$85	6,000	$325	2,510	$779
Call Center	23,000	$22	6,000	$84	2,510	$197
Total	23,000	$107	6,000	$410	2,510	$980

For each program element in a patient recruitment campaign, project the performance of that effort, calculate related costs and prepare performance metrics. These projections estimate the success of the recruitment effort. Examples include number of inquiries, referral ratios and number of enrollees. These numbers can help add meaning and convince management of the value of various media efforts. Tables Three and Four give examples of performance projections by program and anticipated return-on-investment figures. While it may be easy to see that one method of outreach is far more cost-efficient than another, rarely will that one method reach a sufficient number of individuals to achieve the total program goal. Typically, the first fifty percent of patients enrolled will cost less that fifty percent of the total promotional budget. Often, the final twenty percent of enrollees may require up to fifty percent of the total recruitment budget to identify and recruit.

CONTRACTING

In the competitive environment of current patient recruitment practices, contracting is becoming an increasingly popular and essential budget management tool. Through strategic use of contracts, sponsors, investigators, sites and communications agencies work synergistically to achieve a common goal. Contracting can ensure the most effective placement and use of funds and provide a dynamic environment for executing budgets.

Contracts that Work

The most successful contracts include several factors.

Scope of Service

Establishing clear expectation of activities tied to recruitment is essential. It is not enough to simply hold sites responsible for recruitment goals. In the decentralized budget model, what portion should be contracted? Will sponsors pay sites for each patient they screen or only for patients enrolled? What if a site has to handle 200 calls to enroll twenty patients? In this case, payment per enrolled patient is a disincentive to achieve the volume of inquiries needed to complete recruitment.

Process for Change

Change is inevitable in the clinical trial process. Recruitment does not always follow the plan laid out, management makes changes, sites are added or dropped. The most successful contracts build in a process for handling these changes. With a process in place, money can be added if patients are added, or shifted from print advertising to radio based on new knowledge of the target audience. The process for change should include a mechanism for proposal, justification, review and approval and should identify parties responsible for all steps.

Ownership

Contracts must cover the question of who owns the work. Most companies want to own the materials produced for a recruitment campaign. "Perfecting" complete ownership of work can be extremely expensive. The copyrights for a stock illustration or photograph could easily be $40,000. Licensing the use of the same artwork for a distinct period of time might be a fraction of the cost. The same is true of software, fonts and other elements. Advertising is not typically covered as work for hire. However, the agency or artist producing advertising can be asked to assign the copyright to another entity.

Risk-Reward Contracting

Risk-reward contracts are tools for sharing the financial risk of recruitment for clinical trials and for managing budget concerns. As the stakes increase, risk-sharing agreements tied to a variety of objective and subjective goals are becoming more commonplace. Five basic models of risk-sharing contracts are described here.

Withholding: This model involves the buyer withholding certain payments until the supplier meets set objectives. That may include recruiting a set number of eligible patients into a clinical trial or increasing the sales of a particular drug by a preset amount. A withhold contract represents a risk-only approach that ensures the company does not pay until the supplier meets objectives. There is little incentive to suppliers, beyond gaining a new client, to accept such a contract, as it offers no reward other than payment for services if they meet objectives.

Bonuses: This model is the inverse of the withhold contract and is a more widely accepted risk-sharing agreement. It is a rewards-only approach that provides incentives to the supplier to meet or exceed expectations. That approach could include tangible expectations, such as recruitment of a specified number of patients into a program by key milestones set at the start of the program. Less tangible measurements could also serve as measures for bonuses, such as overall product awareness or even the working relationship established between the supplier and project manager.

Volume Discounting: The principle behind this model is that the vendor is guaranteed a certain volume of business and, in turn, the purchaser receives a lower per-unit cost. In other words, by committing to a guaranteed amount of business, the purchaser is able to take advantage of a lower cost and avoid spending the additional money required to find and establish relationships with multiple vendors. The supplier has a tangible commitment and is able to spend less time and money winning the business and more time servicing it.

Utilization Management: This model evolved from volume discounting. The guiding principle behind most risk and reward agreements is the notion of controlling utilization and increasing efficiencies. So that both parties undertake some element of risk and reward, utilization management is based on the principal of controlling overall costs to the client while providing increased unit pricing to the vendor. In those instances, the vendor is responsible for process control and education and for finding new and inventive ways for improving procedures and efficiencies to drive down overall costs.

Capitation: Examples of the capitation model include a cost-per-inquiry on a direct response program, cost-per-marketshare point gained, or cost-per-sales increase. A cost-per-patient arrangement is ideal for clinical trial suppliers, as the trial sponsor can easily measure patient enrollment.

Elements of these various risk-sharing models can be deployed in patient recruitment contracting between sponsors and CROs, SMOs, individual investigators, communications agencies, and call centers. The most successful risk-sharing arrangements are built on existing relationships where trust, clear communications and shared business goals are in place.

CONCLUSION

Creating a patient recruitment budget and considering contracting options is becoming ever more essential in the highly competitive and rapidly growing field of clinical trials. To successfully plan and execute patient recruitment budgets and contracts, there are several essential considerations. Creating a study profile and projecting a recruitment funnel form the framework on which to build the budget. Recognizing the importance of timing in creating a budget cannot be overemphasized in its affect on the scope and size of expenditures. When actually drafting the budget, all elements must be considered and the possibility of future changes incorporated into a contingency budget. Selling the budget to management is a critical step, the success of which often can be influenced by preparation and presentation of performance metrics, both before and after budget approval. To support and strengthen budget initiatives, strategic contracting is vital for reinforcing recruitment performance. By following a thoughtful, strategically sound budget plan into the clinical trial effort, recruitment becomes an increasingly integral part of the process and is much more likely to contribute to the drive toward successful drug and device development and marketing.

AUTHOR BIOGRAPHY

Bonnie Brescia is an agency principal and co-founder for BBK Patient Recruitment. With over twenty years of experience in the development and orchestration of complex communications campaigns and programs on the regional, national and worldwide stage, BBK Patient Recruitment, under Ms. Brescia's direction, has come to be known not only for innovative healthcare communications solutions, but also for insightful analysis and forecast of current and future trends affecting healthcare marketing.

Ms. Brescia is a member of several healthcare associations, including the Advertising Club of New England, and is the chairman of the New England Council Board of Governors for the American Association of Advertising Agencies (AAAA). She also serves as a member of the Drug Information Association, the Massachusetts Medical Association and the Medical Marketing Association as well as serving the role of sustaining member of the Massachusetts Medical Device and Industry Council.

Additionally, recent articles authored by Ms. Brescia include:

- Pharmaceutical Executive. "Creating Risk-Sharing Relationships with Marketing Organizations." June 1999.
- Medical Marketing and Media. "Patient Recruitment Comes of Age as a New Communications Discipline." April 1999.

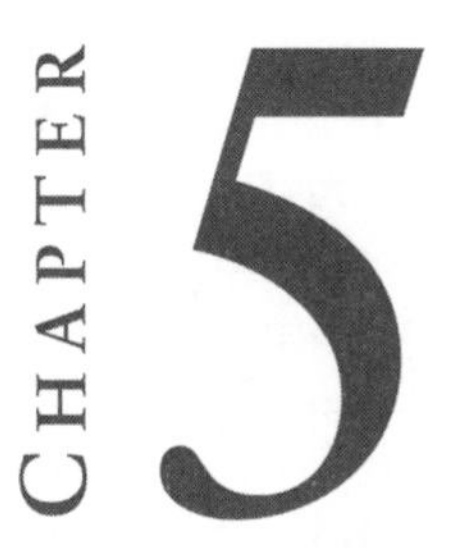

Planning and Evaluating Patient Recruitment Strategies: The Proof Is In the Metrics

Diana L. Anderson, Ph.D., Rheumatology Research International

Accelerating clinical drug development is a top priority. Sponsors, CROs, SMOs, academic medical centers, independent sites and ultimately the public have a vested interest in faster development of innovative drugs. Delays are costly, competition is keen and patent protection ticks away day by day. Consequently, the pharmaceutical industry is highly motivated to find documented methods of speeding the process.

One approach used by sponsors is to select outsourced partners who take responsibility for meeting enrollment targets within the agreed upon timeframe, and have a track record to prove it. These partners often use sophisticated recruitment programs to reach patient enrollment goals, which according to Barnett International, a consulting service for the pharmaceutical industry, accounts for 22% of the clinical development timeline.[1] Assuming clinical drug trials in the United States cost $8 billion annually, the patient enrollment piece translates into a yearly expenditure of $1.76 billion.[2] With stakes this high, it is incumbent upon those managing patient recruitment campaigns to develop metrics, or statistics that quantify their ability to recruit, enroll, randomize, and retain patients, and to demonstrate how their actions contribute to study acceleration.

In the young study conduct industry, the development of metrics that validate the success of professional approaches for patient recruitment and enrollment is just beginning. There is a growing body of anecdotal evidence highlighting the accomplishments achieved by specific strategies for enrollment, but there is neither a body of literature, nor industry standards to benchmark metrics. This leaves the door open for early players to define the field as metrics become an increasingly important tool used by specific patient recruitment vendors, SMOs and high-performing sites to distinguish themselves.

Table 1 **Required Processes for Outsourced Partners of R.W. Johnson**

→ Time from final protocol to enrollment of first patient	8 weeks
→ Time for enrollment of patients	6 months (target)
→ Time from last patient completed to database closure	4 weeks

Table 2 **Metrics Developed by Amgen**

Metric	Time
→ Time from final protocol to enrollment of first patient	12 weeks
→ Time from first patient enrolled to last patient enrolled	Varies by study
→ Time from last patient completed to database closure	Less than 8 weeks
→ Final statistical analysis to final report	8 weeks

Some sponsors are expressing interest in presentations of metrics from outsourced CROs, SMOs and independent sites. In addition, a number of sponsors are creating internal metrics to benchmark their own performance as it relates to study acceleration, and then seeking outsourced partners able to conform to these prescribed guidelines. Eugene Richardson, Director Global Strategic Alliances of R.W. Johnson Pharmaceutical Research Institute, a subsidiary of Johnson & Johnson, says, "We are very metrics driven. We've dramatically accelerated our timeline, starting from writing a protocol, through patient recruitment, to submitting a new drug application (NDA). For example, our time from last patient out to final database release dropped from seventeen weeks to less than four weeks. This was accomplished over a two-year period starting in October 1998 by focusing on two processes. We looked at improving the process from draft protocol through database release; and secondly, we sought to speed the time from database release through final report. We've developed timelines for our processes that we require of the CROs and sites that we select. When I make presentations to a CRO, I make them aware of what our metrics and submetrics are and what our expectations are for their performance." (Table One) Richardson also comments that during the site selection process, he expects sites and SMOs to provide metrics that document their ability to recruit and enroll patients in studies in the same or similar therapeutic areas. This information is critical to R.W. Johnson's site selection process.

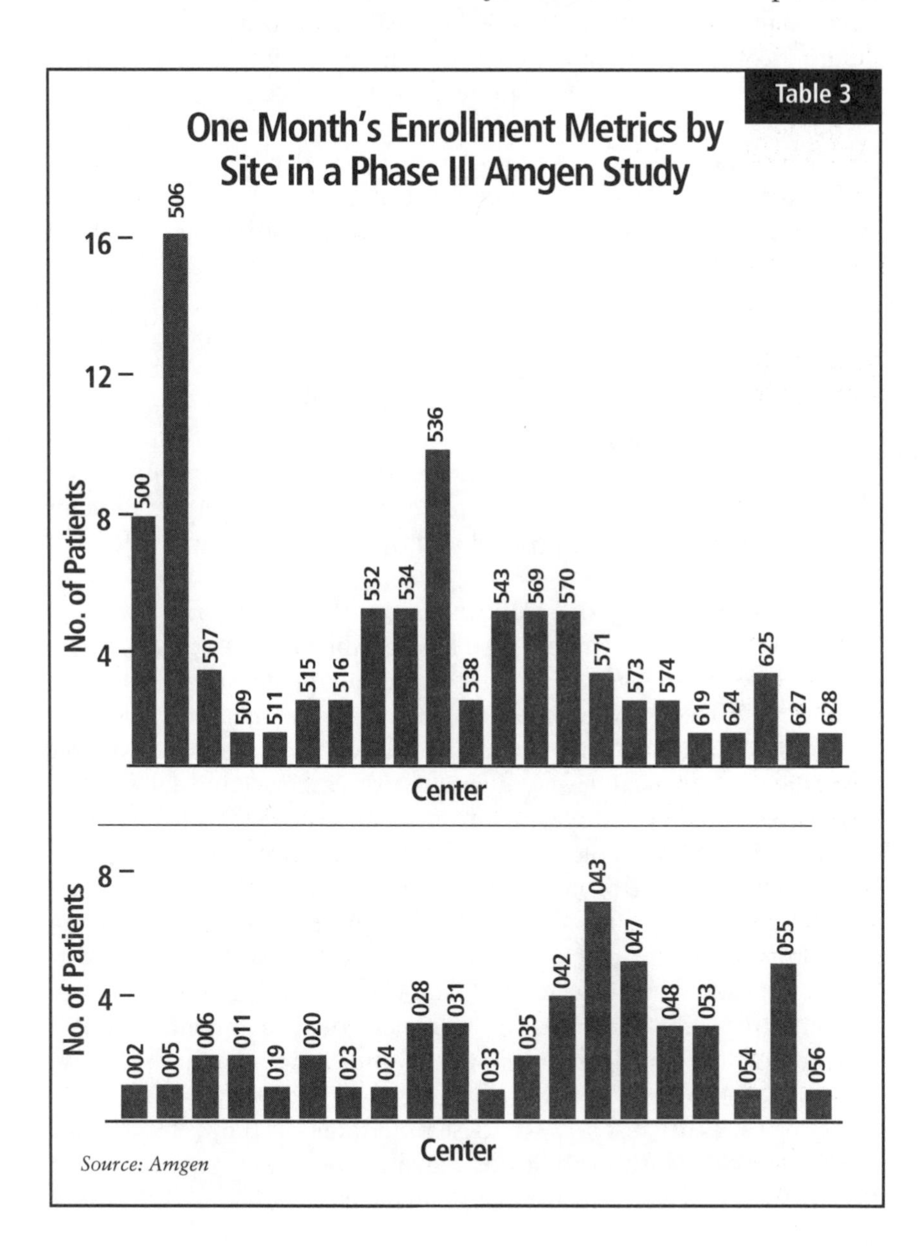

Hassan Movahhed, Director of Clinical Affairs at Amgen, Inc., says the company has spent several years exploring the types of internal metrics that are useful and achievable. Amgen's metrics for several clinical development steps are seen in Table Two. To encourage sites to reach these timelines, Amgen posts study-specific newsletters on secured web sites, detailing how enrollment is progressing, and features sites and investigators participating in the study. Movahhed says, "This is a tool to improve relationships with sites, creates some healthy competition, and helps all parties to know each other's expectations for the study." (Table Three)

In the process of site selection, Amgen first identifies investigators with experience and success in conducting trials in specific therapeutic areas, and then looks at sites' metrics documenting their ability to initiate studies quickly, recruit, enroll, and randomize patients, and submit clean data to the sponsors on time. While these metrics provide insight into the quality of site operations, it may be difficult to evaluate their usefulness when a sponsor does not know how realistic the entrance criteria are for a new study. Movahhed says, "Often we don't have enough data to help us determine the difficulty in recruiting for a specific study. We have to think more carefully about the numbers of patients we need to screen, the types of recruitment strategies that could be successful and the budget for those efforts."

Procter & Gamble Pharmaceuticals has established metrics for some clinical development activities, and has variable timeframes for others. Set timelines exist for time for protocol development; time from protocol development to study startup; time from last patient completed to database lock; and time from data cleanup to final report. Metrics for some other clinical development activities are variable due to trial-specific issues. For example, time from final protocol to enrollment of first patient has a variable timeline. The variability stems from the fact that in one study, the protocol may be finalized, but the drug may not yet be ready to ship. In another, the drug is ready, so the time from final protocol to enrollment of first patient could potentially be shorter. So, for each study, Procter & Gamble develops an internal metric for time from final protocol to enrollment of first patient, and also benchmarks the time from last patient completed to database closure.

Generally, sites are not privy to these timeframes as they refer to steps that are not the responsibility of the sites. By comparison, meeting the timeline for patient recruitment and enrollment is clearly the sites' responsibility. As such, it is part of the protocol; it is discussed at site assessment visits, and is presented at the investigator meeting.

Procter & Gamble reviews metrics prepared by sites that point to their ability to recruit and enroll patients within prescribed timelines. This is part of the company's interest in having sites become more proactive in the way they screen, enroll and randomize patients. Procter & Gamble cautions, however, that it may be difficult to judge the usefulness of metrics for competitive studies as a predictor of success for the study at hand, especially if the nuances of the entry criteria are unknown to Procter & Gamble. Similarly, if the study at hand is for a new indication, metrics presented for different indications may be less important than evaluating the experience of a strong investigator at a site under consideration.

Bruce Linkov, Associate Director of Pfizer, Inc.'s Clinical Business Support Unit, explains that at the beginning of the site selection process, Pfizer develops a lengthy questionnaire to evaluate prospective sites. The questionnaire probes such issues as the number of studies previously conducted in the therapeutic area, and what the site was expected to accomplish in those studies. According to Linkov, Pfizer recognizes that each study is unique, and one study may have a protocol design that is easier or more difficult to enroll than another. "That's why I look at metrics with a grain of salt because the study design in question may be more complex than those conducted by the site in the past. Also, at this point in time, metrics are often not readily available at most sites or academic medical centers. SMOs are more likely to have started keeping metrics."

Pfizer's internal metrics vary from therapeutic area to therapeutic area, but the company clearly states timelines for each specific study, such as the expected enrollment pattern, within the contract. The company does have internal metrics across therapeutic areas but they are rough guidelines based on how studies have progressed in the past. "Metrics are just a guide because it always comes back to the issue of the complexity of each individual protocol," says Linkov. Issues such as time from final protocol to enrollment of first patient are considered to be under Pfizer's control, not the sites', since it may involve drug availability and readiness of case report forms.

Several key factors are driving the need for a documented professionalized approach. First, as mentioned in Chapter One, is the fact that the number of new clinical research starts have been growing steadily. (See Table One, Chapter One) Secondly, the average number of subjects per new drug application (NDA) is 3,900 and growing 7% annually.[3] Thirdly, according to CenterWatch, a U.S. based publishing and information service for the clinical trials industry, a mere 4% of the U.S. population participates in clinical trials annually.

In a competitive environment, attracting more subjects to studies requires a multi-step approach for recruiting, followed by the measuring of the success of the recruitment campaign. In developing the approach, the therapeutic area of interest must be taken into consideration. Designing a successful recruitment campaigns for depression may require different tools than crafting a campaign for urinary incontinence. The need to use various tactics coincides with the growing awareness among sponsors that recruitment and enrollment is too critical to leave in the hands of sites lacking marketing personnel and marketing experience in the specific therapeutic area. The days of sponsors simply handing a lump sum of recruitment money to sites, and hoping that they can implement the best way to use it are numbered. It might be more productive for sponsors to give money to sites known to recruit successfully, and/or to an outside vendor that specializes in and assumes accountability for site enrollment.

OVERVIEW OF A SIX-PART PLAN

One approach to successful patient recruitment, enrollment and collection of resulting metrics involves the use of a targeted six-part plan. (Table Four) This plan is a system enabling sites to document accountability for their patient recruitment commitments. The program is particularly useful if the sponsor has decided to centralize recruiting efforts by outsourcing to a CRO/SMO or to a vendor specializing in patient recruitment, as the data will be collected centrally.

Table 4 **Six-Part Plan**

STEP 1:	Determine need for recruitment plan
STEP 2:	Build a team to handle the budget
STEP 3:	Negotiate a separate recruitment budget
STEP 4:	Develop a specific contract for recruitment
STEP 5:	Create a system to handle the recruitment funds and to track the results
STEP 6:	Analyze outcomes data

The plan starts with **Step One**, which is determining the need for a recruitment program. When submitting a proposal for a potential project, the vendor assembles a separate proposal for patient recruitment. Sponsors are beginning to accept this concept, and are buying into the idea of having at least advertising language in place that has been approved by the Institutional Review Board (IRB). Once accepted, the plan can be further fleshed out.

Movahhed of Amgen says, "We absolutely believe in sites having a recruitment plan in place from the beginning of the study. Good recruitment plans should not be done after the fact to correct broken plans, or to make up for the fact that not enough patients could be recruited from an internal database. Also, we discuss patient recruitment initiatives at investigator meetings."

Linkov of Pfizer voices a similar sentiment. He says, "It is critical to think about the media campaign early. We design our own patient recruitment plan in house when we start a new protocol, and budget for it. We make a determination as to the amount of help that each site needs for patient recruitment. Some sites are more adept and more organized than others. Often we will discuss our plan with the more adept sites and ask for suggestions. Then we can merge our plan with theirs. The biggest mistake is to do recruitment as a rescue effort because by the time you need a rescue effort, months and months have already gone by."

Step Two addresses the development of a patient recruitment plan using a team approach. Once the need for patient recruitment has been established, it is critical to gain an understanding of the project at hand, and from that understanding, build an appropriate team responsible for developing and implementing a successful plan. If a sponsor elects to outsource this work, it is imperative that that vendor does not function independently of the clinical and project management teams. The most successful approach involves convening this group regularly throughout the course of the study. Oftentimes, this takes the form of weekly conference calls with representatives of project management from the sponsor and CRO and/or SMO, and the patient recruitment vendor.

Step Three puts the plan in motion. It involves negotiating, whether internally managed within the pharmaceutical company and/or with the sponsor/CRO, for an upfront budget that will be specifically earmarked for recruitment strategies. Calculating a meaningful budget results from specifics of the recruitment plan, historic expenditures, and revisiting previous metrics for similar studies. Later, when the recruitment campaign begins, the process of matching expenses with the effectiveness of various initiatives will lead to identification of strategies that are media cost-efficient and cost-inefficient. Items to be tracked include physician referral, database, radio, television, print media and direct mail. Chapter Six provides in depth detail in regard to budgeting.

Step Four examines the need to develop a specific contractual agreement for patient recruiting. In the recent past, study contracts tended to tack on a somewhat arbitrary figure for advertising, without any elaboration. For example, a contract might have contained a line item stating "$2500 per site for advertising" without any hint as to how this dollar figure was chosen, or how the money should be spent. As recruitment becomes more sophisticated, there is movement away from this vague, undefined approach to one that is highly specific, in writing, detailed, realistic, and agreed upon prior to study start-up. An example of specific contract language is seen in Table

Table 5 Sample Basic Contractual Language for Patient Recruitment

XYZ shall provide services in connection with the implementation and conduct of the ABC trial Protocol #0000 (the "Project") for 100 US investigator sites. XYZ will commence the Project on or about said date. The specific services provided by XYZ include, but are not limited to the following:

1. XYZ shall manage the subject accrual for 100 preapproved investigational U.S. sites for the Project.
2. XYZ will manage the subject recruitment budget for all U.S. sites; oversee subject recruitment at each site to facilitate meeting enrollment quotas.
3. XYZ will oversee subject recruitment initiatives for all U.S. sites with a budget of said value.
4. XYZ will manage subject recruitment materials submission to a central IRB (if appropriate). XYZ will be responsible for obtaining IRB approval for all the subject recruitment materials. Once approved, these materials will be provided to all sites to be placed in regulatory binders. Sponsor shall be responsible for all IRB fees on a pass-through basis.
5. XYZ Project Manager will monitor enrollment weekly and communicate results to assigned Project Director and Subject Recruitment Director via enrollment and screening tools. Results will also be communicated weekly to Sponsor.
6. XYZ shall maintain communication with all U.S. sites to insure subject accrual and to help answer any non-protocol related questions that may arise during the Project from the sites.

Five. With a formulated plan in place, it is possible to roll the plan out at the investigator meeting, and begin implementation when other study conduct activities are also ready to start-up.

Step Five involves the creation of a system to handle the recruitment funds and to track the results. These data should be provided to the sponsor on a weekly basis. Tracking refers to a number of factors, and allows identification of which strategies provide successful subject referral. (Table Six) The patient recruitment management group should collect this data from the site. A site's willingness and ability to collect these data in a timely manner could become a benchmark to help sponsors differentiate well-organized, experienced sites from less effective ones. It also suggests a baseline level of responsibility for recruitment efforts that the site or recruitment management team is willing to accept.

Tracking Data—Weekly Status — Table 6

1. Calculating the number of scheduled patients
2. Computing the number of pending appointments
3. Determining the number of patients qualified
4. Tallying the number that did not qualify
5. Calculating the number that qualified but not participated
6. Determining the number of randomized patients
7. Tallying the number that completed the trial

Step Six looks at analyzing outcomes data. Once a study is completed, and the last patient has finished the trial, developing metrics that attest to the relative success of a campaign is an important exercise for measuring outcomes of the marketing efforts. The bottom line is comparing the number of patients that completed a study at sites using an orchestrated campaign against the number that finished a study at sites using other means of recruitment.

A CASE IN POINT

A case study involving simultaneous osteoarthritis and rheumatoid arthritis trials highlights the successful use of this six-step approach. In late 1998, site management organization (SMO) with a separate patient recruiting division, started participation in concurrent Phase II studies, both testing the same investigational oral agent. One trial explored efficacy of the compound on pain and function in osteoarthritis patients, while the other studied it for efficacy on pain and function in rheumatoid arthritis patients.

The osteoarthritis study required a three month enrollment period, and initially, the SMO was selected to manage and recruit patients for seventeen of the selected fifty-three sites. Although the target enrollment for the seventeen SMO sites was 114 patients, the SMO actually enrolled 155, thereby exceeding the goal by 36%. (Table Seven) Halfway through the enrollment period, the sponsor approached the SMO to assume responsibility for recruitment for the remaining thirty-six sites. At the time of study completion, the SMO had enrolled 280 patients for the thirty-six sites. The original target was 252 patients, but the SMO exceeded that goal by 11%.

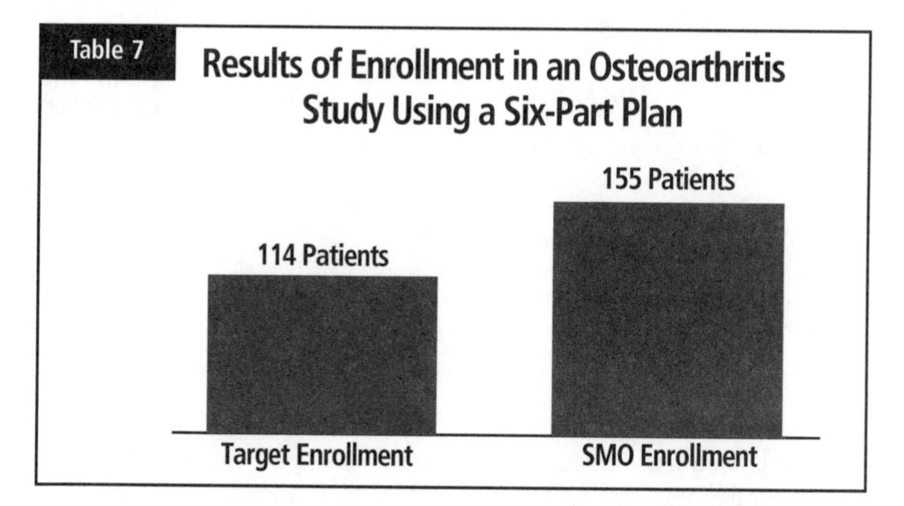

A total of fifty-eight sites were selected for the rheumatoid arthritis study that was conducted in the United States and Canada. The SMO managed and recruited for nineteen of the fifty-eight sites. The enrollment target for the nineteen sites was 133 patients, however the SMO enrolled 180, overshooting the goal by 35% (Table Eight). In addition, the sponsor eventually granted the SMO the responsibility for recruitment at the remaining thirty-nine sites, and the company exceeded that goal of 273 enrollees by three patients.

In order to reach and exceed the sponsors' goals, the SMO started by assembling a team responsible both for the development of a detailed marketing plan and the ultimate success of the study. The team

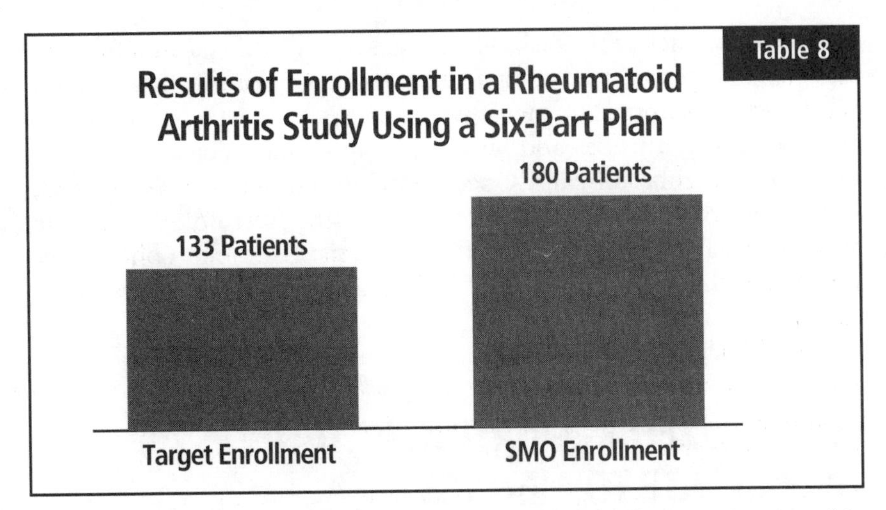

devised a comprehensive approach as seen in Table Nine. During this process, the SMO recognized that there might be a need to employ slightly different tactics to recruit in Canada as compared to the United States. This included establishing a toll-free 1-888 number for Canadian prospective patients. This telephone number was answered in Ontario, Canada, and all of the Canadian recruitment materials carried this number. Additionally, some of the recruitment advertisements contained graphics targeted to the Canadian marketplace.

To implement the plan, a detailed budget that specified anticipated costs of recruitment was negotiated. These costs were spelled out in the resulting contract.

From the beginning of the studies, a system was created to handle the recruitment funds by establishing separate accounts for each study. To follow the results of both studies, the Manager of Patient Screening

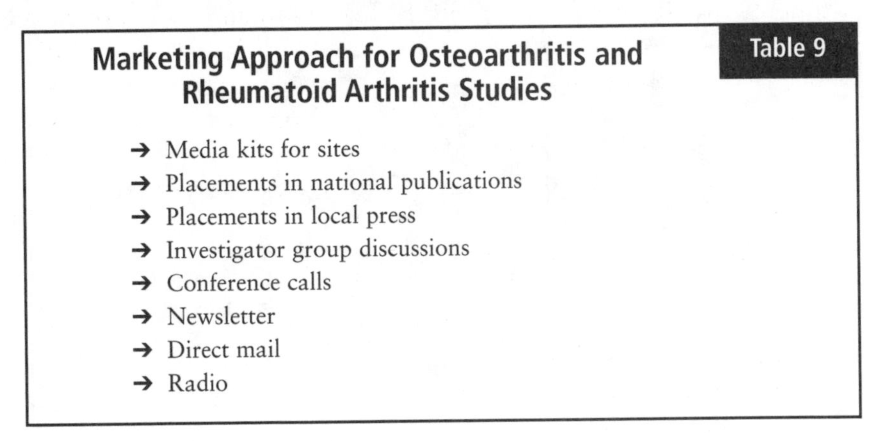
Table 9

Marketing Approach for Osteoarthritis and Rheumatoid Arthritis Studies

- ➔ Media kits for sites
- ➔ Placements in national publications
- ➔ Placements in local press
- ➔ Investigator group discussions
- ➔ Conference calls
- ➔ Newsletter
- ➔ Direct mail
- ➔ Radio

Services was assigned the tasks of tracking the call screens and the associated costs. She began to compile data, looking beyond the number of calls coming from specific media sources. This included computing the number of screen passes and scheduled appointments as a percentage of the total number of calls. Once these calculations were completed, she presented them to the Director of Patient Recruitment and the Project Manager for review and final analysis. Using this comprehensive approach, enrollment targets were not met but were exceeded.

An expanded version of this case study is presented in Chapter Seventeen.

CENTRALIZED RECRUITING INITIATIVES AS THEY RELATE TO METRICS

Centralized recruiting refers to a central campaign created to generate interest by potential patients in a specific study. Because this effort is centrally managed, generally by a firm specializing in patient recruitment, all recruitment data generated by the various media placements can flow centrally into the recruitment firm. This arrangement is an ideal format for collecting metrics, as described in steps five and six of the six-part plan.

The patient recruitment team should start collecting data from the initiation of the campaign. Baseline metrics for a study may include calcu-

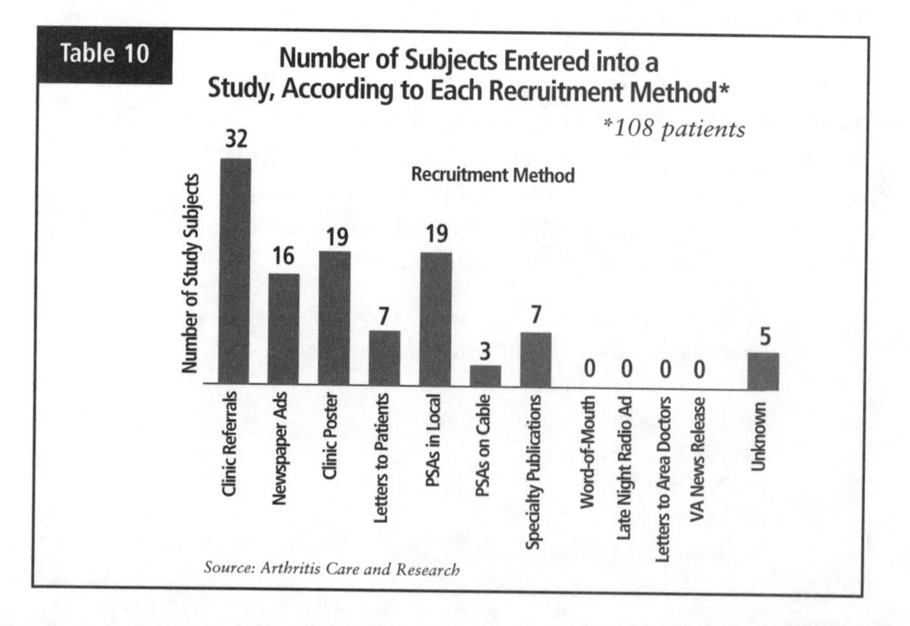

Table 10 Number of Subjects Entered into a Study, According to Each Recruitment Method*

Source: Arthritis Care and Research

lating the number of patients enrolled and randomized per site as a result of the various media efforts, and the costs of advertising per phone screen. Table Ten shows the results of a media campaign to recruit 108 patients in a trial studying the effects of exercise on the knees of osteoarthritis patients.[4] Table Eleven shows the advertising costs per phone screen for a rheumatoid arthritis study. Charts as simple as these can distinguish between successful and unsuccessful tactics, and can help sites determine which strategies to use in the future for similar indications. Additionally, information such as costs per call, and the time needed to screen each call can help sites justify to sponsors why they are requesting a specific budget figure for patient recruitment.

For a central recruitment campaign to be successful, sites and monitors must understand the process. To facilitate buy-in, it is a good idea to discuss patient recruitment at the investigator meeting. Following the meeting, it is important to speak directly to each and every coordinator so he or she knows that a central campaign is under way, and that his or her opinion is valuable. The coordinator should be encouraged to provide input about the campaign, and should be asked to suggest recruitment tactics that might be relevant to a specific geographic area. This simple yet direct approach can pay dividends by involving the study site as well as effectively placing initiatives.

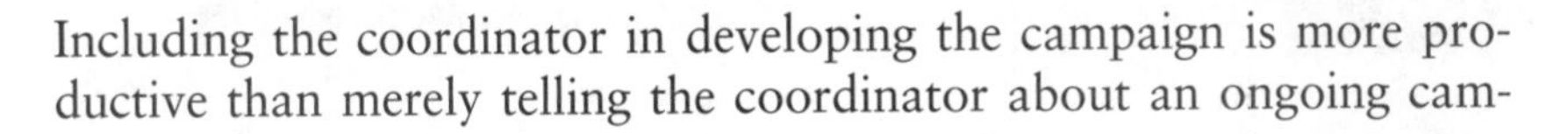

Including the coordinator in developing the campaign is more productive than merely telling the coordinator about an ongoing cam-

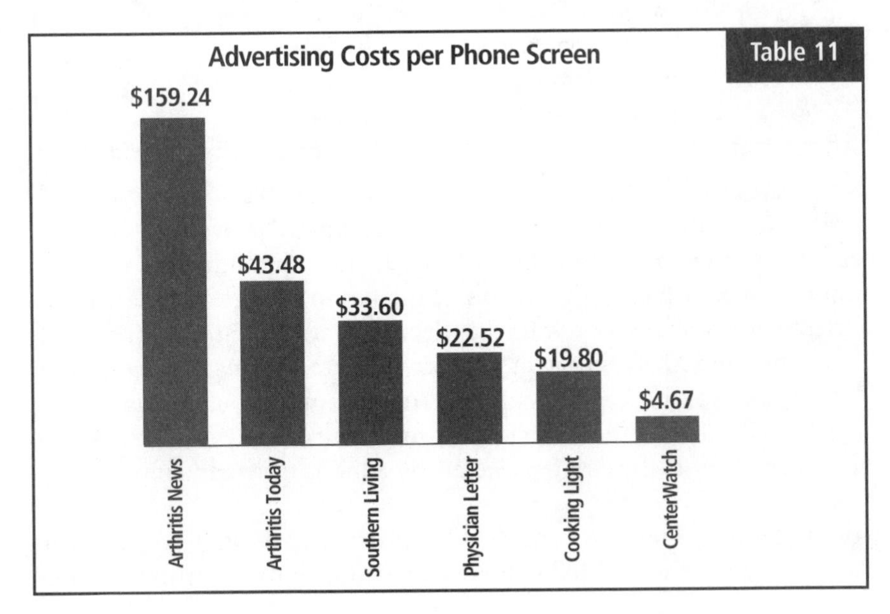

paign. There are instances of sites not even being notified that a central campaign is in place. Certainly, failing to communicate this basic information does little to encourage a spirit of cooperation, and may create an "us versus them" mentality. To maintain enthusiasm for a project, it might be wise to share with the sites the metrics measuring success of the campaign. This can be accomplished via monthly or weekly newsletter, fax, or e-mail. An example of this approach was shown earlier in Chart Three.

METRICS AND THE CENTRALIZED CALL CENTER

As metrics are developed to document the value of a well-planned multifaceted approach to recruiting, the central recruitment campaign may become a more commonly used tool. As part of the central campaign, a sophisticated phone-screening program is often used in the form of the central call center. These centers free sites of the burden of screening hundreds, or thousands of recruitment calls. Sites will, of course, retain responsibility for patient enrollment, randomization, and eventual study completion, but designing and tracking the marketing campaign, and handling numerous phone screens will be left to marketing professionals.

Table 12 Some Metrics Collected by American MediConnect

- ➔ Capturing total number of responses to media
- ➔ Comparing media type vs. media type
- ➔ Calculating ratio of preliminary phone screen passes to fails
- ➔ Comparing performance of sites
- ➔ Computing dollar cost per recruited patient

American MediConnect Inc. is one of the pioneers in centralized patient recruiting. Started in 1985, the company provides a centralized call center to screen calls and to schedule appointments for preliminary screen passes. In addition, the company offers an array of recruitment services, including collecting patient data in a central databank, and analyzing it in a client-preferred format. Some of the data details specifics about the effectiveness of various media placements, and suggests the direction for future media buys. Table Twelve shows some of the metrics collected by American MediConnect.

Joseph Sameh, President and CEO, says that early in a recruitment campaign, American MediConnect provides daily information. He explains that initially, a sponsor would not want to wait a whole week before collecting data because the site could be spending thousands of dollars that are not optimizing the overall effort, and would not realize this soon enough to redirect those dollars.

American MediConnect also collects metrics comparing site performances. This information can help sponsors identify underperforming sites. For example, if a site delays in scheduling in comparison to other sites in the study, this paints a picture of that site's performance.

The concept of a central company developing recruitment metrics for a large multi-center phase III study should be compelling to sponsors. Sameh believes that sponsors are recognizing the added value in having all of the data reside in a central facility, enabling rapid trend analysis. As an example, analysis of the data from all of the sites can identify a very low screen pass rate. Armed with this information, sponsors can apply for protocol amendments. This type of analysis helps sponsors save precious time in their clinical development programs.

For centralized call center efforts to be successful, the central phone screeners must be trained to talk to potential patients in a way that will interest them in participating in the study at hand. Professional phone manner is critical for creating an enthusiasm for the study, which starts with making and keeping scheduled appointments, assuming the patients have passed preliminary screens. Site-based nurses who understand the health problem of a caller can be empathetic and ultimately successful in turning that caller into an enrollee. Unfortunately site nurses often lack the time to screen the many calls coming to the site. This reality, and the ability to house patient recruitment data centrally create the opportunity for centralized call centers. See Chapter Seven for further details on centralized patient recruiting.

PROFESSIONAL TOOLS FOR TRACKING PATIENT RECRUITMENT

Tracking recruitment efforts can become increasingly complex as marketing efforts expand into multiple markets, yet tracking is key to developing metrics. In the early phases of recruitment, those accepting responsibility for centralized recruiting need ready access to media results in order to tally weekly reports of media placement. This is the starting point for computing metrics. As the project unfolds, reports can move from weekly to monthly, and then quarterly. (Table Six)

Advanced Clinical Software, LLC is one U.S.-based company offering a broad-based software package for managing clinical trials at the site level. Their core product, Study Manager™, enables sites to capture data that can lead to the development of metrics. (Table Thirteen) Study Manager creates a database, and through the Study Recruiter module, generates reports that show the rate of enrollment by detailing the number of phone calls and the related media source, followed by randomization, and ultimately the number of patients who complete a study. For example, if one thousand patients responded this month to various media placements for a particular study, Study Recruiter can generate reports showing the number of enrollees, as well as the type of media that resulted in high and low enrollment. Armed with these metrics, recruitment approaches can quickly be refined and redirected to improve media productivity as the enrollment period unfolds. Study Recruiter also has capability for scheduling patient visits, and creating reminder letters for those visits.

The Study Recruiter module is available in a PC version, and a web edition. Using the web version, sites can create their own patient recruitment web sites, enabling prospective patients to enter demographic and screening data online. With the Call Tracker module, the nearest site is notified of the prospective patient, prompting the site to call that person for a more in-depth phone screen.

The demographic data provided by either the PC or web versions connect into the Study Manager database. Patients entered into the database are linked to the specific advertisements or source to which they responded. Recruitment operates through Study Recruiter, while enrollment, randomization and other study functions operate through Study Manager. Also, with Study Recruiter, it is possible to count the number of patients who screened themselves over the Web versus the number who called into a central call center. This comparison highlights which patient recruitment approaches are most efficacious. Currently, far more prospective patients are screened through central call centers than are screened on the web, but over time, this balance is expected to shift more toward web-based activity.

Although recruiters often tend to focus on tallying responses to advertisements, the goal is to develop metrics that identify those approaches

Table 13

Advertising Effectiveness for ONE Site

Media Source	Description	Study	# Calls	# Pre-Screen	# Screen	# Randomized	% Randomized	Event Cost	Cost/Call	Cost per Randomization
950 KJR AM	Evening Spot	93213	14	7	7	5	35.71%	$5,000	$357	$1,000
Telethon Services	Phone Campaign	93213	16	10	10	9	56.25%	$8,500	$531	$944.44
Fox Q13	Lunchtime Ad	2342	19	6	6	3	15.79%	$7,500	$394	$2,500
Seattle Times	1 Mth. 1/2pg. Ad	954-410	12	6	6	4	33.33%	$2,000	$167	$500
Washington Asthma Alliance	Speaking Monthly	954-410	10	6	6	2	20.00%	$1,150	$115	$575
www.nwresearch.com	Web Site Feedback	A-9192	24	10	10	8	33.33%	$5,000	$208	$625
Site Totals			95	45	45	31		$29,150		

Source: Advanced Clinical Software

leading to reaching enrollment targets within the contracted time frame. Frank Kilpatrick, President of Healthcare Communications Group, a provider of patient recruitment services, believes that for sponsors, this is the key metric because timely enrollment is a critical step in accelerating time to peak sales. (Table Fourteen)

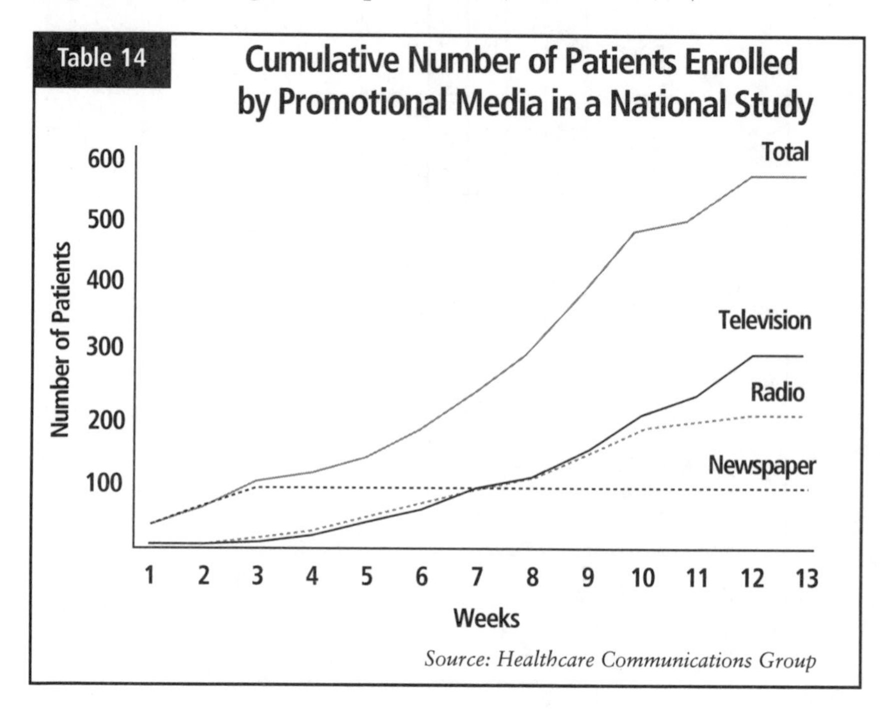

Source: Healthcare Communications Group

Sponsors want more metrics to help them differentiate performance among various sites, but at the same time, sponsors are just beginning to get comfortable with the precise nature of this type of information. Metrics can provide objective data, and can shine a light on productive and unproductive sites.

Metric data can be very useful, but there is more to site selection than evaluating metrics. On one hand, sponsors can use metrics as a quantitative tool to help them identify higher performing sites. On the other hand, sponsors still want and need investigators who are opinion leaders to perform trials. Key investigators often conduct clinical trials with opinion leaders who may not be known for their emphasis on study acceleration. But recruiting those investigators is important for creating awareness of the study compound. Movahhed of Amgen explains that sponsors can meet enrollment timelines through a carefully selected balance of sites with streamlined processes, and sometimes less expedient academic medical centers, which are needed to gain access to opinion leaders.

In the long run, Kilpatrick foresees professionalized recruiting growing in sponsor acceptance because it tends to be more productive while frequently costing no more than the traditional approach of simply handing recruitment funds to sites. For example, Healthcare Communications was brought into a phase II central nervous system study late in the recruitment process to accelerate it to meet the sponsor's enrollment timeline. Within a ten week period, through the use of a comprehensive campaign, Healthcare Communications was able to add an additional 126 patients, enabling the sponsor to meet its enrollment target several months sooner than would have been possible using traditional methods alone. (Table Fifteen)

A key component of Healthcare Communications approach is the Site Practice Management System™ (SPMS), a modular system designed to enhance communications with the sites in an effort to maximize results of the targeted media campaign. SPMS is composed of three modules: Sponsor/CRO Initiation Module; Site Assessment Module; and Site Practice Management System. The Sponsor/CRO

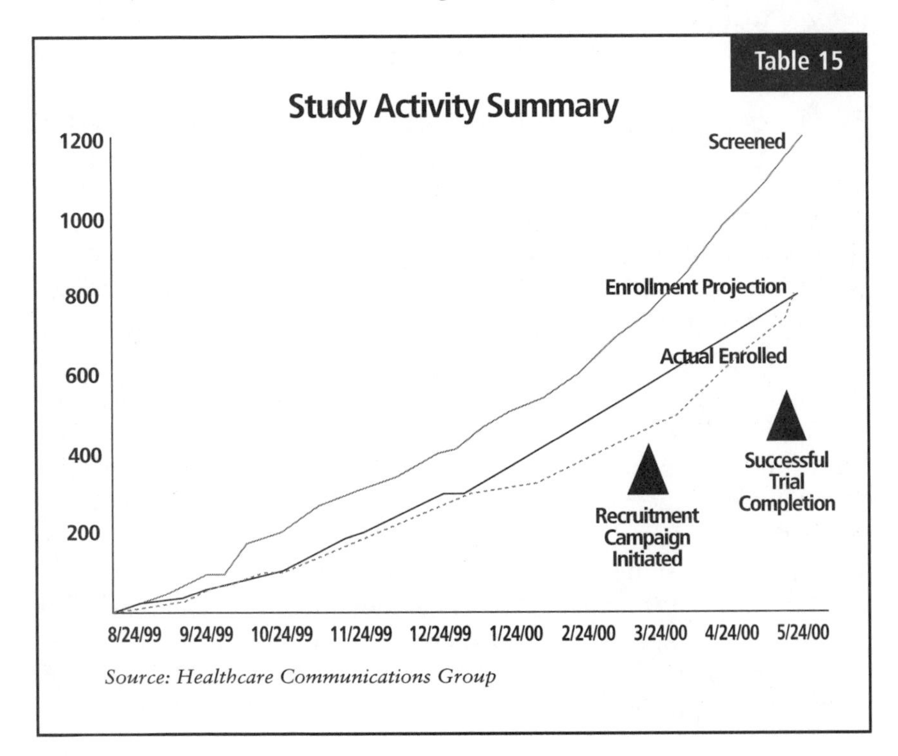

Source: Healthcare Communications Group

Initiation Module focuses on working with the sponsor to establish clear objectives and lines of communication with the investigators and sites to reinforce the sponsor's commitment to accelerated recruitment. The Site Assessment Module uses evaluative instruments to examine the site's workflow, media preferences, management systems and level of motivation for a particular study. The Site Practice Management System refers to the building of trust and a relationship with sites that can only be developed over time. This happens by frequent communication, on-site visits, and as-needed use of temporary administrative personnel.

METRICS—FINALLY

Efforts to professionalize patient recruiting extend beyond tallying the number of responses to yesterday's television commercial. The real focus is on using a comprehensive approach to attract patients who eventually enroll, are randomized, and complete the study in a timely fashion. As these methods unfold during the recruitment period, smart recruiters collect metrics to prove the efficacy of their techniques as they relate to faster enrollment. Quality call centers have already recognized that their higher function is data collection leading to enrollment statistics, not merely totaling the number of screened calls.

As metrics progress, it may be possible to identify the best types of patients to fill a study. For example, are patients coming from their physicians' private practices more likely to complete a study than those recruited externally? What about patients who self-refer? These types of questions will be answered as the collection of metrics matures.

Going forward, knowing which metrics are most meaningful will result from formal and informal strategic relationships between sponsors and their outsourced partners. Metrics cannot be collected in a vacuum. They must suit the sponsors' needs to quantify processes that lead to faster clinical development. Without industry standards, each company is left to devise its own brand of metrics. The hope is that eventually, most players will come to a common understanding of what documentation is needed to move investigational compounds through the developmental pipeline more quickly. Documenting improved recruitment and enrollment techniques is growing in importance, as these two processes represent significant bottlenecks in drug development.

REFERENCES

[1] Pharmaceutical R&D Statistical Sourcebook. May 2000, p. 130.

[2] "Series of Reports Prompted Reforms in Human Research." Edward T. Pound. *USA Today*. June 12, 2000. p. 9A.

[3] DataEdge, LLC. Fort Washington, PA, October 1998.

[4] "A Comparison of Recruitment Methods for an Osteoarthritis Exercise Study." *Arthritis Care and Research*. Brian T. Maurer, et. al. September 1995, Vol. 8, No. 3, p. 165.

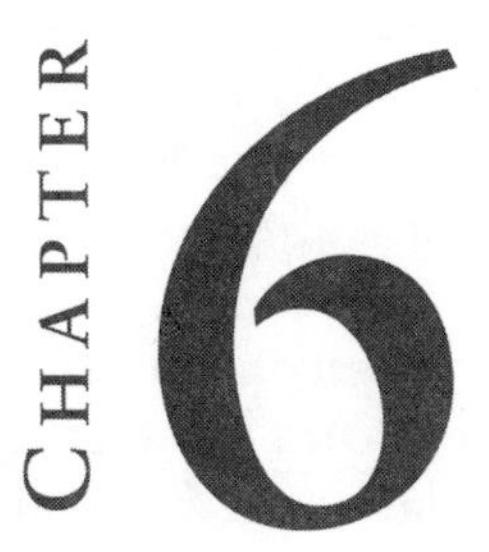

Protocol Design and Patient Recruitment

William K. Sietsema, PhD
Jill Leonard, RN, BSN, ACRN Kendle International, Inc.

Clinical protocols are written in order to provide complete detail on the procedures to be followed and the methods of analysis to be applied to a clinical study. Protocols serve as a guide for all personnel who contribute to their execution so they know exactly what is expected of them, what is permitted, and what is not permitted.

Clinical protocols are used broadly across the field of health care and can apply to traditional medicines (new and old), medical procedures or therapies, and medical devices, as well as nutritional supplements. This chapter uses the term "health care products" to cover all these examples.

The manufacture and sale of health care products is regulated by numerous agencies worldwide, some examples being the United States Food and Drug Administration (U.S. FDA), the Canadian Health Protection Branch (HPB), the Japanese Ministry of Health and Welfare (MHW), and the European Agency for the Evaluation of Medicinal Products (EMEA). Collectively, these and other governing bodies around the world will be referred to as "regulatory agencies."

Any protocol design should first and foremost be based on good science. That is, its objective should be to answer a specific question or set of questions pertaining to tolerability, efficacy, safety, or compliance. For this reason, a clear statement of the questions (or objectives) to be answered makes an excellent starting point from which to design and write the protocol.

The results of a clinical protocol frequently impact the marketing claims or "label" of a health care product and care must be taken in choosing the patient population to study and the clinical endpoints to measure. It is likely that the wording of the claim or label will directly take into account the patients studied and the clinical endpoint measured. For instance, if a new health care product is tested in patients between the ages of 60 and 90, the allowed claim will be "this product has been tested for use in patients between the ages of 60 and 90." Extrapolation to younger age ranges would not be allowed without data to suggest a comparable benefit in younger patients. Similarly, if the measured endpoint in a dermatological disorder is number of skin lesions (but not the size of lesions), the claim must read, "reduces the number of skin lesions" but cannot specify any change in lesion size. Accordingly, much effort has to be expended to choose a patient population and clinical endpoints that are coherent with the pharmacologic activity of the compound and will provide the most favorable marketing claims.

This chapter first examines some of the forces that tend toward the use of a narrow versus a broad patient population. It then describes elements of a protocol that can influence rates of patient recruitment. Finally, the last half of the chapter is devoted to case studies that provide examples of protocol elements that can be modified to impact patient recruitment.

NARROW VERSUS BROAD PATIENT POPULATION

There can be statistical advantages to selecting a narrowly defined patient population for a study. A narrow population could be patients in a narrow age range (for instance, postmenopausal women 45 to 55 years of age) or a narrow disease severity (men with benign prostatic hyperplasia with prostate-specific antigen no more than 50% above the normal range). A narrow patient population generally has less variability than the general population. As a result, standard deviations are smaller and the sample size is reduced, allowing the study to be conducted with fewer patients. Alternatively, the sample size can be larger but the reduced variability increases the power to demonstrate a statistically significant difference between treatment groups where the anticipated difference between treatments is small.

There are, however, disadvantages of using a narrow patient population. One of these is that it may be more difficult to recruit patients if the inclusion/exclusion criteria are too restrictive.[1] So even though fewer patients are required, the study may take longer to enroll. In some cases, extremely narrow patient populations may be impossible to enroll. For example, finding patients with rheumatoid arthritis who are completely naïve to Non-Steroidal Anti-Inflammatory Drugs is virtually impossible. Another potential disadvantage is that use of a narrow population may result in product labeling that is restricted to the population actually studied.

More commonly, clinical research strives to use broad patient populations. This is fueled by a desire to have marketing claims with as few restrictions as possible and a need to investigate health care products under conditions of generalized use. To summarize, the right balance has to be found between using a narrow patient population to reduce variability and increase statistical power, and a broad population, to obtain unrestrictive labeling.

ELEMENTS OF PROTOCOL WHICH IMPACT PATIENT RECRUITMENT

The time required to develop a new drug is dependent on the time required to design and execute a clinical program, including the time required to recruit patients. It should be intuitive that the characteristics of a protocol influence the ease of recruiting patients. Getz and deBruin use the term "realistic protocols" to define those protocols which target patient populations that are not overly difficult to recruit.[2] Many researchers find it difficult to achieve the right balance between requiring a highly defined patient population for study *versus* a realistic patient population that is possible to recruit in a reasonable period of time. When the right balance is not achieved, recruitment difficulties can result.[3] The following sections discuss key protocol elements that have the greatest influence on patient recruitment.

Length of Study

Studies with active treatment periods lasting up to twelve weeks seem to be the most acceptable to patients with an ongoing or chronic disease. Studies that require longer than twelve weeks therapy (such as HIV or hepatitis B, C) require an increasingly difficult commitment from most patients. Acceptability of study length is strongly influenced by chronicity of the disease, so a one-year study may be more agreeable to the patient if the agent being tested is for a disease process such as hypertension or arthritis.

Choice of Control Groups

Inclusion of a placebo group almost always makes recruitment more difficult. The difficulty is related to the duration of the study, as short studies with placebo groups are more acceptable than long studies with placebo groups.[4] The probability of being in a placebo group should also be factored into the study. If there are six treatment groups, one of which is the placebo, there is only a 17% probability of being assigned to the placebo group whereas if there are two treatment groups (one placebo) there is a 50% chance of receiving placebo. Patients think carefully about these probabilities and are less likely to volunteer for the study if they perceive the risk as too high.

The ability to "escape" to a rescue medication can be an important factor in placebo-controlled study designs. Patients have a greater level of comfort if they know they can take a rescue medication if they do not receive adequate relief from their assigned treatment group. Importantly, it can be helpful to choose a rescue medication that is more potent than the agent being tested. This gives the patient a level of comfort that if relief is not realized with the treatment group to which they are assigned, they can escape to a potent medication with proven efficacy. For instance, in a study measuring the effectiveness of an NSAID analgesic for mild to moderate pain, the rescue medication could be a mild opiate such as a codeine/acetaminophen combination.

The positive control(s) being used in a clinical study can also influence patient participation. Positive controls that are well known and trusted encourage patient participation whereas positive controls that are unknown or that are associated with undesirable effects inhibit patients from volunteering.

Inclusion/Exclusion Criteria

Age

Recruitment of patients under the age of 18 is made more difficult because the patient must have guardian consent to participate in the trial. Parents and guardians are generally reluctant to allow their children to be exposed to the risks associated with a clinical trial. However, if the illness being treated has no adequate therapy, parents and guardians are usually more willing to take such risks.

Recruitment of patients who are of working age can also be difficult if the trial interferes with their work schedule. In order to help recruitment, sites can be encouraged to have office hours in evenings and on weekends to specifically accommodate these clinical trial patients. This may also help in recruitment of patients under the age of 18 in order that they not miss school.

Patients over the age of 65 frequently have more spare time to contribute to clinical trials but it may be more difficult for them to travel. Accordingly, it is worth providing some financial assistance to elderly patients who would like to participate but have difficulty traveling. Cab fare or a pick-up service can be very helpful in this regard.

The very elderly can also be difficult to recruit. For patients with impaired cognition, it is also necessary to have a guardian sign the consent form. Often the guardian is a child of the patient and may not want his or her parent to be at risk in a clinical trial.

Because of the complicating factors, it is probably best to use as broad an age range as possible in any clinical trial if the condition being studied is not restricted to a certain age group. Not only does this speed recruitment, it also results in a less restrictive claims structure. If there is a need to balance age ranges in the trial, it may be helpful to stratify by age between treatment groups.

Degree of Disease

Patients with mild diseases are generally willing to participate in a clinical trial, their motivation being a desire to contribute to the scientific good. As the disease becomes more severe (and perhaps life-threatening), patients prefer to be treated with a well-established and predictable medication rather than risk being in a placebo group. However, if the patient has a disease for which satisfactory treatment does not exist, there is again a greater willingness to participate in a trial if the test medication may offer a benefit that is not obtainable in any other way. This can be one of the most powerful motivating factors for a patient considering volunteering for a clinical trial.

As always, the broadest acceptance of disease severity speeds patient recruitment and provides the most generalized marketing claims. But this must be balanced against the need to have a well-defined patient population with an acceptable level of variability so that valid statistical conclusions can be drawn.

Concomitant Illnesses

Most clinical trials exclude severe concomitant illnesses so as to avoid biasing the apparent side effect profile of the new medication. This is good statistical practice as it reduces variability and confounding factors. However, taken to extremes, these exclusions can hamper patient recruitment and protocols that have several pages of exclusion criteria can be very complex and difficult to follow. One option is to charge the investigator with the task of avoiding patients with concomitant illnesses which may interfere with the clinical trial measurements, which may place the patient at undue risk, or which otherwise may make the patient unsuitable for the study. Most clinical trial investigators charged with such a task demonstrate sound judgement and fairly balance the interests of the trial sponsor with those of the patients.

Medication Exclusions

In the quest for the perfect patient population, some pharmaceutical companies seek to enroll naïve subjects, or subjects who have not previously been treated for their condition. This creates great challenges for enrollment[5], especially in Western countries in which patients are likely to receive medication at the earliest stages of disease. Enrollment is faster with protocols that broadly allow exposure to previous medications, albeit with an appropriate washout period.

Concomitant medications create a similar challenge but there is a stronger rationale for restricting other medications used during the trial. It is reasonable to exclude concomitant medications, which impact the efficacy endpoints of the trial since these may lead to ambiguous results. However, enrollment will be facilitated if the protocol allows concomitant medications, which have little or no impact on the efficacy measures.

Certain disease states, however, are characterized by polypharmacy, or the simultaneous use of multiple pharmaceutical agents. New agents are typically studied first as an adjunct to existing therapy rather than as a "stand-alone." Examples include treatment of HIV, epilepsy and rheumatoid arthritis. In these conditions, either an ideal therapy does not exist, or the disease state is inadequately controlled with existing therapies. Just as it is difficult to recruit treatment-naïve patients, recruitment of patients with a chronic disease that is sub-optimally managed can be very challenging.

Procedures Performed

It is understandable that certain procedures are viewed less favorably than others by patients. The following information summarizes some key categories of procedures that are viewed unfavorably by patients. It is important to note that these procedures do not inhibit recruitment if they are part of the normal standard of care for the disease. They are only inhibitory if the trial requires additional procedures to be performed, above and beyond normal care.

For many of these procedures, any discomfort to the patient can be partially offset by small compensation to the patient each time a procedure is performed. The acceptability of these payments differs from country to country and with the type of trial. For instance, patients participating in phase I studies receive some monetary reimbursement in almost any country. Payments for phase II and III trials are also common in North America whereas in many European countries, payments in phase II and III trials may not be allowed.

Blood Draws

Many patients dislike having blood drawn but most patients tolerate having a few blood samples taken, particularly if the blood samples are needed to properly diagnose, monitor and treat the disease. Frequent blood draws, such as are required for pharmacokinetic sampling, are a deterrent for many patients. This can be offset by offering compensation for each blood draw (in countries where this is permitted), as is common practice with patients in Phase I trials.

Invasive Diagnostic Procedures

If not otherwise required to diagnose or monitor the disease, invasive procedures can have a negative impact on enrollment. One example of this is an endoscopic examination of the stomach lining in ulcer studies. This can be a very unpopular procedure and greatly inhibits patient enrollment unless it can be offset with financial incentives to the patients. Colonoscopic procedures are not as unpopular but still inhibit enrollment.

Pelvic exams in women are generally tolerated as part of routine medical care but if a trial calls for numerous or frequent pelvic exams (more than every six months), this may have a negative impact on recruitment unless indicated by the disease state being studied.

Arthroscopy is another example of a procedure which is generally unpopular with patients. Few patients are eager to volunteer for a trial that requires one or more arthroscopic examinations.

X-rays are not generally accompanied by discomfort but many patients or their physicians may be concerned about the amount of ionizing radiation to which they are exposed. This is especially true among well-educated patients if the trial calls for repetitive radiographs of the chest, which often are accompanied by significant exposure to radiation. Consent forms are required to clearly state the risks associated with participation in a trial and this will be apparent to the properly consented patient.

Biopsies

Biopsies are a form of an invasive procedure and generally are unpopular both among clinical trial patients and investigators. Biopsies should be avoided where possible in pivotal trials and are most effectively obtained in smaller non-pivotal studies.

Certain minor biopsy procedures such as a skin punch biopsy have a small inhibitory effect on recruitment and consent is easier to gain, but more invasive biopsies of tissues or organs have a very strong negative impact on trial recruitment. Patients object to biopsies not only due to the pain that often accompanies the procedure, but also because of the increased risk of infection associated with a biopsy.

Surgery

Trials that investigate an experimental surgical procedure as a replacement for an existing therapy could face difficult recruitment. Most patients avoid surgery unless they perceive that the risks of surgery are balanced by the potential gains. If an adequate non-surgical therapy exists, almost all patients elect the non-surgical approach.

Medication Withdrawal

Many clinical trials call for withdrawal of a patient's medication before allowing him or her to begin the test medication. This can be unpopular with subjects if it causes them to go through a phase of discomfort.

Different types of withdrawal procedures exist. The simplest procedure is to withdraw the medication and allow a sufficient number of half-lives to pass so that the medication is essentially cleared from the patient's system. Five half-lives is generally regarded as adequate.

A less popular withdrawal procedure is to discontinue the medication and wait for the patient's disease state to flare or get worse. Sometimes the patient is only eligible for the trial if the disease does get worse. This may be done to ensure that the patient was in fact benefiting from the original medication and is therefore likely to show a response to the test medication. In a sense, this has the advantage of enriching the trial population with responders. However, it still remains an unpopular procedure with patients and does inhibit patient recruitment.

CASE STUDIES

Human Immunodeficiency Virus

Clinical trials involving individuals with Human Immunodeficiency Virus (HIV) Infection are primarily of two types; those that evaluate treatment for HIV infection and those that evaluate the treatment of Opportunistic Infections (OIs) associated with advanced immunodeficency. Recruitment of patients varies greatly based on the type of study involved. The advent of Protease Inhibitors and Highly Active Antiretroviral Therapy (HAART) has resulted in a drastic decrease in the incidence of OIs in the developed world. While this development is a great marker of progress, it has made the study of OI treatment in an expeditious fashion all but impossible. For this reason this case study will focus on the treatment of HIV disease.

HIV treatment trials can be organized into three categories based on prior Antiretroviral (ARV) experience. Antiretroviral naïve trials generally enroll subjects with no previous HIV treatment. These patients are very difficult to find, since diagnosis with HIV is immediately followed by ARV treatment. In some cases, ARV treatment is initiated on the suspicion of HIV infection prior to the results of diagnostic tests. Trials that evaluate experienced patients recruit a wide range of subjects, from patients who are currently taking their initial ARV regimen to those who have taken multiple agents in each of the three classes of medications available by prescription (Nucleoside Reverse Transcriptase Inhibitors, Non-Nucleoside Reverse Transcriptase Inhibitors and Protease Inhibitors). Finally, the third category of trial evaluates salvage regimens and tends to enroll patients who have experienced repeated virologic failure on multiple regimens.

Enrollment into HIV treatment trials is a very unique situation. In spite of the fact that we are 18 years into this epidemic, there is still great stigma associated with the diagnosis of HIV infection and AIDS. This stigma often results in delays in testing and treatment, and in an individual's disclosure of their HIV status.[6] Newly diagnosed individuals are dealing with a potentially life-threatening illness, often without social or family support. Throughout the 1980s this was predominantly a disease of gay, white individuals. However, in the last ten years there have been great shifts of the infected population to women, African-Americans and injection drug users. Currently, African-Americans account for 56% of all new HIV diagnoses.[7] African-Americans have historically shown much distrust in medical institutions, especially following the Tuskegee Incident, and thus have shown little interest in participating in clinical trials.[8] These issues reflect some of the global challenges of recruitment into HIV treatment trials.

Protocol design and entry criteria have been identified as major barriers to recruitment and enrollment of patients into HIV/AIDS clinical trials.[9] Since many trials target antiretroviral naïve patients, the challenge is to identify individuals who are newly diagnosed and have yet to begin ARV therapy. At a time when therapy is recommended for patients with HIV viral loads >10,000 copies/mL, there may be a narrow window of opportunity to identify and recruit these patients. Providing some flexibility in the protocol definition of ARV therapy naïve (< 2 weeks of AVR therapy) may facilitate recruitment and should not increase the incidence of viral resistance in this patient population.

It is often quite difficult to enroll patients in trials that evaluate experienced subjects who have failed a specific agent or combination, and broadening the target population may result in more rapid accrual. For instance, a study targeting patients who have failed one specific protease inhibitor will be much less successful in accruing patients than a study targeting patients who have failed any single protease inhibitor. When virologic failure is defined in a study by a restrictive viral load range (between 10,000 and 50,000 copies/mL), it will enroll patients much more slowly than one that defines failure as >10,000 copies/mL. Clearly the second study has a much larger potential patient pool.

Restrictive laboratory criteria can cripple enrollment, especially in trials that recruit patients with advanced HIV disease. Excluding patients with a WBC <2,500 would be unreasonable in this population because leukopenia is common. However, a neutrophil count that is adequate for patient safety (>750) is critical. Likewise, excluding patients with positive hepatitis serology will make recruitment difficult, since 20% of HIV positive patients are co-infected with hepatitis C and an even greater percentage have positive hepatitis B serology. In this same population of patients, allowing a higher threshold for exclusionary liver function tests will favorably affect study accrual (allowing > 5 X rather than > 3 X upper limit of normal for ALT/AST).

When evaluating various combination therapies, it is very helpful to minimize the complexity of the regimens and decrease the pill burden for the patient. This is not always feasible; however, one may be able to use an open label rather than a double blind, placebo-controlled design. The word "placebo" is often misinterpreted to mean that patients will only receive inactive drug, and is looked upon unfavorably by patients. The number of pills that patients are required to take when participating in an HIV treatment trial can be daunting, and a pill burden >20 pills/day can make patients twice as likely to decline participation than a pill burden of < 10/ day.[10]

When designing an HIV treatment trial, the scheduled evaluations should only be as rigorous as required to answer the questions being asked. Adding evaluations, questionnaires, or procedures to a study because it would provide data that are "nice to have" should be carefully considered. Additional laboratory tests increase the volume of blood drawn; additional procedures and questionnaires increase the length of the visit; and increasing the number of visits can be detrimental to patient recruitment. An HIV trial that is conservative in blood collection may require 7-10 blood tubes collected at baseline, which can be ominous to patients. Additional laboratory tests can in some cases increase the number of tubes to 20 or more. A patient who is fully informed prior to consenting to a rigorous study might decline participation for that reason alone.

Patient perceived incentives for participation should be built into the design of HIV clinical trials. One such incentive would be providing all the medications for the regimens involved in a trial, rather than just the targeted drug. Increasingly, protocols require that patients obtain access by prescription to some of the therapies included in a protocol-defined regimen. This is probably the result of the expense of providing complex regimens to patients in trials. The inherent risk of this is at least slow accrual, and at most enrollment of a skewed population of patients. Low-income patients may be unable to afford these medications and may therefore be excluded from the trial. The end result may be that the data cannot be generalized to all infected populations.

Studies that provide more than the standard of HIV care are attractive to patients. It may no longer be enough incentive to provide routine viral load testing. One might consider providing resistance-testing (genotypic and/or phenotypic) results in real time. Designing a study that utilizes resistance data to determine a subject's secondary or rescue therapy would be a strong argument in favor of participation for many patients. In the same vein, studies that provide less than the standard of care are acceptable to neither patients nor Ethics Committees.

Rheumatoid Arthritis

NSAIDs and Flare Designs

Clinical trials in rheumatoid arthritis differ depending on the type of new agent being studied.[11,12] Many recent trials have examined the effectiveness of new non-steroidal anti-inflammatory drugs (NSAIDs). These agents provide rapid symptomatic relief by reducing pain and swelling but they do not change the long-term course of the disease. Virtually all patients with rheumatoid arthritis take an NSAID and it is common to switch from one NSAID to another either to find improved efficacy or to avoid some side effect.

Disease-modifying anti-rheumatic drugs (DMARDs) focus on the underlying mechanisms and do not provide the same rapid symptomatic relief as an NSAID, but eventually reduces pain and inflammation by inhibiting the underlying disease processes. Most patients with rheumatoid arthritis have tried several DMARDs over the course of their disease.

For clinical trials which examine the effectiveness of a new NSAID, it is popular to use a "flare" design to select patients who are NSAID-responsive. For a flare trial, patients are asked to discontinue the use of their current NSAID and are given up to a week or two to flare. Patients who were benefiting from their NSAID experience a disease flare (their baseline arthritis assessments are worse than at the screening visit) and are selected to participate in the clinical trial. Patients who do not flare are presumed not to be NSAID-responsive and are not used in the trial. This approach has the benefit of providing a population enriched for their NSAID-responsiveness but it requires patients to go through a period of discomfort before they can enter into the clinical trial.

Two aspects of the flare design are viewed unfavorably by the patient. First, some patients will be excluded from the study. Patients who do not flare are disappointed and frustrated at having been subjected to the first stage of trial procedures and then found ineligible. The second and more concerning aspect is that patients must go through a period of significant discomfort before being assigned to one of the treatment groups in the trial. Both of these aspects make recruitment more difficult.

For discomfort during the flare, it is helpful if the protocol allows the patient to use a short-acting analgesic agent (or rescue medication) such as acetaminophen. This helps the patient get through the flare period and to the point of randomization. However, it is important that the patient not be experiencing any analgesic effects when the flare is assessed. It is common to restrict rescue medication during the 24-hour period preceding the arthritis assessments at the time of randomization.

An alternative to the flare design is to define minimum entry criteria for the arthritis assessments. In this case, patients are not required to flare but instead are required to have a minimum level of disease activity. Generally this design still requires a washout period but patients don't have to get worse, they just have to demonstrate the minimum level of disease activity.

DMARD Trial Designs

When testing a new DMARD agent, it is often desirable to examine its effects in the absence of other DMARDs. This is difficult because many DMARDs either have long half lives or a long pharmacodynamic effect, so washout periods can be four weeks or longer. Trials that require DMARD washout are typically difficult to enroll because patients do not wish to be without their DMARD. One way to address this is to allow patients to continue NSAIDs at a stable dose level throughout the washout period and the rest of the clinical trial. Most DMARD trial designs allow this continuation of NSAIDs at a stable dose level.

Alternatively, one can allow patients to continue their existing DMARD(s) during the trial. Although this model does not permit evaluation of a new test agent's effects in isolation, it can be justified on the basis that none of the available DMARDs is very effective. Accordingly, a new DMARD which is highly effective should not have difficulty proving its value against a background DMARDs that provide only minimal to moderate effectiveness. Additionally, it is much easier to justify the use of a placebo control group if all patients are permitted to continue on a stable background of NSAID and traditional DMARD medications.

Limiting Quantities of Background Medications

In order to reduce the variability that would accompany the use of background medications, trials often provide an upper dose level that cannot be exceeded. For instance, methotrexate is a widely used DMARD for rheumatoid arthritis. It is one of the more effective DMARDs so its use is often limited to doses that do not exceed 15 to 20 mg per week. Similarly, corticosteroids are often used chronically in rheumatoid arthritis. As a background medication, corticosteroid doses may be limited to no more than 10 mg per day. The allowance of these background medications but at limited dose levels facilitates recruitment.

In NSAID trials, concomitant use of other NSAIDs is generally prohibited. However, many patients use aspirin for its anti-coagulant effect. Since aspirin is itself an NSAID it is important to be sure that patients are not taking anti-inflammatory doses. Fortunately, anticoagulant effects are optimized with doses less than 100 mg per day. It is acceptable to permit the use of low-dose aspirin without risking interference with the anti-inflammatory effects of a new NSAID.

Cancer Pain

Cancer pain trials in terminally ill patients can be very difficult to perform because such patients prefer to be left alone during the final stages of their disease. Patients may be unwilling to admit to pain, feeling that their physician may be less aggressive in treating the primary disease. There is often the sense that pain is ennobling and must be borne with fortitude.

It is virtually impossible (indeed unethical!) to include a true placebo control arm. However, if adequate rescue medication is allowed, a placebo arm may be possible. In this case, it aids enrollment to choose a rescue medication which is highly efficacious (such as morphine) and to allow the patient to use the rescue medication at any time during the trial. In this case, one expects placebo patients to use rescue medication frequently so it would be appropriate to have the frequency of use of rescue medication as a primary endpoint.

Another trial design that recruits well in patients with severe cancer pain is a morphine-sparing design. For this type of trial, patients are kept on a background of morphine and the test agent (or placebo) is added to the morphine regimen. The primary endpoint is the amount of morphine used, so if the test agent is effective, there is a decrease in morphine usage. This design has the advantage that patients are never required to suffer; so reasonable recruitment rates are feasible.

Trials in patients with mild pain due to cancer are not as difficult to enroll, but there is still reluctance by patients to participate in a trial if they expect to experience discomfort. Recruitment will be much easier if the trial permits the use of a rescue medication at any time the patient chooses. As discussed above, it is also helps recruitment to offer a rescue medication with a higher level of efficacy than the test agent, so the patient knows that a highly effective rescue medication is available if needed. Knowing that the rescue medication is available may even help patients delay the need to rescue even when they are feeling discomfort.

Hormone Replacement Therapy

Several regulatory guidelines have been written for studies on hormone replacement therapy (HRT) for women.[13,14] There are a number of elements in these guidelines, which make recruitment difficult.

One of the claims allowed for HRT products is the relief of menopausal symptoms, especially hot flashes. The guidelines from the U.S. FDA specify the use of women having at least 60 hot flashes per week, whereas the European "Points to Consider" document suggests starting with patients with 35 or more hot flashes per week. Both documents suggest that one or more placebo-controlled studies are needed to validate a claim for menopausal symptoms and that the trials should be about 3 months in duration.

Due to the unpleasantness of menopausal symptoms and the need for a placebo control group, this is a difficult population to recruit. The regulatory guidances provide little flexibility in study design, but there can be some flexibility in allowing patients to withdraw from the trial. Most patients would not want to be on placebo for three months, but might be willing to risk a placebo group if they are allowed to withdraw for lack of efficacy. It might be reasonable to ask patients to remain in the trial for at least a week, but if they find their symptoms to be intolerable, to escape to a rescue medication such as a marketed HRT product.

The regulatory guidances also discuss the need to co-administer a progestin component along with an estrogen component. This is necessary for the long-term health of the endometrium since continued administration of unopposed estrogen can lead to endometrial hyperplasia and increased risk of endometrial cancer. The European and U.S. guidances both discuss the need to understand the dose-relationship between the progestin and estrogen components of an HRT therapy. The U.S. guidance document suggests that a progestin placebo group must be used to establish the baseline rate for endometrial hyperplasia in a group receiving the estrogen component alone (often called an unopposed estrogen group). This makes for a very difficult enrollment challenge because women are not be eager to volunteer for a study knowing they may risk developing endometrial hyperplasia if they are assigned to the unopposed estrogen group. The EMEA document does not suggest that an unopposed estrogen group is necessary and this is sensible since numerous studies with unopposed estrogens have been conducted and there are therefore much comparative data to estimate background rates. There is recent evidence that the U.S. FDA is softening their requirement for an unopposed estrogen group and may allow alternative trial designs. This is not stated in any guidance document but can be negotiated with the U.S. FDA on a case-by-case basis. An unopposed estrogen group should be avoided in any clinical trial due to ethical concerns and because it will make recruitment very difficult.

If the issue of an unopposed estrogen group does not add sufficient difficulty to HRT trials, they are made even more difficult by the need for endometrial biopsies to observe the effect of HRT regimens on the endometrium. Endometrial biopsy is the only validated method for establishing with certainty the state of the endometrium. Transvaginal ultrasound allows an assessment of endometrial thickness but does not permit identification of cell types characteristic of hyperplasia. Both the U.S. and European guidance documents strictly imply the need to obtain endometrial biopsies from patients at baseline and after one year of therapy. Biopsy results are generally the primary endpoint for establishing the ability of a progestin component to protect the endometrium.

Endometrial biopsies are unpopular. In North American trials, recruitment will be improved if some reimbursement of, for instance, $100 to $200 is offered to women for the discomfort associated with an endometrial biopsy. This practice is not well received in a European environment, where one must rely on the personal assurances of the investigators and study coordinators to convince trial participants that their participation in a study is a valuable contribution to science and will benefit other women.

Osteoporosis

Regulatory approval of a new therapy for osteoporosis requires very long clinical trials. The guidance document from the U.S. FDA recommends that a sponsor demonstrate a reduction in osteoporotic fractures in trials of five years duration.[15] Product approval can be granted on the basis of three-year data if selected criteria are fulfilled. The EMEA guidance document suggests a trial length of three years.[16] The long-term nature of these trials makes it very difficult to recruit patients and even more difficult to retain patients for the entire trial period.

Trials to demonstrate fracture reduction can be especially difficult because observing the trial endpoint (fractures) depends on choosing a population at increased risk of fracture. In order to accomplish this for trials of vertebral fracture, sponsors often choose patients who have one or more pre-existing vertebral fractures and low bone mineral density. Even with this approach, sample sizes of 500 to 750 subjects per treatment arm are necessary. To find these patients it is necessary to screen volunteers for bone mineral density as well as for the presence of vertebral fractures. These are expensive screening procedures and the rate of screen failure is high.

To demonstrate efficacy against hip fractures, sponsors can choose patients who have low bone mineral density and who have one or more risk factors for fracturing a hip. Risk factors include poor gait, balance, and cognition, as well as having already fractured one hip.

As with HRT trials, the regulatory guidances don't leave much room for flexibility in trial design. The trials must be for three to five year duration and in order to keep the number of patients down to a manageable size, it is necessary to select patients with a high risk of fractures. Further difficulties can be avoided if the protocol is written so as to avoid numerous exclusion criteria. It can also be helpful for recruitment if some social aspects are built into the trial design. For instance, women in the age range 60 years and higher often have unmet social needs. Group luncheons held monthly or quarterly as part of the clinical trial can have a positive impact on enrollment as well as retention.

Another protocol element that can help retention is to provide some feedback to the patient on how the test agent is working. This can be particularly helpful since many therapies for osteoporosis don't make the women feel any different so they don't know whether the test agent is providing benefit. Biological markers are available that provide evidence that the test agent is working. If selected biological markers are measured regularly during the trial and the results presented to the patient, this provides encouragement to continue participation.

An important aspect of long-term osteoporosis trials is to evaluate the health or quality of newly formed bone. This is only partially addressed with bone mineral density measurements. A much better picture of bone quality is obtained by taking bone biopsies from a few patients at selected intervals during the trial. Bone biopsies can be painful and are not favored by patients so it is more desirable to obtain biopsies in a small subset of patients and to not require biopsies from any patient. Where possible, patients should be reimbursed for discomforts associated with a bone biopsy. Most North American IRBs should consider a payment of $100 to $200 per biopsy reasonable. European Ethical Committees may prohibit such payments.

If the anti-osteoporotic agent being tested has hormonal qualities, it is necessary to examine its effects on the endometrium. Qualitative effects can be gauged with transvaginal ultrasound but most regulatory agencies also expect to see data from endometrial biopsies, at least in a subset of patients. The impact of endometrial biopsies on patient recruitment for osteoporosis trials is similar to those for HRT trials as discussed above.

AVAILABILITY OF AN OPEN LABEL EXTENSION STUDY

Patients are generally apprehensive about participating in a trial with a placebo control group. One approach that may ease their concerns and facilitate recruitment is to offer an open label study once their participation in the double-blind portion has been completed. Thus, patients who enter a double-blind trial know that even if they are assigned to the placebo group, they will eventually have an opportunity to receive the test medication in an unblinded fashion.

An open label extension can be an important part of any development program due to the need to collect long-term safety data on a new substance. The ICH E1 guideline[17] indicates that for approval of a drug intended for long term therapy, the sponsor should provide data on at least 100 patients for one year, 300 to 600 patients for at least six months, and exposure overall to more than 1,500 patients. An open label extension is an excellent way to fulfill the six month and one year requirements.

A range of criteria can be established to determine which patients are allowed into an open label extension. The most stringent would require that a patient complete the whole trial period before being allowed into the extension. However, this may be too strict and it is also possible to offer the extension to patients who complete at least a few days of therapy and then withdraw due to lack of efficacy. In this way, patients who received placebo can enter the extension without having to remain on placebo for the entire double-blind period.

Patients who withdraw from the double-blind portion due to an adverse event which may be drug related should probably not be allowed into the extension since it could expose them to further hazards if the adverse event were indeed drug related.

CONCLUSION

Selected elements of protocol design can have a profound impact on patient recruitment. The key is to achieve a balance between the need for a narrow population to optimize statistical considerations and the need to recruit rapidly from a broad population. Each disease state has its own special issues related to protocol design and patient recruitment, but with careful consideration, an appropriate balance can be achieved and recruitment will proceed at a suitable rate.

REFERENCES

[1] International Conference on Harmonization Document E9; Guidance on Statistical Principles for Clinical Trials. Adopted by the ICH on February 5, 1998, www.ifpma.org/ich5e.html#Population.

[2] "Speed Demons of Drug Development." Getz KA and de Bruin A. Pharmaceutical Executive. July 2000, pp. 78 to 84.

[3] "Merck Substance P Delay Attributed to Patient Recruitment Difficulties." The Pink Sheet. June 19, 2000. p. 25.

[4] International Conference on Harmonization Document E10; Choice of Control Group in Clinical Trials. Issued for comment by the ICH in May 1998, www.ifpma.org/ich5e.html#Population.

[5] "Recruiting Human Subjects: Pressures in Industry-Sponsored Clinical Research." Report issued by the Office of Inspector General in the Department of Health and Human Services, June 2000. OEI-01-97-00195. Available at www.dhhs.gov/progorg/oei.

[6] Chesney, Margaret A. and Smith, Asley W. "Critical Delays in HIV Testing and Care: The Potential Role of Stigma." American Behavioral Scientist, (1999). 42(7):1162-1174.

[7] HIV/AIDS Surveillance Report: U.S. HIV and AIDS cases reported through December 1999. Issued by the Center for Disease Control and Prevention, 11(2).

[8] *Health Care Inequities Lead to a Mistrust of Research*. Durso TW. The Scientist 11(4):1 (1997).

[9] *Strategies and Barriers for Recruitment and Retention in Clinical Trials*. Issued by the Adult Patient Care Committee, AIDS Clinical Trials Group. Finalized 1997.

[10] *Patient Recruitment into ACTG Clinical Trials: A Pilot Survey*. (1997) Adult Patient Care Committee, AIDS Clinical Trials Group.

[11] *Guidance for Industry: Clinical Development Programs for Drugs, Devices, and Biological Products for the Treatment of Rheumatoid Arthritis (RA)*. Issued by the U.S. FDA February 1999, www.fda.gov.

[12] *Points to Consider on Clinical Investigation of Slow-Acting Anti-Rheumatic Medicinal Products in Rheumatoid Arthritis*. Issued by the Committee for Proprietary Medicinal Products December 1998, www.eudra.org.

[13] "Guidance for Clinical Evaluation of Combination Estrogen/Progestin-Containing Drug Products Used for Hormone Replacement Therapy of Postmenopausal Women." This is an informal communication by the U.S. FDA's Division of Metabolism and Endocrine Drug Products. It does not have a specific issue date but was approved for distribution by the Division Director on March 20, 1995. It can be obtained at the FDA web site at www.fda.org.

[14] "Points to Consider on Hormone Replacement Therapy." Issued by the Committee for Proprietary Medicinal Products November 1997, www.eudra.org.

[15] "Guidelines for Preclinical and Clinical Evaluation of Agents Used in the Prevention or Treatment of Postmenopausal Osteoporosis." Issued by the U.S. FDA April 1994, www.fda.gov.

[16] "Note for Guidance on Involutional Osteoporosis in Women." Released for consultation by the Committee for Proprietary Medicinal Products in September 1999, www.eudra.org.

[17] International Conference on Harmonization Document E1; The Extent of Population Exposure to Assess Clinical Safety: For Drugs Intended for Long-Term Treatment of Non-Life-Threatening Conditions. Finalized by ICH in October 1994, www.ifpma.org/ich5e.html#Population.

AUTHOR BIOGRAPHY

William K. Sietsema, Ph.D., was educated at the University of Colorado (B.A. Biochemistry 1977) and the University of Wisconsin (Ph.D. Biochemistry 1982). Mr. Sietsema's first industry employment was with Mobay Chemical Corporation in Kansas City where he studied pesticide metabolism. He joined Procter & Gamble Pharmaceuticals in 1984 where he studied drug metabolism for three years before joining the Skeletal Research department. From 1987 until 1993 Mr. Sietsema was program manager for P&G's bisphosphonate risedronate (Actonel) and during that time he helped pioneer the use of mass media for recruiting clinical trial patients. In 1993, he transferred back to basic research at P&G and was Section Head for Bone Metabolism Research. In 1996, Mr. Sietsema joined Kendle as Assistant Director of Clinical Research and was responsible for managing the osteoarthritis and rheumatoid arthritis development program with a new COX2 inhibitor. During that time, he helped design and implement two very successful mass media patient recruitment campaigns to attract clinical trial subjects. Mr. Sietsema's current title is Senior Director of Clinical Research at Kendle, where he spends much of his time designing protocols and development programs for new medications. In addition to his expertise in development of new drugs for treating inflammation and skeletal disease, Mr. Sietsema has a background in pain, hormone replacement therapy, drug metabolism, bone histology, histomorphometry and biomechanics. He is a member of the American Society for Bone and Mineral Research, the American College of Rheumatology, the Inflammation Research Association and The Endocrine Society.

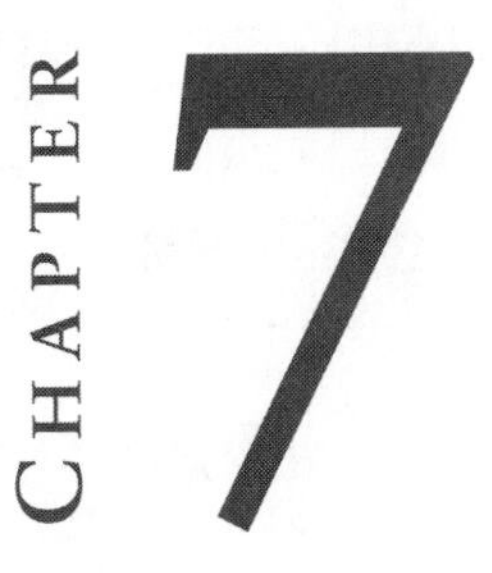

Media Strategies and Tactics for Clinical Trial Patient Recruitment

Linda B. Kreter, Pharmaceutical Research Plus

OVERVIEW

What to Say, How to Say It, Where to Say It, When to Say It

Everyday we are exposed to so much print, radio and television advertising; we might be tempted to assume that media strategies and tactics for patient recruitment are quite simple. However, if you consider the protocol specific goals and objectives of a media strategy for clinical trial patient recruitment, it can be as complex and sophisticated as the protocol itself.

With the ever-growing need for clinical trial volunteers (Chapter One), media strategies and tactics for patient recruitment are becoming more common if not mandatory. This chapter will provide a fundamental overview of what considerations are necessary to implement an effective media strategy for both multi-site studies as well as single site campaigns. This chapter will focus on the print, radio and television formats as Internet based patient recruitment will be covered in chapter nine. It will be important to note that a media strategy is simply one part of the entire patient recruitment campaign; hence this chapter should be used in conjunction with the other, equally important, components outlined throughout this book. The primary objective of a media strategy for patient recruitment is to create interest in the particular protocol that leads to action (usually a phone call to inquire further). Other chapters in this text will outline the important steps and processes necessary to convert this interest to enrollment.

The remainder of this chapter will pragmatically address the obvious questions surrounding a media campaign as well as provide more specific questions and tools to help devise the most efficient campaign for a specific protocol.

What to Say

Though stated earlier that the objective of a patient recruitment media strategy is to create interest in clinical trial participation, thorough compliance with the regulatory environment surrounding clinical research must be exercised. A recent report on clinical trial patient recruitment from the Inspector General of the United States Department of Health and Human Services states: "Recent investigations and complaints reveal disturbing recruitment practices."[1] The Food and Drug Administration provides guidelines for acceptable patient recruitment advertising.[2] Furthermore, the Institutional Review Board (IRB) overseeing the protocol will need to approve all final advertising materials as well as any scripted call guides or other materials that interface with potential study subjects. It is important to be certain to obtain all approvals for all advertising materials from both the IRB and sponsor company in writing and maintain files for these very important authorizations.

How to Say It

It is also critical to balance the regulatory considerations mentioned with the limitations of the media vehicles available. For example, a television advertisement will most likely be held to thirty seconds, a print ad might only be 15–25 words and a radio ad will have no visual content. The challenge will be to engage the target audience while maintaining compliance with regulatory requirements. IRBs will require review of the "final cut" advertisements to assess the connotations of the final advertisement. For example, a television script may have acceptable text, but if upon viewing the ad, the actors and scenery misrepresent the clinical trial opportunity, it will most likely not be approved. Another very important component of "how" is quality. The biopharmaceutical industry is revered for substantial quality standards and any advertisement to participate in the drug development process should mirror the high standards of the industry and the sponsor.

Where to Say It

The target audience, and the scale of the program and budget dictate the mix of print, radio and television. Each of these media formats will be examined in more detail but suffice it to say that there will be a different media mix for targeting benign prostate hypertrophy patients (males 40+) than for adolescent ADHD (Attention Deficit Hyperactivity Disorder) patients (males and females 12–17 and their guardians). Each format has strengths that can be leveraged for certain target audiences as well as weaknesses that can be minimized in most situations.

When to Say It

It is critical to understand the media habits of the target audience selected in order to maximize the desired response and investment. When is the target audience most likely to intersect with the creative message? Morning drive time (radio?), afternoon talk shows (television?) or Thursday's Health insert in the evening newspaper? It will also be valuable to understand some of the basic tenets of each format before embarking on a media driven patient recruitment strategy. For example, when listening to the radio we select a station, but when watching television, we select a show. In other words, our loyalty and predictability are based on completely different variables for the two formats. Depending on how specific the target audience is, "when" positioning the advertisement may be the most important parameter of the campaign.

MEDIA STRATEGY CONSIDERATIONS

The following model, used by Pharmaceutical Research Plus, Inc. has been developed to help customize the media strategy for each protocol, each media market and even each investigator site participating in the campaign. The model consists of a series of questions to assist in illuminating the key drivers for a campaign as well as a Call Volume Analysis Table that illustrates the scale of the program across each site, each market, and each protocol.

CASE EXAMPLE

For purposes of illustration, protocol 123 is a pivotal phase III, placebo-controlled study seeking 650 completed patients at 25 U.S. sites. The sponsor would like a media plan to provide aggressive accrual for 450 of the 650 completed patients. The following questions will be important to answer, to analyze and to understand before investing in media driven patient recruitment.

Step One: Clarification of Sponsor Goals & Experience

- Is the media strategy prospective or for an ongoing trial? This will help indicate whether the strategy can be designed in concert with site selection and protocol finalization or if working within an existing environment is required.

- What is the targeted patient volunteer? (Disease, inclusion/exclusion criteria, etc.)

- What is the current and ideal patient accrual timeline (patients/site/week)? The sponsor's past or current experience will indicate protocol challenges, realistic expectations and how aggressive the media strategy should be.

- How many patients should the media campaign contribute overall and per site? Private practice enrollment should be considered as well as budgetary limitations.

- How many sites will be involved in the protocol?

- What are the specific locations of each of the sites involved in the protocol?

- Will the media campaign need to coordinate with other, local recruitment efforts?

- What is the IRB affiliation (local or central) for the sites involved in the campaign?

- What is the average weekly screening rate per site? How many patients can each site handle per week? Are visit 1 appointments long and involved?

- Is there an enrollment cap per site?

- Is the investigational medication approved for other indications?

- Is the sponsor conducting concurrent protocols in the same markets that could also benefit from the media campaign?

- Who are the patients targeted? Inclusion and exclusion criteria including age, gender, ambulatory, chronic vs. acute conditions.

- How effective will a phone screen be in determining protocol eligibility? Are the inclusion and exclusion criteria objective considerations that can be ascertained over the telephone or is patient eligibility going to be primarily based on "physical" medical evaluation and lab data?

- What are the perceived enrollment rate limiters?

- What is the budget for the entire patient recruitment program?

- Has the sponsor assessed the indirect and direct cost of enrollment delay?

- Has the sponsor assessed the indirect and direct value of early or timely enrollment completion?

- What is the sites' motivation to enroll patients into a protocol in a timely manner? Is the compound exciting? Is the grant competitive? Is the sponsor well established in this therapeutic area?

- What is the patients' motivation to participate in the protocol? Are there alternative therapies?

- Does the sponsor have a feel for how the 80-20 rule (will 80% of the patients enroll at 20% of the sites?) will apply to patient recruitment and site performance?

- What is the anticipated phone screen attrition rate?

- What is the anticipated site screen attrition rate?

- What is the anticipated patient drop out rate?

- What system is in place to handle the phone inquiries generated from the media campaign?

- What is the planned start date for first patient enrolled?

- Would acceleration of the enrollment timeline create challenges for study drug availability or other logistical constraints?

- Is the protocol scheduled to run through a major holiday season? Are there other seasonal considerations for the protocol (flu, allergies, pediatrics and school year).

Answering, analyzing and understanding these questions will assist in developing protocol specific goals and objectives for the media component of the patient recruitment strategy. The next step is to construct a protocol specific call volume model that predicts each step of a study subject's progression from initial interest through protocol completion.

Call Volume Analysis for Protocol 123

Step/Process	Percentage	Total Calls (25 site)	Total Calls Dr. Jones (1 site)
Total Calls		13,203	528
Phone Screen	80%	10,562	422
Pass Screen	40%	4,225	169
Interested	85%	3,591	143
Schedule V1	80%	2,873	114
Show V1	75%	2,155	86
Consent	90%	1,939	64
Med. Qualify	65%	1,261	58
Pass Run In	70%	882	37
Randomize	85%	750	26
Complete	65%	450	18

**Please note that call volume models will vary significantly from protocol to protocol. It should also be clear at this point that the "volume" in the above call volume model would necessitate a sound call center strategy (Chapter Seven). The best media strategy will be moot if the patient recruitment strategy does not have the resources in place to process potential study subject questions and interest.*

Step Two: Estimating the Interest Level (via inquiries) Required for the Needed Recruitment

Armed with this protocol specific information, a media strategy can be constructed that will accomplish the goals and objectives of this protocol on a global, market and site level.

For protocol 123, the media strategy will need to generate approximately 13,200 targeted phone inquires globally, approximately 530 targeted phone inquires per site and approximately 1600 targeted phone inquiries for the sample market, Atlanta.

In order to accomplish this objective, it would be necessary to devise a market-by-market media strategy that considers the three principle formats of print, radio and television.

Television

The first step in accessing television audiences is producing a regulatory compliant advertisement to be digitally distributed the stations selected. The objective of the advertisement is to motivate the viewer to take action. This objective is in contrast to "branding" advertising that is seeking to create an image and awareness. To produce a television quality advertisement, it is necessary to contract with a professional studio and perhaps a myriad of other subcontractors depending on the complexity of the advertisement. Production costs range from $4,000 dollars to more than $200,000 again, depending on the complexity. It is important to remember that the advertisement created will represent the pharmaceutical industry, the sponsor company, the clinical trial, the disease state and the investigators.

The majority of novice produced patient recruitment television advertisements feature a clinic setting with staff in white lab coats. The unanimous recommendation of most public relations firms would advise to do anything but a clinic setting with white lab coats, etc. if you are trying to recruit patients. Focus on the patient and their symptoms.

As far as advertisement content, clearly state:

- The Target Audience (age, gender, disease state)
- General Study Information

- Major Inclusion and Exclusion Criteria
- Contact Information for Further Inquiry
- A call to action

Once the television advertisement is produced and approved, you will need to develop a media placement strategy that will achieve projected goals. Each year more than 12,000 products and services are advertised on the Nation's 200+ million active television sets[3], thus television is known as the "reach" format. To be on the right television sets at the right time, qualitative and quantitative analysis of the viewership data available from the 20+ television media research firms will need to be conducted. Request data that stratifies viewers by age and gender. Some firms may specialize in the demographics that are targeted. With the research conducted and a strategy in place, be prepared to make weekly, if not daily, refinements to the strategy based on market nuances and unexpected events (major news event or weather event) and in response to callers' source information.

The price for a particular "spot" or "buy" can vary as much as 30% based on the clout of the buyer and their ability to negotiate. Local, spot buys also fluctuate by more than 30% from one quarter to the next. These price fluctuations are a function of supply and demand and viewer habits. Evaluate the investment based on "cost per objective" (targeted, interested caller) instead of "cost per spot." As discussed earlier, "when" and "where" advertising is placed is much more important than "how many" placements are made.

Be sure to relay the media placement plan and all subsequent refinements to the call center handling the inquiries so that they may staff appropriately. Also, be sure to set up a communication plan that will allow the media strategy and placements to be refined based on call center feedback and media source information.

Radio

Production of radio commercials can take place within most radio stations themselves or outside firms are available to manage more complex commercials involving original music, sound effects and non-station staff talent. Typical radio spots also run for sixty seconds allowing for more detailed messages about the clinical trial.

There are over 10,000 radio stations nationwide and radio is ubiquitous in our cars and workplace.[4] This is why radio is known as the "frequency" format. Another differentiating characteristic of radio from television is that listeners choose a station instead of show as viewers do with television. If you are considering radio as part of a media strategy, it is necessary to consider the same qualitative and quantitative analysis of a particular station's audience. As is known from individual's personal listening habits, there are stations that one frequently listens to and stations that one never listens to. Which stations will the target audience be listening to and when will they be listening? If the target audience works, drive time may be the placement time for an advertisement. Talk radio also has a fragmented audience across each daypart. The best strategies will have both vertical (across several dayparts) and horizontal (across multiple stations) placements. Again, be sure to coordinate the placement strategy with the selected call center.

Print

While print is consistently the most expensive format for clinical trial patient recruitment (cost per objective), it can be the format of choice for certain situations (small, isolated markets) and audiences (more mature demographics or niche conditions with specialty publications). Print production is relatively easy and there are more than 1,600 daily newspapers in circulation throughout the Country.[5] Additionally, there are specialty newspapers, magazines and publications that may reach the specified audience.

Readership analysis by publication, page and section are available from a variety of market research firms. This data will go well beyond simple circulation statistics and will be important in helping the decision of:

- Which publication?
- Which section?
- Which page in the section?
- Where on that page?
- What size?
- What day?

Be sure to coordinate the publication's deadline with the IRB approval process as well.

VALUE-ADDED POTENTIAL FOR ALL FORMATS

Each of the media formats discussed can play a vital role in reaching the clinical trial patient recruitment objectives. Each of these formats also offers the potential to further maximize investment through value added enhancements. Examples of value added enhancements include:

Television

- Sponsorships of related news segments, "Today's medical minute has been brought to you by..." Also called a television billboard
- Station sponsored promotion of community awareness event, Health Screening
- News coverage, feature news segment on location

Radio

- Sponsorship of show portions, especially for medical talk shows
- Abbreviated study announcements, segue ways between segments by announcer/DJ
- Station sponsored, on location, awareness events
- Feature discussion, special topic for talk radio or morning DJ team
- News coverage

Print

- Editorial mention
- Bonus placements in sister publications, if publications fit target demographic

SUMMARY

Clearly, media strategies and tactics can dramatically assist clinical trial recruitment efforts. With proper planning during the strategy phase and diligent execution during the tactical phase, trials may be enrolled swiftly and cost effectively. The examples shown here consider the development of an effective media strategy that is both efficient and cost-effective, takes site capacity and resources into perspective, and provides a strong framework for the other components of a well-defined recruitment strategy will assist in assessing future programs. It is critically important to view your end user (the prospective study volunteer) and to direct your message with dignity, adherence to guidelines and to the potential benefit from learning and participating in important scientific research. Volunteers who better understand clinical trials, their own medical conditions and take charge of at least one aspect of their personal health are empowered in today's impersonal healthcare world.

APPENDIX 1

Glossary of Terms

Affiliate–A station contracted with a network and carrying that specific network's programming during certain hours. (Example: ABC, CBS, NBC, FOX, WB, UPN and PAX)

Arbitron–The Arbitron Company is an international media research firm providing information services that are used to develop the local marketing strategies of the electronic media, and of their advertisers and agencies.

Audience–The non-cumulative potential audience for a single advertising message. The total number of people reached by a particular medium.

Audience Composition–The demographic profile of a medium's representative audience.

Average Frequency–The number of times the average household or person is exposed to an advertising schedule by media carrying the schedule within a specific period of time.

Clear Channel–A radio station operating at a maximum power of 50,000 watts on an exclusive frequency.

Commercial/Spot–Broadcast terminology for a commercial message.

Daypart–Any of the time segments into which a broadcast day is divided, by audience composition and/or broadcast origination time, (e.g., for TV: AM News, Daytime, Early Fringe, Early News, Prime Access, Prime Time, Late News and Late Fringe; for Radio: AM Drive, Mid-Day, PM Drive, Evening and Overnight).

Demographics–The study of the numerical characteristics of the population. Common demographics are: age, gender, income, occupation and education.

Designated Market Area (DMA)–A Nielsen area concept similar to Arbitron's ADI, embracing the counties in which the TV station obtains the highest proportion of the viewing audience.

Direct Response Advertising–An advertising message that calls for a prompt purchase commitment directly to the manufacturer by the reader, viewer or listener.

Efficiency–Ratio of cost to audience.

Exposure–An individual's physical contact with an advertising message or medium.

Fixed Position–In broadcast, rates that are negotiated which are not pre-emptible and cannot be moved or bumped.

Flighting–A campaign scheduling pattern characterized by period of advertising effort followed by periods of inactivity.

Gross Rating Points–The sum of all individual ratings of all elements in a broadcast advertising schedule. One rating point equals 1% of the total potential audience for a given medium, also refers to the product of reach and exposure frequency. R x F=GRP. Persons or households estimate expressed as a percentage of the appropriate estimated population.

Impression–The total of all the audiences delivered by a medium. It is calculated by multiplying the number of people who receive a message by the number of times they receive it.

Local Rate–Rate charged for local (sometimes referred to as retail) advertising. Generally much lower than national rate.

Makegood–When the advertising purchased is pre-empted, omitted in error, or run in an unfit condition, the medium offers, at no additional charge, comparable or better airtime at a later date.

Metro Survey Area (MSA)–Generally corresponds to Standard Metropolitan Statistical Areas (SMSA's) as defined by the U.S.

Government's Office of Management and Budget (OMB). Generally speaking, radio geography.

Newspaper Designated Market (NDM)–The market area served by the newspaper, as defined by the publisher.

Nielsen (A.C. Nielsen Company)–An organization that, among other marketing research, conducts television audience measurements.

Penetration–1) Percent of set-owning households that subscribe to Cable TV. 2) The percent of set-owning households to total households in a given area. 3) The degree to which a medium or vehicle has obtained area coverage. 4) The effectiveness to advertising's impact on the public.

Rotator (or Broad Rotator)–A spot that gets equal rotation both horizontally as well as vertically within the time limits specified. (i.e. radio, Monday through Sunday, 6 a.m. to midnight, 7 times, would mean one runs each day, starting with 6–10 a.m. on Monday, 10–3 p.m. on Tuesday, 3–7 p.m. on Wednesday, 7–midnight on Thursday, 6–10 a.m. on Friday, 10–3p.m. on Saturday, 3–7 p.m. on Sunday.)

Spot Length–In television, the normal unit is thirty seconds; fifteen and ten second's are accepted. In radio, the normal unit is sixty seconds; thirty and ten second's are accepted. 35% of network TV spots are fifteen seconds. A fifteen second in television is 70% to 80% as effective as a thirty second. Fifteens generally cost 60-80% of a thirty second spot in TV. In radio, most stations are unit rated. You pay the same for a thirty as you would a sixty second. Some stations charge 80% of a sixty for a thirty second spot in radio.

Total Audience–In broadcast, the number viewing/listening to all or part of a program for not less than five minutes for a ten minute program or longer, for a least one minute if the program is less than ten minutes long. Also refers to the unduplicated readership of a periodical. Readers per copy multiplied by circulation equals total audience.

REFERENCES

[1] "Recruiting Human Subjects." June Gibbs Brown. Inspector General, OEI-01-97-00195, June 2000.

[2] FDA website: www.FDA.gov. "Guidance for Institutional Review Boards and Clinical Investigators." 1998 Update.

[3] FCC website: www.FCC.gov.

[4] *Ibid.*

[5] SRDS Headquarters, 1700 Higgins Road, Des Plaines, IL 60018.

AUTHOR BIOGRAPHY

Linda B. Kreter, President and Chief Executive Officer, is the founder of Pharmaceutical Research Plus and incorporated the company in 1994 with funding from Pharmaceutical Product Development, Inc. In September 1995, Ms. Kreter purchased full ownership of the Company and today remains the primary shareholder. Prior to founding Pharmaceutical Research Plus, Ms. Kreter was Director of the Pharmaceutical Division of TeleSpectrum, Inc. in Annapolis, Maryland, and duties included sales and marketing, as well as project management of medical marketing and communications programs. Ms. Kreter was also a programmer at NASA's Goddard Space Center in Greenbelt, MD and a hospital sales representative for Norwich-Eaton and Proctor & Gamble, in Chicago and Philadelphia, respectively. Ms. Kreter received a BA in Biology from Smith College in Northampton, Massachusetts.

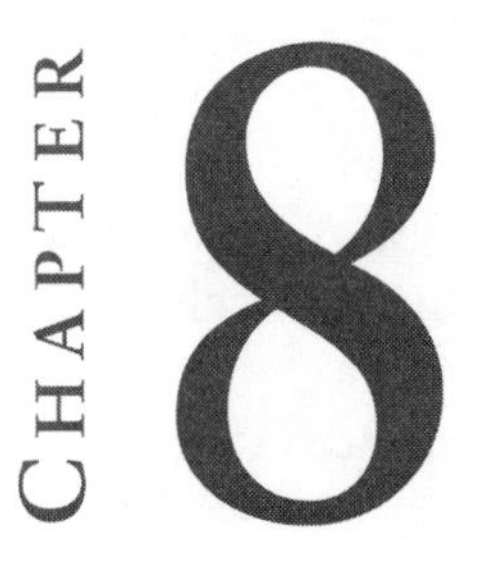

Centralized Patient Recruitment and The Use of Call Centers

Sarah Ebner, PhoneScreen, Investigator Support Services
Joseph Sameh, PhoneScreen

Faced with slow patient accrual, an increasing number of pharmaceutical companies are turning to centralized call centers. From patient recruitment prescreening and scheduling to retention, compliance and drug reminder calls, these centralized facilities can bring efficiency and expedience to a complicated process.

Increased reliance on call centers is primarily due to delays in the drug development process as a result of insufficient or slow patient accrual. Offering 24-hour availability and quick access to centralized analytical information, the call center relieves study coordinator's burden. The combination of professional staffing and state-of-the art medical communications technology helps reduce the bottlenecks of patient recruitment.

The use of central call centers is increasing in many industries. By 2001 more than 75% of the 2,000 largest global companies will outsource some function of their help desk, an annual growth of more than 35 percent.[1] The world-wide call center services market totaled $23 billion in revenues in 1998 and is projected to double to $58.6 billion in 2003. Outsourcing is the largest segment of the market, at $17 billion in 1998 or 74% of the total market, with expectations of reaching $42 billion in 2003.[2]

In healthcare, typical call center services include:

- clinical study support
- physician and hospital answering service
- centralized appointment scheduling
- nurse triage services
- direct-to-consumer advertising
- help desk
- insurance eligibility and reimbursement
- field service support
- product insert support
- pre-surgical assessments

Clinical researchers are recognizing the contributions call centers can have on accelerating the patient recruitment process. This trend is evidenced by the creation of "partnerships" with pharmaceutical companies and call centers. In addition to pharmaceutical companies, partners include clinical research organizations (CROs), media and public relations companies, web-based recruitment organizations and site management organizations (SMOs) as well as independent research sites. The call center has become an essential part of the clinical research team from the early stages of the trial through study completion.

CALL CENTER ROLE IN CLINICAL RESEARCH

Call centers can provide a variety of services to serve and inform the patient recruitment, referral, retention and compliance processes. Descriptions of services currently available are provided below.

Patient Recruitment: Standardized scripts are developed for each study to educate the patient vis-à-vis the nearest site location, length of the study, frequency of (diary) reporting, number of required visits, whether medication will be involved, whether there is any financial remuneration, and paid expenses. Operators are guided by an automated script which provides operators with all available study information. Current regulations suggest that all information provided should be approved by governing IRB's.

Site Referral: The most basic patient recruitment service available through call centers is a simple messaging service. This function is limited to collecting names and telephone numbers from prospective subjects who are calling in response to advertisements, public service announcements (PSAs) and web advertising. This patient contact data is forwarded to the nearest site for follow-up. Even when serving in this minimal function, essentially as the "first step" in the screening process, the call center can be effective in alleviating the study site staff from disruption of their other duties. Benefits also include a lower number of "lost calls" due to a rapid response to the incoming calls. Sites conducting advertising response often process overflow calls using their voice mail systems, which results in delayed follow-ups and lost recruitment opportunities.

Appointments: Call centers may also be utilized to schedule and/or confirm appointments. Call center staff also coordinate with the appropriate site scheduling methods so that the schedule information is consistent and there are no overlapping appointments. Confirmation of a appointments is completed by a telephone call, an e-mail message or a standard letter, depending on subject preference.

Retention: Call centers are also well suited to work on projects that may involve hard-to-reach patients or studies where little interaction between site and patient is experienced between visits. This increases the efficacy of the study especially in long term studies. Call centers can help provide that communication link so essential to the retention of patients in long-term studies.

Compliance: The call center staff also can serve to remind patients about taking their medication and answer other questions study participants may have. The call center format lends itself easily to contact the patient on a regular basis at the patients' convenience to ensure that they are keeping a diary and/or assist them in doing so. Continued communications with patients is used to ensure diary compliance, medication compliance and helps to ensure that individuals continue to stay involved throughout the study.

Adverse Events: The 24-7 availability of call center staff is used to serve as a "hot line" for any problems patients may experience during a trial. Not only does this assuage the possibility of health consequences for the patient but it also increases the integrity of data for the study.

Site Reports: Patient data sheet on each patient who has met the criteria for the first level of qualification is faxed or e-mailed to the site by the call center or can be posted to a secure web site. The patient data sheet includes the name and contact information of the call center, the name and address of the site office nearest to the patient, contact data and demographic information (i.e., age, marital status) of the patient and his or her replies to the qualifying medical questions including previous health history.

Management Reports: Using various technological approaches, call centers can provide statistics and reports to provide insight regarding enrollment rate, reasons for disqualification, site performance including patients enrolled per site, contact or scheduling lag time, patient demographics, media type and channel effectiveness, disqualification analysis, sites, geographic area, and/or inclusion or exclusion criteria, cost per patient call, per patient enrolled.

These reports are generated for use by the call center, the site manager, the media buyer the sponsor project manager and others monitoring the trial. Summary reports inform management decisions by providing the critical statistics and metrics. Careful review and mining of call center data can prove to serve identify and ultimately implement needed corrections to recruitment programs. In many instances, ad copy in text, media selection and in some cases even protocols. Data can impact sponsor decisions such as site performance, media strategy, internal procedures, and many other critical success factors.

Table One illustrates a typical call center process.

Call centers can assist considerably in providing information about the effectiveness of advertising by collecting cost-per-call data. This and other valuable information is often not captured at the site due to time constraints. The call center can easily keep records of the number of calls received related to advertising in each medium and market. This data can be reviewed and compared vis-à-vis the cost for a specific print advertisement and/or broadcast media advertising. The sample reports following this chapter are:

Patient Screen Report: Daily report detailing patient responses to screening questions and appointment times. A patient screen report for each prequalified caller will be faxed or e-mailed to the appropriate research site (depending on site preference). (Appendix One)

Daily Call Volume and Referral Report (Appendix Two)

Call Center Functions*

Table 1

Pre-screen candidates and provide site information using standardized scripts

Initiate outbound calls to prospective subjects

Receive inbound calls from prospective subjects responding to an advertisement, broadcast media commercial, or Public Service Announcement

Request call back from prospective subjects who are a web-based referral

Schedule appointments for qualified candidates

Maintain electronic respondent records

Provide management level reports

Call response

Media response

Media effectiveness

Media cost per call

Disqualification analysis

Pass-fail ratios

Site performance

Lag time to first contact by research site

Lag time to screening appointment at research site

Site comparison of patient accrual

Study performance

Aggregate patient accrual

Patient referral status

Consult with trial manager regarding response challenges

Follow-up with medication and/or diary reminders

Follow-up with other required patient communications

Maintain ongoing patient communication for long term studies

*Call centers can provide one or all of these functions or any combination that is required/needed by the client.

Media Response: Provides data on the number and source of responses from advertising. (Appendix Three)

Call Activity by Market Media: Provides several data types such as prequalified leads, unqualified leads and total calls by media for a multi-site recruitment project. (Appendix Four)

Disqualified Call Analysis: Demonstrates reasons for disqualification from disease-related criteria to logistical problems. (Appendix Five)

Site Lag Time: Shows patterns in delays to schedule screening visits by site for a multi-site recruitment effort. (Appendix Six)

CALL CENTER AND THE INTERNET

Web Recruitment: Web sites are often used a as a "first stop" in the patient recruitment and screening process. Once a brief questionnaire is completed, those individuals who meet the most basic criteria can be instructed to contact the call centers either by providing toll-free phone number(s) or e-mail may be used so the call center can contact them at their convenience. Further screening can be accomplished at this time with the end result of scheduling the initial appointment. Since the call center provides live, interactive interviews, the format allows for more questions to be asked than can be effectively asked at a web site.

According to IDC industry experts, global spending for customer relationship management services, including call centers and online computer help desks, are expected to exceed $40 million in 2000. These experts also predict that this figure will double during the next four years. Customer relationship management services are defined as "a variety of services used to design and operate customer-care systems that help companies attract, retain, service and expand customer relationships to generate business and improve the consumer experience." Retention and compliance support will be managed using this type of technology as the internet becomes present everywhere.

Web Reporting: Internet connections between the sponsor of the patient recruitment program and the call center can serve well as a method of immediate communications regarding appointments, progress of the recruitment, problems encountered or identified. As web technology is still in its early stages and continues to evolve, its use and applications will expand significantly during the next few years.

Integrated web and call center services can manage the entire online communication process, linking study subject, a call center agent and study sites. For example, the call center staff member can provide new content to the prospective candidate, provide access to web information, provide answers to questions through web chat and push information to subject over the web.

As technology continues to advance, current users of existing call center technologies, as well as those considering call center options, will be able to leverage their network investments to deliver unprecedented levels of operational efficiency. Simultaneously, the investment will provide these users with a converged networking infrastructure capability that will enable them to handle even greater emerging multimedia applications. The next generation of call centers is being developed to support communications over a wide range of media: the public telephone network, corporate Intranet and the Internet. Call center staff members will be able to provide support from remote offices, home or on the road.

COMPARISON WITH INDIVIDUAL SITE RECRUITMENT EFFORTS

Traditionally, recruitment efforts have been dependent on investigator site efforts to develop advertisements, place advertisements, prescreen callers, manage patient databases and schedule appointments. In this traditional method, successful recruitment depends almost exclusively on the ability of a CRC (Clinical Research Coordinator) to manage the recruitment process. This traditional method also does not allow for more than one call at a time to be handled with live coverage on a twenty-four hour basis. Call center services are scalable; call centers are able scalable to accommodate the peaks and valleys of call volume.

Retention, compliance and appointment reminder calls are not always made with the regularity that they should be. Follow-up may also greatly be compromised due once again to the necessity of contacting each patient in a timely manner. These routine communication functions are often times outside the scope and core competency of most research sites. (Table Two)

Table 2 **Comparison of Use of Call Center Versus Individual Site-Based Patient Recruitment**

Service	Site	Call Center
24/7 availablity	Low	High
Likelihood of acquiring data	Low	High
Ability to report	Moderate	High
Likelihood of reporting	Low	High
Central analytical capacity	Low	High
Ability to standardize scripting	High	High
Likelihood of standardize scripting	Low	High
Ability to process large number of calls	Low	High
Management reporting capability	None	High
Ability to manage multiple priorities	Low	High
Intimate knowledge of protocol	High	Low
Ability to do thorough screening	High	Moderate
Ability to schedule callers immediately	High	Moderate

PREDICTING CALL VOLUME

The use of a mass media advertising campaign to generate telephone calls is one of the factors that make the centralized call center cost-effective. A media agency that specializes in clinical trials understands how to produce eye-catching advertisements that meet IRB guidelines. Plus, the agency, or a partner media buying firm, can select the right combination of broadcast stations and print publications to reach the target population efficiently.

Inevitably, the pool of potential patients for a clinical study diminishes in size progressively as it progresses through the various phases of the screening process and informed consent process. The key to planning such a program is a phenomenon known as the "funnel effect." The universe of individuals affected by the disease state being studied may be quite large; but the number of patients ultimately randomized is much smaller. A number of factors cause the funnel effect:

- Not all of the advertising reaches the potential patients;
- Many of the potential patients who see the advertising aren't interested in participating in a study;
- Of those who respond, many live too far from a research site, while many others fail the telephone prescreening;
- Many of the callers who pass prescreening fail to go to the research site for their first appointment; and
- Some of the patients who pass the prescreen end up failing a more detailed screening process when they arrive in person at the site.

Working as a team, the ad agency, media firm and call center apply these factors based on knowledge gained from previous experience, as well as demographic studies and information known about the incidence and nature of the disease state in the study. They are thus able to calculate the size of the target population for the media message.

The application of the factors can vary widely. There is postulation that if a trial offers benefit for an active medical problem, the ratio of enrollment as compared to screened patients is 1:5. If the trial relates to the prevention of a disease, the ratio of enrollment to screened candidates for the trial drops to 1:40.[3]

The data in the chart is best reread from the bottom up. The goal for the project is 267 randomized patients. Based on prior experience with this therapeutic area, it was estimated that only one-fifth of the prescreened patients referred to sites would pass the more rigorous site-based screening. Thus, 1,069 patients must visit the sites.

It is estimated that as many as 20% of the prospective study subjects would not to keep their appointment. Thus, the call center would need to make appointments for 1,337 people.

The media/call center team estimated that 20% of those responding to the advertising would pass prescreening. The call center would need to receive 6,683 calls. For this study, about six percent of those reached by advertising could be expected to respond. To produce the six percent response, the campaign message would need to be viewed three times by 111,375 people. The remaining rows at the top of the chart show how the media/call center team determined that advertising in media markets totaling 33 million people would be required to produce the goal of 267 randomized patients.

Total population in the selected DMAs within age range required by study	33M	
Population with diagnosis under study	1.485M	4.5%
Population with diagnosis meeting other study criteria	22,750	15%
Media reach (assumes 3 exposures needed)	11,375	50%
Call response rate	6,683	6%
Qualified responders (passing telephone screening and scheduled for screeing appointment at the research site)	1,337	20%
Attend screening appointment at research site	1,069	80%
Randomized patients	267	25%

DEVELOPING A PROPOSAL FOR CALL CENTER INVOLVEMENT

Despite the many organizational advantages that call centers offer, they would not be used if they did not make economic sense. Evaluating the cost is more complicated than simply requesting a rate sheet. The typical pharmaceutical company or advertising agency provides the call center with a detailed request for proposal (RFP) to ensure that all parameters are covered in an effort to establish a firm, realistic bid.

The RFP should provide information on many factors that will have an impact on the call center fees, including:

- Recruitment goal or target (number of randomized patients)
- Deadline by which the goal must be met
- Number of sites and geographic reach
- Inclusion/exclusion criteria
- Planned recruitment methods
- Per-site recruitment goals
- Predicted patient accrual rates
- Site media preferences
- Appointment scheduling scenarios
- Obstacles to recruiting, retention and compliance
- Foreign language requirements
- Fulfillment (mailing) requirements

The RFP should examine of the call center's therapeutic experience and history of involvement in healthcare telecommunications. A section on technical capabilities should include the following points:

- Number of incoming telephone lines
- Access to T1 high capacity lines
- Access to full-time Internet connection
- Ability to accept/place telephone calls in all area codes and time zones
- Ability to assign specialized toll-free numbers (e.g., 1-800-GI-STUDY)
- Computer-based customized scripting capability
- Type and structure of database
- Data backup and security
- Emergency electrical supply
- Security at the call center facility
- Ability to deliver management reports in real-time

The call center's depth of personnel expertise is another critical element that must be evaluated in the RFP Factors include:

- Hiring qualifications for operators
- Ongoing training
- Training for specific studies
- Average length of employment; turnover rate
- Educational and experiential background of project management team

CALL CENTER COSTS

There are both hard as well as soft costs involved with patient recruitment. The budget range for a particular project is quite varied depending on a number of factors. Among these expense categories are personnel, direct expenses, and travel expenses in addition to interactions with a central recruitment group and with an IRB.

Fixed Costs and Management Costs

- Programming the telephone system for the specific requirements of the study
- Securing appropriate toll-free numbers
- Writing the call guide script
- Interfacing with Internet components
- Database and report set-up
- Attendance at investigators meeting
- Foreign language translation services, if required

Ongoing Variable Costs

- Study-related training of operators
- Cost per call, if applicable
- Cost per minute of time spent on the phone, if applicable
- Cost of completing data entry after the caller disconnects
- Guaranteed per-seat charge (may be necessary if exact broadcast times of commercials is not known)
- Report generation
- Project management
- Regular conference calls with research coordinator and/or study sites
- Printing and postage costs for mail fulfillment

CALL CENTER REGULATIONS & IRB REVIEWS

Call center screening of study subjects is not covered in the code of federal regulations. The FDA "Information Sheets" 1998 update provides guidelines encouraging IRB review of "Receptionists Scripts." This document states: "The first contact with a prospective study subjects make is often with a receptionist who follows a script to determine basic eligibility for the specific study. The IRB should assure the procedures followed adequately protect the rights and welfare of the prospective subjects."

The Department of Health and Human Services, Office of the Inspector General (OIG) report on "Recruiting Human Subjects" released in June 2000 details concerns about the physician impartiality in the patient recruitment process.[4] As a third party, call centers are able to maintain impartiality and adhere to standardized scripts to maintain consistency in the telephone interaction.

Current regulations do not thoroughly cover the growing services provided at call centers. Guidance or regulations must be developed to better govern the expanded role of call centers in patient recruitment.[5] Current call center technology allows for recording (with approval of all parties) to confirm (if needed) that the patient has agreed to participate in a given trial and that the patient's demographic and medical history information can be retained.

SUMMARY

Use of a call center consistently has led to an earlier detection of problems and correction of such problems. For example, it may become evident that a site is not providing sufficient patients. With sophisticated data analysis provided by a call center the weak performance of one or more sites may become evident more quickly. Conversely, it may become necessary to add sites to a certain geographic area or areas because of high enrollment and volume. The same holds true about expanding or reducing recruitment activities at existing site or sites. Additional support staff may be added to process the additional patient load. By being able to respond quickly to this type of observed need, it greatly increases the trial's effectiveness and efficiency.

One example, a national study experienced a 94% disqualification ratio, leading to serious delays in enrollment. Review of the call center's screening data revealed that a study-required medication was not being taken by more than a quarter of the callers. The sponsors of the study determined that this medication should be provided to the callers who otherwise met all of the criteria in order to qualify them. The call center was then assigned to recontact the group of individuals who were previously disqualified from participating in the study and provide them with information about how to obtain this medication.[6]

We have attempted to explain patient recruitment can be addressed by a call center operation. Any similarity of data shown or discussed within this chapter to actual trial studies is purely coincidental.

REFERENCES

[1] Meta Group, November 1998.

[2] IDC, June 1999.

[3] Spilker, Bert. Cramer, Joyce. "Patient Recruitment in Clinical Trials." Raven Press, 1992. p. 22.

[4] Weschler, Jill. "HHS Recommends Subject Recruitment Changes." Applied Clinical Trials, August 2000. p. 20-23.

[5] *Office of Evaluation and Inspection, Recruitment Human Subjects: Protections in Industry-Sponsored Clinical Research*. OEI-01-97-00195 (OEI, Boston, MA, June 2000).

[6] AmericasDoctor.com and Phone Screen. Case Study. 1999.

AUTHOR BIOGRAPHIES

Sarah Ebner is the President of Investigator Support Services, Inc. and Director of Sales for Phone Screen. Ms. Ebner holds a Master of Business and a Master of Public Health from the University of Illinois at Chicago.

In 1992, Ms. Ebner founded Investigator Support Services (ISS) as a business consulting service for independent research sites. Today, ISS provides both consulting and business development services to a select group of private practice and hospital-based sites, as well as, Phone Screen, a subject recruitment and compliance call center. Phone Screen, founded in 1985 by Joe Sameh, provides sponsors with call center services to expedite patient recruitment, retention and compliance.

ISS communicates with industry sponsors and CRO's to identify new business opportunities for its clients. Through a broad range of marketing strategies, ISS develops long-term relationships with Sponsors and clients to facilitate timely initiation and completion of clinical trials.

Joseph Sameh began his career in medical operations management in 1976. As business manager, Mr. Sameh led the expansion of a sports medicine practice into a multi-site operation. Subsequently, he served as operations and business manager for a variety of medical specialists.

In 1985, Mr. Sameh founded American Mediconnect, Inc. Mediconnect is a communications application service provider (CASP) meeting the demand for high-quality patient-to-provider communications. The company's system uses both the traditional phone network as well as Internet-based methods of communications with a highly scalable and reliable infrastructure.

Mediconnect created its Phone Screen℠ service in 1994. Phone Screen℠ has become a recognized leader in the field of patient recruitment, retention and compliance/persistence services.

The service centralizes telephone screening and retention of potential clinical trial study subjects, helps shorten the recruitment cycle, provides valuable data to inform advertising and clinical decision making, and makes available extensive knowledge in recruitment in key therapeutic areas. The Chicago-based company operates around the clock, processing more than 9,000 calls per day.

Mr. Sameh and Mediconnect have been featured editorially in numerous national trade publications and he has lectured at many educational conferences.

Appendix 1

14-Jan-00 Site: CHICAGO (312) 980-1234

Pediatric Depression Study Patient Screen Report

PS ID# 154 Referral Source: Newspaper screened by: Amy Date: 1/13/00

Demographic Information

Patient: Robert G. Jones DOB 12/07/1990
Caller: Tammy W. Jones Relationship to child: PARENT
Address: 1145 Elston Ave, Chicago, IL 60618
Phone: (773) 555-5555
Additional Phone: 773 628 7563 this is mother's work phone

Study Questions

Previous Study: No

Questions related to symptoms of Depression

Depressed/sad at least 2 Wks:	Yes
Decreased interest in activities?:	Yes
Appetite changes	No
Sleep Disturbances:	Yes
Irritability:	Yes
Fatigue/loss of energy:	Yes
Drop in Grades:	No
Worthlessness/guilt:	Yes
Impaired Thinking:	Yes
Thoughts of Death/suicide:	Unsure Attempt Suicide: No

List Rx meds: **None**

List Otc meds: **advil–for knee pain**

Meds Allergies?: No
Any previous use of SSRI: No Willing to allow future use of SSRI?: Yes

Any Significant Medical condition: ADD–not currently undergoing Treatment.

Any history of seizures:	No		
Difficulty Swallowing Pills:	No	Abnormal Thyroid Function?:	No
Side Effects Meds:	No	Anorexia:	No
Abused/used Drugs/alcohol?:	Unsure	Bulimia:	No
Organic Brain Disease:	No	Bipolar in family?:	No
Bipolar Disorder:	No	Borderline personality disorder	No
Psychotic Depression:	No		

Is child seeing therapist Not currently (family counseling/not since thanksgiving)

Appointment Information

Appt scheduled?: YES 01/17/01 9:00 am
Addl. notes: Mother has been treated for depression.
Child was diagnosed w/ADD in 2nd grade–took ritalin for short while–but son wanted to go off. Mom was not sure if ADD correct diagnosis, recognizes some behaviour that she is familiar with from her own experience–being depressed at times

Daily Call Volume and Referral Report

Daily Call Volume	6/26/00
Incoming Calls	36
Screened	28
Disqualified	18
Pre-qualified	10
Pass Ratios	36%

Location	Investigator	Daily Referrals	Cumulative Referrals
Albuquerque, NM	Hacksaw	3	59
Atlanta, GA	Hall		53
Atlanta, GA	Hanson		51
Butte, MT	Hill		9
Greer, SC	Hope		65
Hollywood, FL	Harris	4	67
Minneapolis, MN	Heinz	1	70
Ogden, UT	Hinman		21
Phoenix, AZ	Hilliard		24
San Antonio, TX	Hirsch		29
San Antonio, TX	Harrow		10
San Antonio, TX	Hinton	1	25
Tampa, FL	Himmel		65
Tucson, AZ	Hicks		37
Vero Beach, FL	Horton	1	21
Total		10	606

Phone Screen
3232 N. Elston, Chicago, Il 60618

Appendix 3

Media Response

Site Information		Print		Radio		TV		Other	Total	
Investigator	City	Ad Runs	Referrals	Ad Runs	Referrals	Ad Runs	Referrals	Referrals	Ad Runs	Referrals
01-Brooks	Tampa, FL	2	23	1	10	2	28	4	5	65
02-Davis	Tempe, AZ	1	8	0	0	0	0	2	1	10
03-Finegold	Chicago, IL	2	24	0	0	0	0	3	2	27
04-Findlay	Pittsburgh, PA	3	25	0	0	2	74	2	5	101
05-Gable	Kansas City, KA	4	32	2	20	0	0	1	6	53
06-Emerson	Winston-Salem, NC	2	16	3	21	0	0	0	5	37
07-Hall	Buffalo, NY	2	18	1	18	0	0	0	3	36
08-Henderson	Redondo Beach, CA	3	28	0	0	0	0	2	3	30
09-Johnson	Fort Worth, TX	2	14	0	0	2	45	1	4	60
10-Lindberg	Detroit, MI	2	9	1	11	0	0	0	3	20
11-Pearl	Rochester, NY	1	12	1	12	3	42	4	5	70
12-Rose	Cleveland, OH	0	0	1	25	1	65	4	2	94
13-Taylore	Wuakesha, WI	1	8	0	0	1	47	2	2	57
14-Young	San Antonio, TX	2	17	1	18	1	30	1	4	66
TOTAL ADS		27		11		12			50	
TOTAL PASSED			234		135		331	26		726

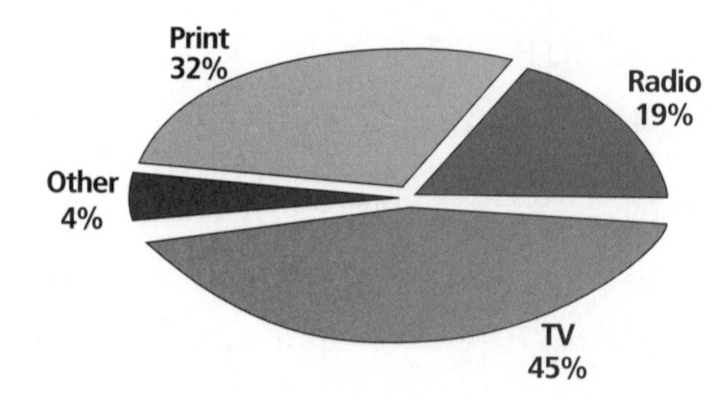

Media Response by Date Range and Investigator

	Date Range: 9/10/00-9/16/00	Radio		Newspaper		TV		Friend/ Family		Internet		Physician		Other		Total Calls	Total Referrals	Referral Ratio (%)
	Investigator	Calls	Ref*	Calls	Ref*	Calls	Ref*	Calls	Ref*	Calls	Ref*	Calls	Ref*	Calls	Ref*			
~	DQ pre- site selection*	5	0	3	0	0	0	0	0	1	0	0	0	0	0	9	0	~
111	Ayers	10	8	4	2	0	0	4	3	3	2	4	3	3	1	28	19	68%
122	Bowdon	4	2	0	0	0	0	0	0	0	0	0	0	3	2	7	4	57%
133	Cathcart	4	3	3	1	0	0	0	0	0	0	0	0	2	0	9	4	44%
144	Davis	3	1	0	0	0	0	0	0	0	0	0	0	0	0	3	1	33%
155	Lowell	0	0	0	0	0	0	0	0	0	0	0	0	0	0	0	0	~
166	Murphy	5	4	4	2	0	0	1	1	0	0	2	1	1	1	13	9	69%
177	Smith	0	0	0	0	0	0	0	0	0	0	0	0	0	0	0	0	
	Total	31	18	14	5	0	0	5	4	4	2	6	4	9	4	69	37	54%

**Ref=Prequalified, referral forwarded to site*

Cum. Totals 8/1/00- 9/16/00	
Calls	Ref*
26	~
120	87
115	81
80	44
22	12
0	0
44	25
0	0
407	249

Identifies call levels according to media tactic as well as distribution of referrals. Includes referral ratio and cumulative totals columns.

Appendix 5

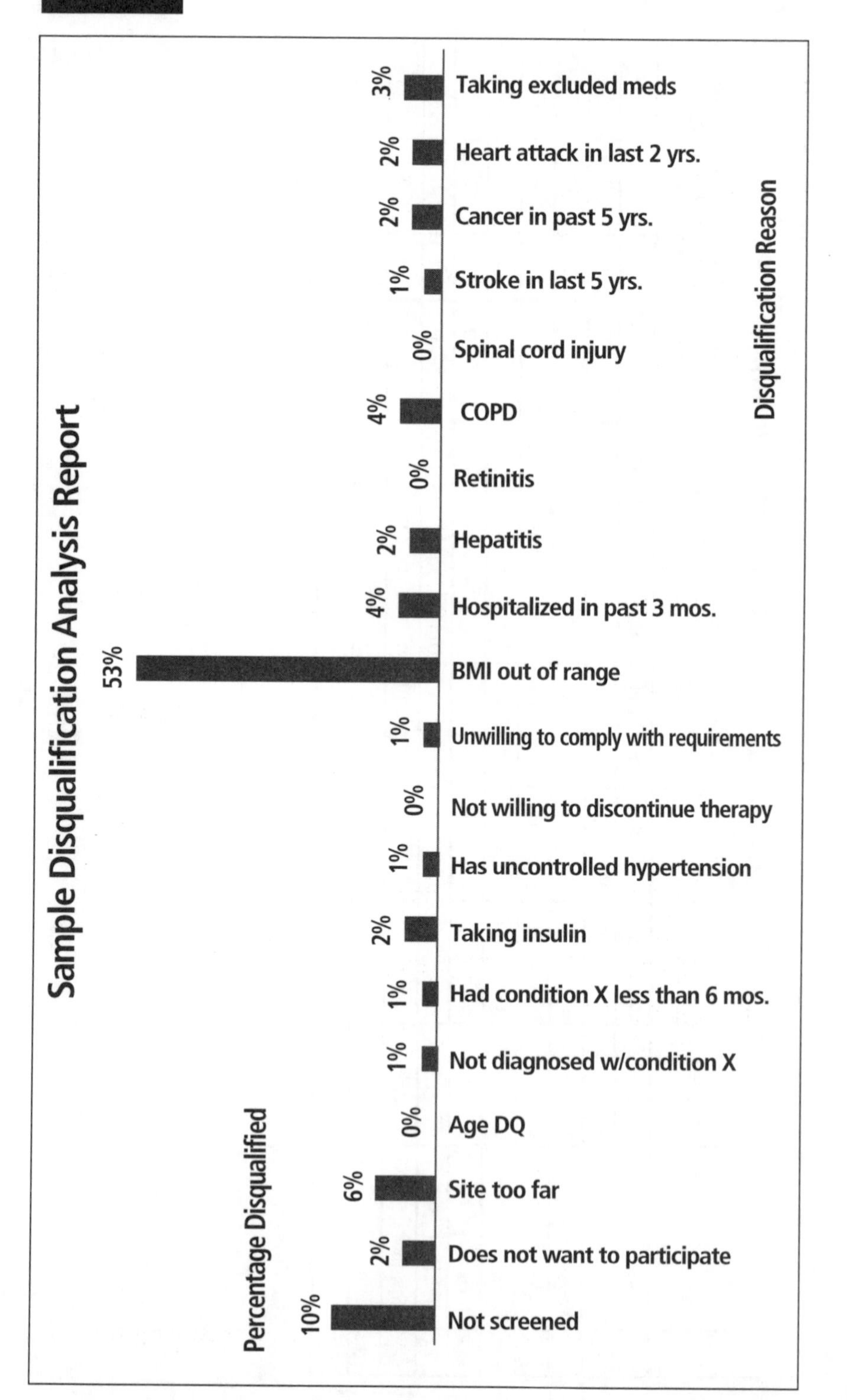

Sample Disqualification Analysis Report
Disqualification Reason
Percentage Disqualified
3% Taking excluded meds
2% Heart attack in last 2 yrs.
2% Cancer in past 5 yrs.
1% Stroke in last 5 yrs.
0% Spinal cord injury
4% COPD
0% Retinitis
2% Hepatitis
4% Hospitalized in past 3 mos.
53% BMI out of range
1% Unwilling to comply with requirements
0% Not willing to discontinue therapy
1% Has uncontrolled hypertension
2% Taking insulin
1% Had condition X less than 6 mos.
1% Not diagnosed w/condition X
0% Age DQ
6% Site too far
2% Does not want to participate
10% Not screened

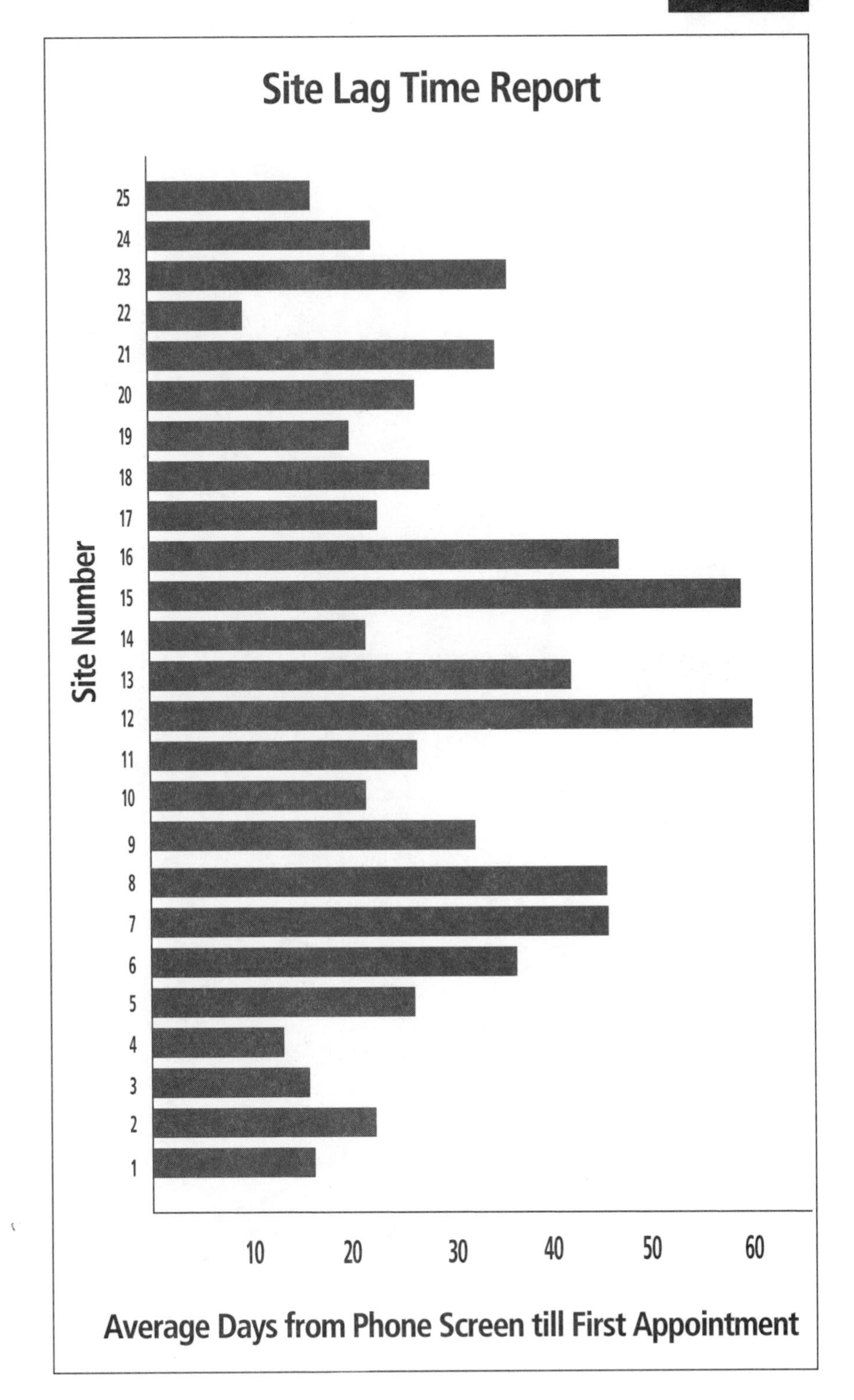
Site Lag Time Report
Site Number
25
24
23
22
21
20
19
18
17
16
15
14
13
12
11
10
9
8
7
6
5
4
3
2
1
10
20
30
40
50
60
Average Days from Phone Screen till First Appointment

Recruiting Patients on the Internet

Whitney Allen, David Heck and Daniel McDonald, CenterWatch

In the past several years, the Internet has gained credibility as a viable patient recruitment resource. Although the incidence of Internet usage to recruit patients is relatively low at this time, clinical research professionals—in sponsor and CRO companies as well as in investigative sites—have begun to see dramatic increases in usage. For example, a survey conducted by the Association for Clinical Research Professionals (ACRP) in December 1999 found that less than 15% of clinical research professionals are routinely using the Internet to recruit patients. By 2001, however, almost half

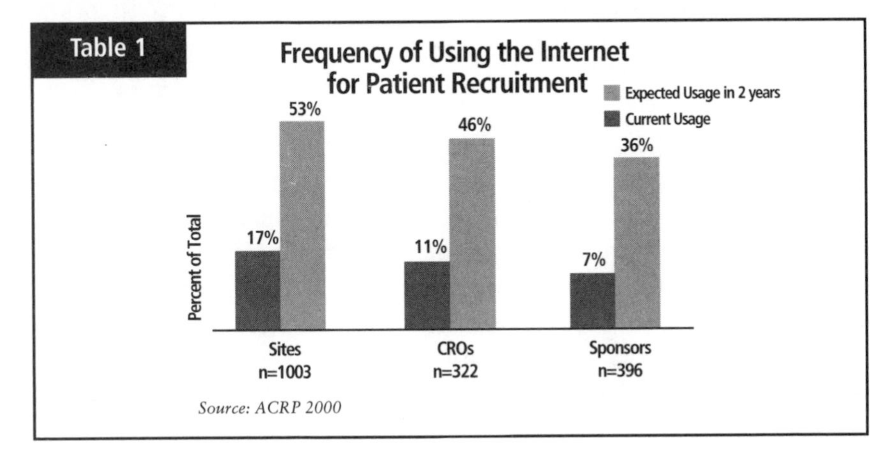

Source: ACRP 2000

of survey respondents believe they will be regularly recruiting patients via the Internet.[1] Similarly, in a survey conducted by CenterWatch among sixty-one sponsor and CRO companies, only one-third of companies used the Internet to recruit patients for at least one trial in 1997. Two-thirds of companies reported using the Internet for this purpose for at least one clinical trial in 1999.

EXAMPLES OF EFFECTIVENESS

The question remains as to how effective a patient recruitment tool the Internet is. The following case examples show that posting the trial on the Internet significantly increased the number of responses received. These three case examples present extremely favorable outcomes for recruiting patients on the Internet. While they are all real life examples, it should be noted that they document ideal scenarios that might not be attained by each trial. At present, the Internet has a minimal but growing impact on patient recruitment as the clinical research industry grapples with the most effective way to use this tool.

Case Example #1

A top-twenty pharmaceutical company recently completed a pivotal trial of an investigational treatment for depression among forty research centers. The company used a variety of recruitment methods including chart reviews, physician referral, newspaper, radio and the Internet. At the conclusion of the study, the sponsor determined that 16% of the 1,000 randomized patients who completed the trial came from listing that trial on the Internet. The sponsor had spent approximately $63.00 per enrolled patient through the Internet—less than half the per-patient spending for several other recruitment approaches implemented.

Case Example #2

A large phase III rheumatoid arthritis study among thirty investigative sites had fallen several months behind the planned patient accrual rates. The sponsor decided to post the clinical trial online. In the first three months, participating sites reported receiving more than two thousand e-mails and phone calls from patients responding to the Internet trial listing. A total of eighty patients were screened, and twenty were randomized into the trial. The sponsor determined that the costs to enroll patients through the Internet came to $95 per enrollee—a cost-effective level relative to other approaches that were used.

Case Example #3

As one of its recruitment methods, the sponsor of a dermatology study involving twenty-four investigative sites posted the trial on the Internet. Over a period of two months, sites received a total of 1,253 visits, 340 e-mails and 93 phone calls from potential patients. The sites screened thirty-four of those responders and enrolled eight patients into the study. Estimated cost per patient totaled $60.

INCREASING IMPORTANCE OF THE INTERNET

The Internet now plays an active part in the lives of most North Americans. NUA Internet Surveys and Nielsen NetRatings report that an estimated 124 million people—45% of the U.S. population—are using the Internet regularly.[2] Based on a recent survey, Jupiter Communication reports that 96% of all browsers use the Internet to routinely send and receive e-mail messages; 72% of users browse the Internet to research a topic; and 51% use the Internet for daily news and stock quotes. Only 10% of browsers report that they regularly shop for products and services on the Internet.[3]

In 1997, an estimated 26% of all browsers used the Internet to find health-related information. In 2000, the volume of browsers increased exponentially, and nearly half (47%) of all browsers now say that they use the Internet routinely to find health-related information. In response, more than twenty-two thousand web sites have now been created to provide consumers and professionals with health and medical information.[4]

According to Media Matrix,[5] baby boomers and seniors—a significant pool of clinical trial participants—are the fastest growing Internet population, increasing 18% in 1999. Life-style and health-related sites are especially popular with this segment. Compared to eighteen to twenty-four year olds, baby boomers and seniors spend 6.3 more days per month on the Internet, surf more frequently, stay online longer and check out more web pages.[6]

THE NEED FOR IMPROVED PATIENT RECRUITMENT

According to Keith Ruark, of the consulting firm The Wilkerson Group, the receptivity and awareness of the Internet as an important patient recruitment resource has reached a new peak. "We see several factors contributing to the unprecedented excitement level: A breakdown of traditional practices with respect to who is conducting patient recruitment and how patients are being targeted for recruitment, the growing costs of drug development, and the large strain that recruitment is going to cause in the coming years. As more and more drugs reach critical larger scale trials, pharmaceutical companies will be looking for more effective ways to reach patients while holding down those costs."

Indeed, the pharmaceutical industry spent more than $30 billion on R&D in 1999 alone, with almost 40% going to clinical development.[7] Spending in this area is growing disproportionately by an estimated 13% annually. There are now more than seven thousand drugs in the R&D pipeline worldwide. In addition, a number of incremental new molecular entities (NMEs) have been growing annually by 6% for the past five years. Due to technology advances (e.g., genomics, combinatorial chemistry), the number of NMEs during the next five years are expected to grow by more than 10% annually.[8]

Along with burgeoning drug pipelines, pharmaceutical companies typically are gathering higher numbers of evaluable patients for their New Drug Applications (NDAs). It's estimated that more than four thousand patients are evaluated for a given NDA—a 7% annual growth rate in the number of patients per new drug application. (Table Two)[9] As much higher numbers of drugs enter clinical trials,

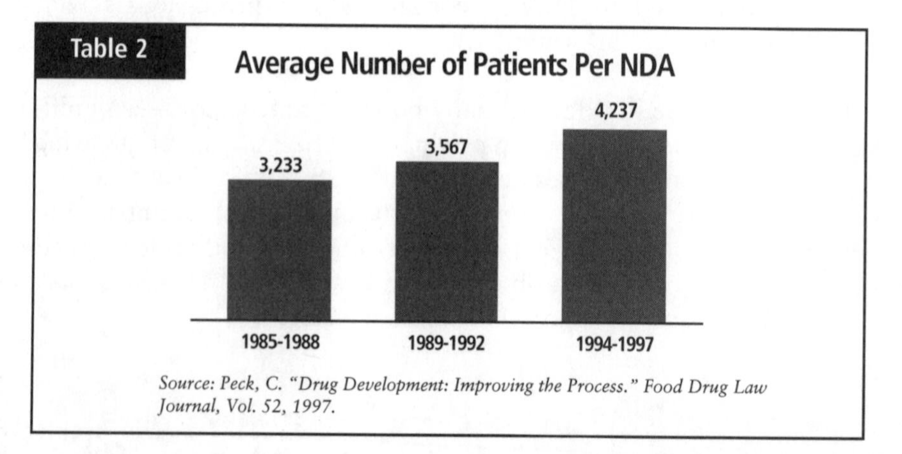

Source: Peck, C. "Drug Development: Improving the Process." Food Drug Law Journal, Vol. 52, 1997.

the challenge becomes even more pronounced. Patient recruitment is already the largest cause of lost time accounting for an estimated half of all delays that occur during the study conduct. In a recent analysis, CenterWatch found that almost 80% of all clinical trials must extend their enrollment periods by at least one month.[10]

Not only is it harder to find patient participants, it's getting harder to keep subjects in clinical studies. Pharmaceutical and biotechnology companies are also pursuing more ambitious research projects today. These programs tend to be larger in scope with more trials and more data to collect per protocol. As a result, many clinical trials conducted today require a larger commitment (e.g., more visits, more procedures) from study subjects.

Currently, only an estimated 10% to 12% of the fifty million individuals in the United States who have chronic illnesses participate in clinical trials, which means that 90% of eligible patients are not entering clinical trials.[11] There are numerous reasons for this low level of participation. Reasons range from poor protocol design (e.g., highly restrictive eligibility requirements) to negative public perceptions and patient distrust in health providers.[12] Others argue that traditional approaches to reaching and informing potential study participants are failing due to changes in attitudes and behaviors that have occurred among both provider and patient communities. These traditional approaches have included physician referral, chart reviews, walk-ins, investigative site-initiated phone calls to patients and study notices and bulletins in waiting rooms or common areas.

"We see a fragmentation of the traditional recruitment approaches. In many cases, the clinical research coordinators are trying to recruit patients, but they are not marketing experts. We see an opportunity to offer a centralized approach and to apply more sophisticated target marketing," explained Ruark. He believes one approach can be provided via the use of the Internet.

Said Eric Coldwell, analyst with Prudential Vector Healthcare Group, "With patient recruitment being the number one limiting factor in clinical trials, [having a web site] provides greater access to potential subjects at a low price point." Coldwell explained that the significant players in clinical research, whether they are pharmaceutical companies, CROs or e-health portals, will have web sites with some way for patients to learn about clinical trials.

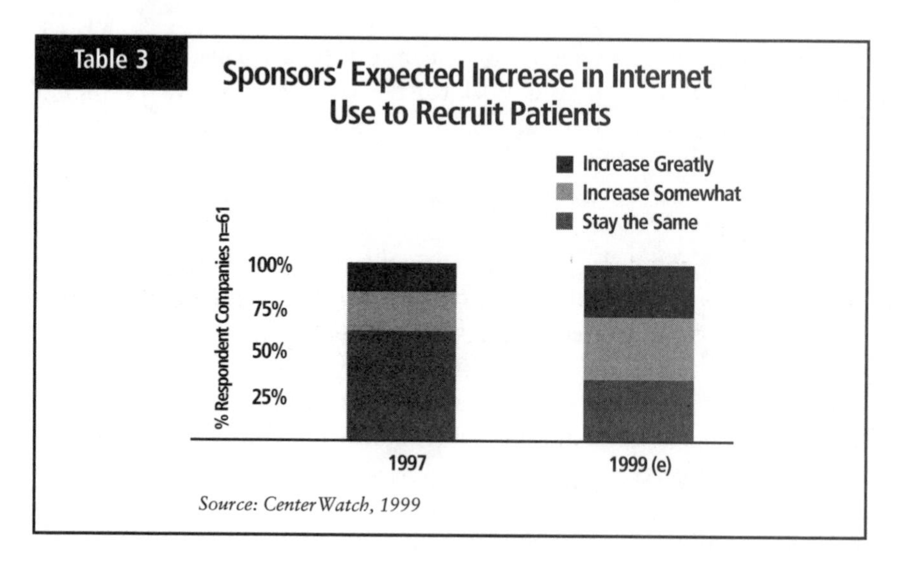

Nevertheless, not all trials are appropriate for Internet-based recruitment. Sponsors and CROs primarily use the CenterWatch listing service for longer-term chronic illnesses (98% of studies). Less than 2% of all posted trials are for acute illnesses.

In addition, at this time a large percentage of trials are posted for those studies where recruitment is the most difficult. More than 40% of clinical studies posted by sponsors and CROs on the Internet are for cancer-related illnesses, 12% and 13% of posted trials are for endocrine disorders and infectious diseases respectively, and 9% of postings are for hematological illnesses.[13]

Investigative sites are using the Internet to recruit patients across all clinical research phases. Sponsors and CROs are primarily using the Internet to recruit patients for phase II through IV projects. To date, almost half of all sponsor and CRO postings on this web site have been for phase III trials (43%), phase II trials comprised one-third of the total, and 19% of posted trials were for phase IV projects. Recently there has been significant growth in the number of phase IV programs listed by sponsor and CRO companies, and this trend is expected to continue.

INTERNET RECRUITMENT PROVIDERS

Six years ago, only a handful of web sites were being used to assist patients in identifying clinical trials. These web sites were primarily listing services. They were largely funded by government agencies or health associations (e.g., the National Cancer Institute, the National Institutes of Health, the American Cancer Society and the National AIDS Foundation).

By the mid-1990s, a number of companies, primarily patient recruitment service providers, began including the web among the various media used to reach potential study participants. These providers tended to be small players in the clinical trials industry.

Early entrants into the field typically used Internet-based recruitment as one of several promotional services. Along with television, newspaper and direct mail, recruitment service providers would also post trial announcements on the Internet.

After attempting to offer Internet-based listings for several years, two companies, Sterling, a sponsor, and Pharmatech, a CRO, scaled back their involvement on the Internet following disappointing levels of usage by sponsors and CROs. Other early entrant companies continue to offer their Internet-based services. These companies include Clinical Solutions, a subsidiary of Nelson Communications; Butler Clinical Recruitment, a subsidiary of Quintiles; and ClinicalTrials.com, a service provided by Pharmaceutical Research Plus.

Now, companies offering a recruitment component use more interactive web-based functions such as chat groups, real-time e-mailing and aggressive and widespread banner advertising. New Internet-recruitment service providers continue to follow the process of directing web-surfing patients to the investigative site or a call center as the entry point into a clinical trial. Several companies, however, plan to have more established and effective support to handle potential study subjects at the investigative site level. These companies place a priority on patient retention in the trials. Their support techniques may include hiring employees dedicated to answering phone calls and e-mails from prospective and current patients. They may also send proactive e-mail reminders to encourage patients to comply with the day-to-day trial requirements.

The structure of the Internet as a patient recruitment resource has divided into two distinct camps, with a few hybrids: (1) Content Providers and (2) Content Aggregators. Content providers tend to be neutral, independent parties—government agencies, associations and publishing and information services companies—where the vast majority of the clinical trial content is generated by their own resources. Content aggregators tend to be large health information destination web sites that tap outside resources for their clinical trial content. Aggregators typically license content from providers in an effort to generate repeat traffic to their large web sites. These content aggregators try to offer content across a wide range of healthcare segments. A few companies fall into the hybrid category, meaning they generate some listings on their own but also license content from external parties.

CONTENT PROVIDERS

At the time of this writing, a list of the most significant web sites generating their own trials listings includes the following:

- clinicaltrials.gov
- nih.gov
- cancernet.nci.nih.gov
- cancerconsultants.com
- clinicalstudies.com
- centerwatch.com

GOVERNMENT REGISTRIES

Government-sponsored web sites continue to dominate the content provider field. In early 2000, the National Library of Medicine announced the introduction of a registry of government-sponsored clinical trials to begin to address the requirements of Section 113 of the Food and Drug Administration Act of 1997. This legislation calls for the National Institutes of Health (NLM), working with other agencies and companies, to coordinate the establishment of various databanks for public access to government- and industry-sponsored clinical trials information for serious and life-threatening illnesses.

Information listed on the NLM registry, or any government-sponsored web site, is classified as public domain. Any organization or individual can duplicate public domain information without permission and without establishing a process for updating such data. Over time, it may become increasingly difficult for government-sponsored clinical trial listing services to maintain the quality and timeliness of their information.

THE CENTERWATCH CLINICAL TRIALS LISTING SERVICE

Since 1995, CenterWatch has been providing its Clinical Trials Listing Service™ to potential research participants and their advocates. The CenterWatch web site is one of the oldest and most comprehensive sites posting industry-sponsored clinical trials on the Internet. During the past several years, CenterWatch has been providing content to a large number of content aggregators including WebMD, Mediconsult, Medscape, AmericasDoctor.com, Acurian and iVillage. At any given time, an estimated 7,000 to 9,000 industry-sponsored clinical trials actively seeking study subjects are listed on the CenterWatch web site.

Since its inception, several thousand investigative sites and more than 350 sponsor and CRO companies have placed their trials directly on the CenterWatch web site. Investigative sites list their trials, depending on their involvement in clinical research. A number of large academic medical centers and site management organizations also list multiple trials. Many small investigative sites typically list no more than a handful of trials at any one time. In contrast, only 26% of sponsors and CROs post their individual trials on this web site. Almost three out of four companies post multiple trials across a variety of therapeutic areas. The average study posted by a sponsor or CRO is relatively large, an average of nineteen geographically disbursed research centers, and is placed on the Internet for almost a year.

An estimated 275,000 to 350,000 people review the CenterWatch clinical trial listings every month. Much of this traffic is reached through the content aggregator affiliations. In March of 2000, for example, more than 330,000 people viewed the clinical trial listings. Based on an ongoing survey conducted on the CenterWatch web site, the majority, 80%, of all visitors are patients and their family and friends. Approximately 20% of all visitors are sponsors, CROs or health professionals.

Visitors to the CenterWatch web site are highly receptive to clinical trials. In a survey of almost 1,200 patients, 67% of those visiting the web site are interested in participating in clinical trials. Almost half of the visitors to the CenterWatch web site have been recently diagnosed with an illness, one out of four patients report that they are seeking an alternative therapy to one they are already taking and 27% of visitors are family or friends of a patient who has been recently diagnosed.

Most individuals who visit the CenterWatch web site (61%) do so once a month. Approximately 14% are visiting the site for the first time. One out of four visit on a weekly basis. The patient population visiting the web site appears to be a unique target audience. Only 23% of visitors to the web site have ever participated in a clinical trial, suggesting that the Internet may prove a valuable means to reaching new study participants. In addition to visitor traffic, CenterWatch now receives and responds to approximately five thousand e-mail messages each month. Of this number, only 2% to 3% are e-mail messages from patients in Europe and Asia.

Approximately 31,000 people or organizations are now registered to receive notices from CenterWatch when a new trial is listed. Almost daily, CenterWatch sends out broadcast e-mail notices over the Internet to inform patients and advocates of newly posted trials. Many of these e-mail recipients, for example, are associations and patient support groups representing large numbers of patient members. The broadcast notices over the Internet extend well beyond electronic boundaries. Numerous organizations including other publishers, support groups and health educators print these notices in their literature and communications to their patient members. Combined with viewer traffic to the online listing of clinical trials, it is estimated that as many as 500,000 patients and their advocates will see these clinical trial listings in electronic or print form every month.

Based on patient traffic logs taken in 1999,[14] sponsors, CROs and investigative sites can expect an average of two to three people per day to view individual trial descriptions for a diabetes or cardiology study. One to two individuals every other day will view a description of a trial in GI or urology. Sites posting various cancer or infectious diseases/immunology trials receive, on average, four visits each day to their trial descriptions.

At the present time, 36% of all patients and advocates viewing trial postings on the web site report contacting a research center. This is encouraging as it represents an increase of almost ten percentage points over the level of follow-up with research centers reported in 1998. Of those potential subjects failing to contact the investigative site: 44% felt they did not meet the eligibility requirements, 41% were not in the appropriate geographic area and 10% reported having trouble contacting the center. Less than 5% claimed it was due to a lack of interest in trial participation. This suggests that as greater traffic comes on to the Internet, and as a larger number of studies are posted, patient follow-up should increase.

THE *META*REGISTER

We're beginning to see the first signs of content providers operating on a global level. The global academic community, together with government-sponsored trial organizations from various countries around the world, have started to put their weight behind a global registry of clinical trials. Aided by recently passed laws in several countries mandating the registry of drug trials for serious and life-threatening conditions, the *meta*Register, as it is called, has gathered steam enough to launch an international initiative.

"Ours is, to an extent, a register of registers held by other organizations," explained Anne Greenwood, managing director for Current Controlled Trials, the company behind the *meta*Register. "Our idea is to be the first place that people might come to find out what trials are ongoing, and then, if they find information that is of interest to them, to point them in the direction of the organization or researcher that knows most about that trial."

After two years of work from 1998 to 2000, the *meta*Register currently includes fifteen registers and 6,370 trial records, mostly from the United Kingdom, the United States, Australia and Canada. The members of its international advisory group span the United Kingdom, Germany, Italy, Australia, the Netherlands and Spain. They also represent the American National Institutes of Health (NIH), the British National Health Service (NHS) and the European Commission. At present, industry is represented by the Association of the British Pharmaceutical Industry and Glaxo Wellcome.

The advisory committee provides Current Controlled Trials with many leads for existing registries, according to Greenwood. At the same time, members of her company also troll the Internet, looking for organizations that list trials. They then approach the organizations and invite them to join the metaRegister initiative.

Current Controlled Trials, Limited, a private company that is part of the Current Science Group, was created for the sole function of running the *meta*Register. It provides the funds so that users can view the *meta*Register for free. In return, Current Controlled Trials plans to derive publishing activities from the project. "We hope that the traffic that we are generating to the site means that we have the beginnings of a potential market for these types of publications," said Greenwood.

The *meta*Register's next big initiative launched in the fall of 2000. Greenwood describes the scheme as the creation of a unique number called the international standard randomized control trial number. "This number will work rather like an ISBN (an international standard book number) which publishers use to identify their publications. A trial at approval stage—probably that would be at the ethics approval stage—we hope would register itself and also apply for a number. And then that number would live with the trial through all its stages and its publications."

Nevertheless, in putting together the *meta*Register, Current Controlled Trials has encountered a number of problems. For one, Greenwood says that it can be hard to convince companies that already have trial listings on web sites to join the *meta*Register. The second big hurdle is the amount of work it takes for an organization to put together a registry. In some cases, Greenwood said, Current Controlled Trials offers to create the registry for the organization.

For those organizations with existing registries, Current Controlled Trials offers two different solutions. One method involves signposting some basic details about the trials on the *meta*Register and then sending users to the original company's web site for full details, explained Greenwood. "The other method is to tunnel into the organization's online site, with their permission, and download the data and let it also be visible in the *meta*Register. For example, the NIH has allowed us to do real time searches of their data. So when people search, they are in fact searching the NIH as well."

"I think there is a big momentum that supports what we're doing," Greenwood said. "Even though we are far from being complete, we are already a really useful resource. Whether or not we ever can claim to have covered all of the trials in the world will be many years down the line."

CONTENT AGGREGATORS

As of this writing, there are an estimated twenty companies, both large health portals and focused e-recruitment solutions companies, many of which are seeking to receive fees for patients enrolled in their clients' clinical trials. A list of the better known content aggregators that have navigated the shoals of Internet-based patient recruitment with varying degrees of success includes the following:

- webmd.com
- onhealth.com
- medscape.com
- cbshealthwatch.com
- allhealth.com
- myskinmd.com
- acurian.com
- thebody.com
- oncology.com
- drkoop.com

They have also been joined in the marketplace by a few companies espousing the hybrid model. VeritasMedicine.com, AmericasDoctor.com and the HealthExchange.org exemplify companies with both internal and external resources for clinical trials listings. At present, companies such as these aggregators and hybrids have yet to find a foothold in the European market.

The new aggregators are focusing specifically on patient recruitment as one of only a few key service areas. They hope to offer web-enabled services to provide more comprehensive patient recruitment solutions including:

- Clinical trial listings licensed from content providers
- Online chat with a medical professional
- Online questionnaires

- Outbound and inbound e-mailing
- Referral services to a network of investigative sites
- Study volunteer compliance assistance

A common pricing model for content aggregators and hybrids involves collecting a small fee for every patient who is screened for a clinical trial and a larger fee for patients who enroll and complete a clinical trial. The fees typically range from $100 to $200 per enrolled patient. Companies offering recruitment services have reasoned that, given the fact that companies pay $350 to $500 to recruit a patient on average, a $150 per enrollee fee is reasonable. The jury is still out on whether sponsors and CROs will pay these fees. According to DataEdge, pharmaceutical and CRO companies typically pay as much as $1,500 overall (combined recruitment, compensation and operating fees) for an evaluable patient across all therapeutic areas. There is a great deal of skepticism about whether these new Internet recruitment service providers will prove their mettle in practice.

THE FUTURE

Coldwell believes that the market for Internet patient recruitment is just beginning and that it is here to stay. "This is an era where there is no standard," said Coldwell. "SMOs and others will need to buy, build or partner for this service. Anything to speed the process, cut costs and access better patient populations. The majority will partner and, as it shakes out, there will be just a handful that will do it where it's a significant revenue generator with significant patient recruitment effectiveness. That will take a few years, but there will only be about ten to fifteen companies that can do this on a sufficient scale."

Focussed content aggregator companies offer a compelling new approach provided they are able to blend quality content with well-executed patient recruitment management. It is likely that content aggregators and content providers will form tighter alliances in the future in order to ensure that timely and accurate content is offered to the potential research participants. This, in turn, will assist in generating and directing traffic to services designed to process and manage study subjects.

Indeed the data have already begun to reveal the importance of the Internet to the clinical trials community. According to CenterWatch market statistics, 71% of all sponsors and CROs say they are accessing the Internet at least once a week. (Table Four) In 1999, the percentage of investigators saying they were regular users of the Internet increased to 37% from 20% in 1997. Of the investigators, 56% say they are online daily. Investigators as a whole average 5.1 hours per week online. Study staff spend even more time online than investigators do. In that group, 48% of study staff say they are regular users, up from 31% in 1997.

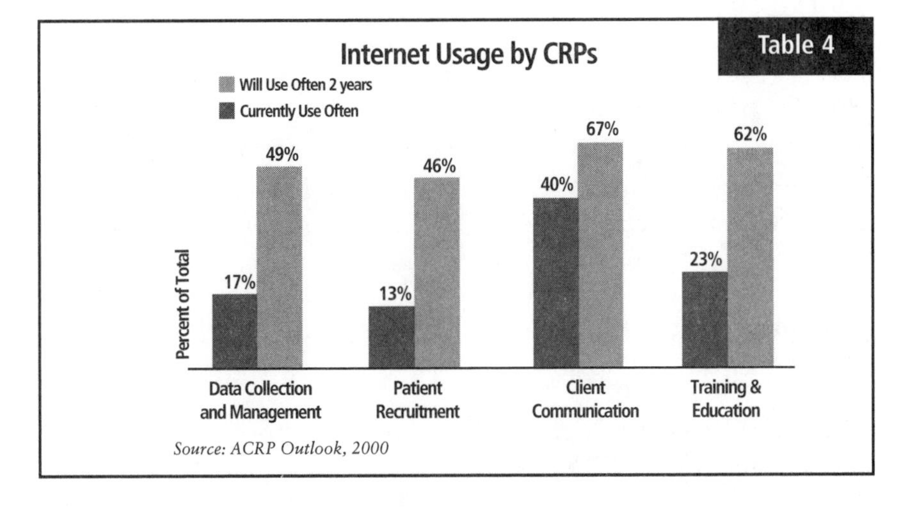

Source: ACRP Outlook, 2000

The distribution of clinical trials information over the Internet continues to evolve, making it an increasingly viable and valuable medium for reaching study subjects. With growing pressure on sponsors, CROs and sites to find, recruit and retain patients in their clinical trials, the Internet has quickly become an important supplement to traditional approaches. The coming years will be very telling ones as the Internet evolves and matures.

The Internet is not the answer to all recruitment prayers. On the other hand, industry experts recommend that the Internet should be considered as another resource among a portfolio of recruitment approaches, such as television, radio and newspapers.

REFERENCES

[1] Future Trends Committee. ACRP White Paper on the Future, Association for Clinical Research Professionals, 2000.

[2] *USA Today*, page 1A. December 11, 1997.

[3] Jupiter Communications. *Wall Street Journal.* December 1999.

[4] *Ibid.*

[5] Media Matrix, 1999 Internet Report.

[6] Ibid.

[7] CenterWatch Editors. "Grant Market to Exceed $4 Billion in 2000." *CenterWatch Newsletter*, 2000. Volume 7, Issue 11. Pages 1, 6-10.

[8] Pharmaprojects. *PARAXEL Pharmaceutical R&D Statistical Sourcebook*. March 2000. Page 33.

[9] Peck, C. "Drug Development: Improving the Process." *Food Drug Law Journal.* Vol. 52. 1997.

[10] CenterWatch Editors. "Grant Market to Exceed $4 Billion in 2000." *CenterWatch Newsletter*, 2000. Volume 7, Issue 11. Pages 1, 6-10.

[11] U.S. Census Bureau. Statistical Abstract of the United States. August 2000.

[12] CenterWatch Editors. "A Word from Clinical Trial Volunteers." *CenterWatch Newsletter*, 1999. Volume 6, Issue 6. Pages 1, 9-13.

[13] CenterWatch Clinical Trials Listing Service.

[14] *Ibid.*

AUTHOR BIOGRAPHIES

Whitney Allen is a Senior Editor at CenterWatch. Currently, she is the managing editor of *CWWeekly*, which covers breaking news in the clinical research industry. She is also the managing editor of the recently launched *CenterWatchEurope*, a quarterly newsletter that focuses on the European clinical research industry. Ms. Allen writes for both business professionals and consumers on topics ranging from gender-specific trials and pharmacogenomics to what patients can expect when participating in a cancer trial. In addition to *A Guide to Patient Recruitment*, Whitney has also served as book editor for CenterWatch's top selling books: *Protecting Study Volunteers in Research* and *The Investigator's Guide to Clinical Research*. Prior to CenterWatch, Whitney worked for the pharmaceutical consulting group at Deloitte Consulting and at Aetna Health Plans. She holds a B.A. from Dartmouth College.

David Heck is Senior Account Manager, CenterWatch Web Services. He works with pharmaceutical companies, biotechnology companies, medical device companies, and CROs in placing their clinical trials on the CenterWatch web site. Mr. Heck has over fifteen years experience in sales and marketing, including six years in patient recruitment. As a patient recruitment consultant and specialist, he focused his energies on implementing strategies, programs and technology to accelerate the patient identification process. David also served as Director of Patient Recruitment with a CRO for three years where he was involved in all aspects of patient recruitment. As vice president of telemarketing with an SMO, David was responsible for implementing an inbound/outbound, centralized telephone-screening center. A well-known author and speaker, David has participated as a panelist and speaker at numerous patient recruitment conferences.

Dan McDonald is the Manager of Internet Services at CenterWatch. He manages the content and services that support the CenterWatch.com web site operations. He works with clinical research professionals to assist them in their web-based promotion and recruitment activities. Mr. McDonald is a well-known speaker at conferences, and he has conducted workshops and sessions on patient recruitment over the Internet. Prior to CenterWatch, Mr. McDonald worked for over four years in various management positions for Marriott International of Bethesda, MD. Mr. McDonald holds a B.A. from the University of Massachusetts School of Management.

CHAPTER 10

The Importance of Market Research in Patient Recruitment

Diana L. Anderson, Ph.D., Rheumatology Research International

A large pharmaceutical sponsor is developing a new compound for treatment of Type II diabetes. The compound is about to move into Phase III clinical trials, and the company will be seeking 2,500 patients. It is widely known that several other competitive diabetes trials are currently underway, all testing investigational agents from the same therapeutic class. A large NIH study is also in progress. How will the sponsor find patients to fill this trial?

Patient recruitment and enrollment are destined to become more challenging as the number of clinical studies grows. There are presently an estimated 50,000 to 60,000 ongoing clinical trials in the U.S. alone[1], and there is every reason to expect this figure to increase based on the rise in R&D expenditures; number of compounds in pipelines; the growing number of patients per new drug application (NDA); and the more complex and global nature of trials. Growth is likely to be accompanied by a rise in directly competitive clinical trials, many seeking access to the same investigators. In addition, there are bound to be more studies aimed at testing new compounds in special populations, which will yield a marketing advantage to the innovator if the studies prove successful.

The traditional patient recruitment model has centered around sponsors' reliance on proven investigators who promise to recruit the agreed upon number of patients from their own resources. In years past, this approach was generally successful as there were far fewer trials than there are presently. Today, a sought-after investigator is likely to have already used an in-house patient database to enroll several ongoing competitive trials, so that investigator may have exhausted his or her supply of potentially qualified patients for new trials. This reality is reflected in the fact that 78% of today's clinical trials fail to meet patient enrollment deadlines.[2]

Some sponsors may not recognize this reality, which challenges their traditional expectation that investigators will be able to achieve all or most of the enrollment target from proprietary patient databases. This raises the question of what other efforts, besides use of these investigator databases, can be undertaken to spur patient enrollment. While answers lie in the development of multimedia patient recruitment campaigns, the searching of large insurance claims databases to determine the likelihood of finding the needed number of patients, or conducting protocol feasibility studies, these solutions are not always obvious to some sponsors. Developing these kinds of solutions can result from market research initiatives designed to pinpoint the best, most efficacious approaches to enhance patient recruitment and enrollment.

Cheryl Miller, Pharm.D., Executive Director of eServices at Scirex Corporation, a contract research organization, says, "In large pharmaceutical companies, researchers developing a compound often have tunnel vision because they eat, sleep and breathe the development of that one specific compound. They tend not to have a sense of the magnitude of the competition facing that compound nor for the fact that sites are likely to be doing many trials, not just this one."

For these reasons, some pharmaceutical sponsors have been slow to adopt the use of market research to explore ways to boost enrollment, or they wait until a rescue effort is needed to employ one. Rescue efforts tend to be costly, and may extend the development timeline because they take time to put together, and must be reviewed by an Institutional Review Board (IRB). If a media campaign is used, for example, it might be worthwhile and cost effective to conduct various types of market research, such as focus groups, or one-on-one telephone or face-to-face interviews to identify strategies for attracting potential patients, particularly for studies with difficult inclusion/exclusion criteria. Knowledge gained through market research can serve to focus the patient recruitment media campaign, particularly if it is in a therapeutic area where a sponsor has limited experience. Using results of market research to develop targeted campaigns coupled with the traditional approach of identifying experienced investigators with access to specific patient populations can be a productive combination.

WHAT IS MARKET RESEARCH?

Market research is a way of finding out what people believe, think, want, need or do. Formal market research is a relatively new endeavor, as it dates back only to the 1920s. The concept began in Germany, and then spread to Sweden and France in the 1930s. After World War II, American companies began adopting market research techniques in business, and it is now a routine component of many industries in the industrialized world.[3]

Conducting market research involves asking questions and interpreting the answers using a systematic, objective approach that focuses on gathering data relevant to a specific marketing issue.[4] It is information that may not be obtainable from existing or "secondary" sources. Original research developed to answer specific questions is referred to as primary research. Secondary research is generally conducted before launching a more costly primary research effort.[5]

Table 1

Market Research Should Be:

- ➔ Systematic
- ➔ Objective
- ➔ Useful
- ➔ Problem-Specific
- ➔ Decision Oriented

Source: The Portable MBA in Marketing

There are many niche-oriented market research firms dedicated to organizing and conducting primary research campaigns. Trade associations, the Internet, market research textbooks, and word-of-mouth referrals from within the industry are good sources for identifying market research companies.

To yield meaningful results, market research must address a clearly defined problem and must be tailored for the intended audience. Characteristics of market research are listed in Table One. For the research to be successful, it is critical to do a careful analysis of the decisions that need to be made.[6] For example, if a sponsor wishes to determine the commercial possibilities for a drug that might be developed for treatment of Alzheimer's Disease, a research goal of simply learning about the size of the market will not allow the researcher to make an informed decision about moving forward with a multi-million dollar drug development program. It might be more useful for a sponsor to conduct market research to determine the kinds of compounds most likely to fit the treatment needs of the various types of Alzheimer's patients. Some questions to be asked might be:

- How long do patients generally live with Alzheimer's?
- Is any approach currently successful?
- Where are Alzheimer's patients most likely to be found—both geographically and in what kinds of settings?
- What is the percentage of patients being treated for comorbid conditions?
- What is the status of competitors' investigational drugs?
- What kinds of improvements in Alzheimer's pharmacotherapy would clinicians like to see?
- Do we have the scientific and marketing expertise in this therapeutic area to be a competitive player?

These kinds of targeted questions can help a sponsor determine the feasibility of moving forward with a development program for a compound to treat Alzheimer's Disease. While some of these questions can be answered through secondary research, questions about competitive investigational drugs, and clinicians' opinions are more likely to be answered through primary research.

The flow chart (Table Two) can help determine if primary and/or secondary market research will be useful.

There are two basic types of research to produce answers to market research questions: Quantitative and Qualitative. Quantitative research provides numerical data, enabling the user to measure the number or percentage of subjects that fall into specific categories. This type of research is structured to gather information from statistically representative samples of the targeted population, and

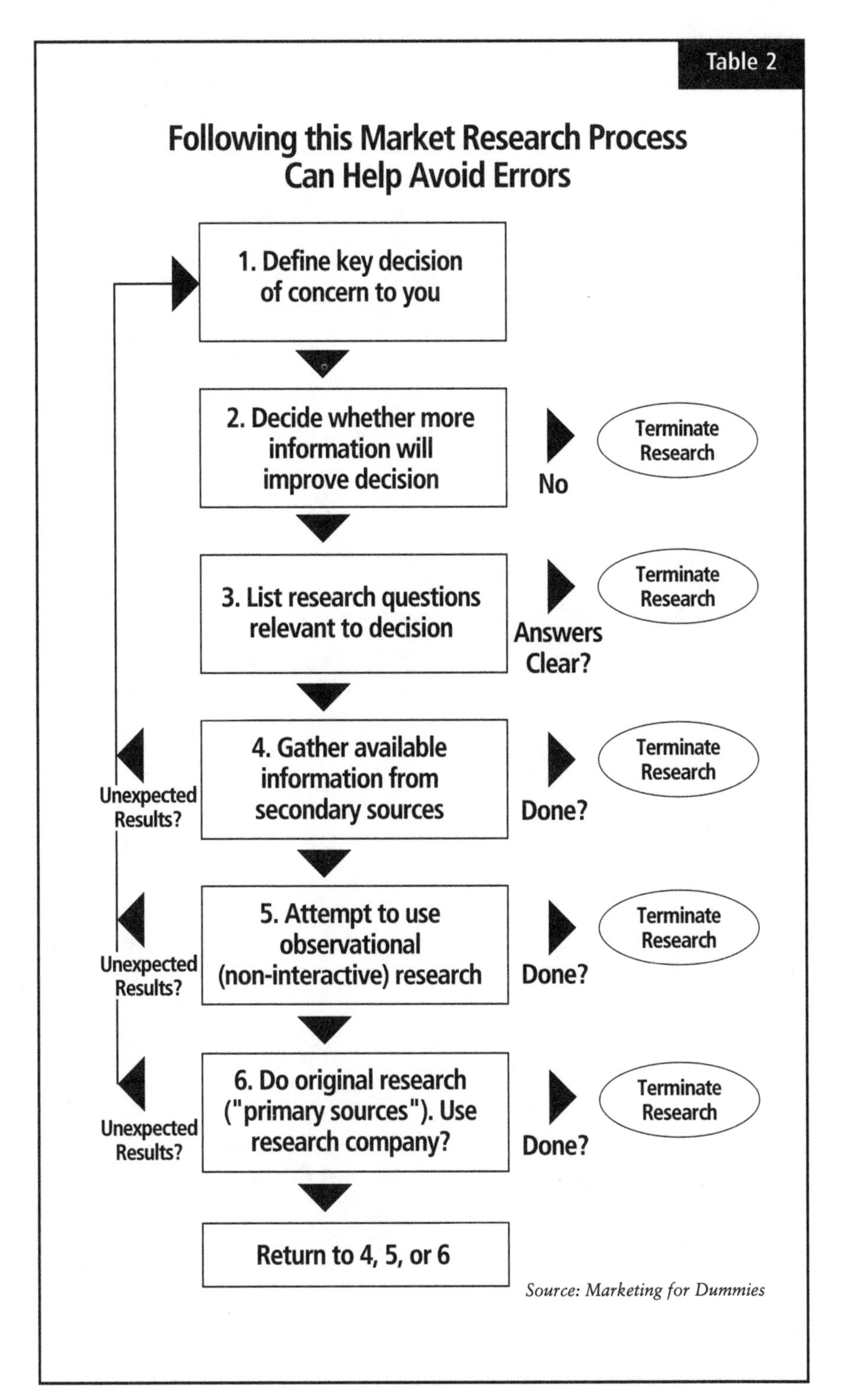
Table 2
Following this Market Research Process Can Help Avoid Errors
1. Define key decision of concern to you
2. Decide whether more information will improve decision
No
Terminate Research
3. List research questions relevant to decision
Answers Clear?
Terminate Research
4. Gather available information from secondary sources
Done?
Terminate Research
Unexpected Results?
5. Attempt to use observational (non-interactive) research
Done?
Terminate Research
Unexpected Results?
6. Do original research ("primary sources"). Use research company?
Done?
Terminate Research
Unexpected Results?
Return to 4, 5, or 6
Source: Marketing for Dummies

helps the user draw numerical conclusions. Every respondent is asked the same series of questions, either by mail, face-to-face interview, telephone interview, or Internet-interview. For example, if a car manufacturer wants to estimate the percentage of Americans between the ages of 35 and 50 more likely to buy a sport utility vehicle than a minivan, that company might conduct quantitative research. In the pharmaceutical industry, a sponsor interested in positioning a new over-the-counter medication might want to know the percentage and profile of respondents most likely to buy its new over-the-counter drug versus competitor A, B and C.

Qualitative research does not provide numerical data, but provides more of an understanding of attitude, perception and opinion. Focus groups are often used in qualitative research because they are, by nature, a structured open discussion providing an exchange of ideas and opinions. Discussion tends to be more free-flowing, and there may be open-ended questions. For example, if a bank notices that older customers use automated teller machines (ATM) less frequently than younger customers, the bank might conduct qualitative research, including focus groups or one-on-one interviews, to develop hypotheses as to why this particular group is reluctant to embrace ATM technology.[7] Information gathered can help the bank decide where to place new ATM terminals.

In the drug industry, a sponsor might want to use focus groups with the targeted population to uncover opinions about specific advertisement messages being developed for a soon to be launched medication. Reactions to Advertisement A, B, C and D could be tallied. Generally, this type of qualitative research is not considered to be statistically projectable to the larger targeted population.

Qualitative and quantitative data can be gathered by a variety of methods as detailed in Table Three.

Table 3 Methods of Gathering Market Research Information

➔ Focus Groups	➔ Internet Surveys
➔ One-on-One Interviews	➔ In-store Surveys
➔ Telephone Surveys	➔ Internet Surveys
➔ Direct Mail Campaigns	➔ Approaching People in Shopping Malls

APPLYING PRINCIPLES OF MARKET RESEARCH TO PATIENT RECRUITMENT

The pharmaceutical industry is beginning to look more closely at using market research to enhance patient recruitment efforts. Simply relying on investigators to fill studies is no longer sufficient, nor is developing a media campaign without some understanding of what would motivate patients to participate in a clinical trial for a drug being designed for a specific illness. From this perspective, conducting market research would seem to be a logical pursuit.

Experienced sites know that market research is not always necessary because certain kinds of studies are easier to enroll than others. Therapeutic areas that can enroll relatively smoothly are obesity and oncology studies. Other areas that may be more difficult to enroll, such as stroke, osteoporosis, various forms of arthritis, and Alzheimer's disease, might benefit from a market research effort designed to explore ways to attract potential patients.

Maureen McNamara, Independent Communications and Patient Recruitment Strategist, explains that only a few sponsors are enthusiastic supporters of the market research process, and have started to become more proactive. She says, "Most don't want to sacrifice the time to do proper market research for patient recruitment. Because many sponsors are still coming to us when they are in a rescue mode, they often don't want to invest the time to conduct structured focus groups."

McNamara believes that focus groups uncover useful opinions, and can be helpful in identifying the best wording, color and layout for a recruitment advertisement. Focus group participants shown several different advertisements might be asked to comment on their immediate reactions. "If prospective patients aren't drawn to a headline, they're never going to read the advertisement. For example, some diabetes patients have compromised vision, and we've learned from focus groups that certain type styles and colors are better than others for successful diabetic recruitment ads. Nuggets such as these can make or break a media campaign," McNamara comments.

Matt Harris, Vice President of the MDS Harris site management organization, says that his company routinely conducts market research to understand the motivations behind why some patients choose to participate in clinical trials. MDS Harris specializes in Phase I trials, which are small safety and pharmacokinetics trials. To do this research, Harris explains that his company constructs advisory panels of people who have previously participated in clinical studies. Harris says, "This tool provides feedback as to why these people participated, and helps us gauge if people they know, or people like them would be willing or reluctant to enter a clinical trial in the future. (Table Four) The research helps us stay on the pulse of the participant community."

Questions Posed at Advisory Panel Discussions in Phase I Projects **Table 4**

→ Why would you or wouldn't you participate in a clinical trial?
→ What can we do differently?
→ If you have participated in a trial, did you enjoy your stay at our facility?
→ What would encourage you to participate in more studies, or prevent you from participating in more studies?

Source: MDS Harris

Although MDS Harris conducts this type of research for its phase I operation, Harris says that market research for phase III studies is very rare. He explains, "By the time a project goes to an investigational site, the sponsor expects immediate deliverables. The tendency is not to do market research."

Janet Gale, Account Director at Age Wave IMPACT, a marketing firm specializing in the baby boomer and senior markets, agrees that there is little time to conduct research and develop a meaningful message to attract patients, but there are some positive developments. "Despite this time crunch, sponsors do seem to be more interested now in refining their message." Gale says that periodically, Age Wave conducts focus groups, using advertising storyboards, and tries to combine knowledge learned from these groups with information available in patient databases. This combination approach helps Age Wave to develop a Responder Model, which is the development of a profile of someone who might have a propensity to participate in a clinical trial. The ideal is to refine the model to the point that it becomes specific for different therapeutic areas. In other words, the profile of a prospective patient for a depression trial may be different than a profile of prospective participant for a study researching treatments for hypertension.

ADDITIONAL FORMS OF MARKET RESEARCH FOR PATIENT RECRUITMENT

There is much more to the world of patient recruitment than soliciting input from consumers to develop targeted media campaigns. The traditional source of patients has always been, and still is the clinical investigator. Few approaches are more interesting to a prospective enrollee than the one he or she hears from a trusted physician. If that doctor has established a good rapport with a patient, and knows of a clinical trial that may benefit that patient, the doctor could suggest that he or she consider being screened for that trial. This suggestion can be made either during an office visit or by contacting the patient by mail.

As mentioned earlier, the limitation of this approach is that the rising number of trials may have depleted a doctor's resources of prospective patients for trials in specific therapeutic areas. In other words, if a doctor is already an investigator in three migraine headache trials with a number of patients from his or her patient database, what is the likelihood that that doctor will have enough patients in his or her practice to complete a fourth migraine trial?

Because the search for patients must expand to accommodate the growth in the number of trials, the industry will demand more cost effective, time-efficient methods of doing so. One approach would be for sponsors to have access to massive insurance claims databases that have been "de-identified," that is, the patient's identifying information has been removed. These types of databases contain healthcare information on millions of de-identified patients, and might enable sponsors to determine if enough patients exist to fulfill enrollment requirements.

In 1999, Quintiles Transnational launched its Informatics Division to develop various Internet-based products to create an overview of the healthcare experience in the United States. By aggregating large amounts of physician visit, hospital, and pharmacy data, it is possible to get a snapshot of the prevalence of certain disease states in various geographic areas.

The division's first informatics product, RxMarket Monitor™, debuted in April 2000, and offers customers Internet access to a substantial database of aggregated, de-identified patient-level insurance claims information. Patrick Jordan, Director of Product Management of the Informatics Division, explains, "This database contains information on 1.5 billion healthcare transactions, representing 100 million patients, approximately one-third of the U.S. population. It is updated daily. It also identifies physicians who have the types of patients in their practices who might fit entrance criteria for various trials. We can use this database to seek out those physicians as investigators for studies of interest."

Jordan points to a client that was experiencing much difficulty in recruiting patients for a pediatric HIV study because of some stringent inclusion/exclusion criteria. By searching the RxMarket Monitor database, Quintiles' Informatics Division was able to show the client that these patients do not exist in a quantity sufficient to reach the sponsor's original recruitment goal. Jordan says, "Having this type of information available upfront can be an eye-opener to sponsors, and can help them with decision making such as protocol design, and ultimately product portfolio design. With traditional methods, it could be several months before a sponsor realizes that enrollment targets may not be achievable because of specifics in the protocol. By using this type of database, this kind of market reconnaissance can be completed within hours."

Currently, Quintiles is working to pair information from its investigator database with its de-indentified patient information in the RxMarket Monitor database. The third piece of the puzzle is to identify the geographic clusters of patients. For patient recruitment initiatives, this information can help sponsors place media campaigns in these targeted locations. Jordan believes that this three-part approach; pairing patients with investigators with geographic clusters, will spearhead the next evolution in market research for patient recruitment.

Additional approaches can be used in conjunction with the searching of large patient databases to determine the likelihood of a study reaching its enrollment target. One useful exercise to perform upfront is the testing of the feasibility of the protocol. Researchers developing a compound are accustomed to designing experiments with very tight inclusion/exclusion criteria in an effort to demonstrate a compound's effectiveness in a clearly defined clinical study. Unfortunately, it is not always realistic to transfer those exact criteria into the real world with hopes of enrolling patients. Jordan says, "Clinicians know what kinds of patients they see everyday, and experienced investigators can often tell you if inclusion/exclusion criteria will prevent a study from enrolling. Clinical experts offer a practical perspective on protocol feasibility."

Jordan describes the sending of fact sheets summarizing a protocol and its inclusion/exclusion parameters to approximately fifty sites to review. Study teams ask the selected sites for quick feedback as to the likelihood of the protocol enrolling as scheduled. Using this qualitative research approach provides the Clinical Development Services Group with a good indication of the ease or difficulty of recruiting for this study. "If one-third of the sites receiving this protocol summary do not understand the study, or foresee enrollment problems, this is useful information to share with the sponsor. We might look for further evidence of the existence of patients for that study by searching our Informatics' database," says Jordan.

A slightly different approach to protocol feasibility studies has been undertaken by Scirex Corporation. On various occasions, the company's Feasibility Group has conducted qualitative market research with investigative sites to identify specific problems in the protocol that are creating difficulty with enrollment. Dr. Cheryl Miller of Scirex says, "Armed with this type of information, we've been able to go back to sponsors with feasibility reports and point out the key challenges in the inclusion/exclusion criteria that sites report as causing the exclusion of most potential patients. If the protocol is designed to test a very specific population, and the reason you need that population is the scientific crux of the protocol, then changing the inclusion/exclusion criteria would essentially be changing the purpose of the study. In those cases, we have to accept the protocol the way it is. For example, if you are trying to test a blue-eyed population, you can't suddenly make amendments to study brown-eyed people."

In 1999, Scirex entered into a $20 million strategic partnership with Diversified Agency Services (DAS), which is part of Omnicom Group, Inc., a worldwide marketing communications company. This initiative is but one example of the merging of clinical research with marketing, in an effort to accelerate all aspects of the clinical development process.

The searching of claims databases, and the conduct of protocol feasibility studies, including qualitative market research, can be useful forerunners to the development of patient recruitment media campaigns. In some instances, they can occur simultaneously in an effort to condense the clinical development timeline.

THE CURRENT STATE OF MARKET RESEARCH FOR PATIENT RECRUITMENT

Patient recruitment accounts for nearly one-quarter of the clinical development timeline[8], a bottleneck that must be addressed in various ways to improve the chances of reaching desired enrollment targets on time. As discussed, patient recruitment initiatives can take the form of an investigator searching his or her proprietary database; a large CRO searching massive claims databases; protocol feasibility studies, the development of IRB-approved media campaigns; or some combination of these methods. Yet background research conducted for this chapter suggests that few sponsors are involved in market research or ask their outsource partners to conduct it either for investigational drugs not yet marketed, or for post-marketing studies seeking expanded indications. If it is being conducted, it tends to be done by patient recruitment companies which are likely to have built the cost of market research into a Request For Proposal (RFP). A few sponsors mentioned that they conduct some market research for patient recruitment but they declined to be interviewed for this chapter.

Lorraine Marchand, Managing Director of Patients1st, a medical research marketing firm, says her company always conducts market research for patient recruitment as this is the essence of the service that Patients1st provides. Knowledge gained from this effort is key to shaping the messages for a media campaign, or in the case of rescue efforts, understanding why some studies are not enrolling. She comments that before a protocol is written, there needs to be an honest dialogue with the sponsor about the realities of finding some of the narrowly defined populations called for in today's protocols. This dialogue should include media advisors, medical advisors and representatives of advocacy groups for the disease in question to raise all of the concerns of the targeted population. (Table Five) She explains that if advocacy groups are involved in the protocol planning stages, they can later become key supporters of certain studies by spreading awareness to their targeted audiences.

Table 5 Communication Issues Addressed in Dialogues with Sponsors about Protocol Development

- ➔ Will people understand the message?
- ➔ What exactly is being offered?
- ➔ What is required of a participant?
- ➔ Is this study ethical?
- ➔ Is the patient's safety being adequately protected?
- ➔ Is all the necessary information being adequately disclosed in the Informed Consent Form?

Source: Patients1st

Marchand says, "Historically, the patient's perspective has never been considered. Pharmaceutical companies conducting studies are just starting to understand that they are trying to market a product to prospective patients, which in this case, is the protocol. Our theory is that the key reason why there is so much difficulty in recruiting and retaining patients for some studies is that the protocol design is flawed in that the customer doesn't like the 'product' or study, and doesn't want to be in it or stay in it. Also, we want to know if the sponsor has considered important factors such as childcare services for participants, round trip transportation for older patients and polite staff at the site who seem to be genuinely interested in the study and in the patients. These issues impact patient retention."

According to Marchand, some CEOs and key medical officers at major pharmaceutical companies are wanting bold, new approaches to patient recruitment, that are well-researched, and multi-faceted because resorting to the same old techniques is not solving patient recruitment dilemmas. (Table Six) Most of the time when her company is contacted, it is for a rescue effort.

Leslie Clark Lewis, Director of Patient Recruitment at America's Doctor, a site management organization (SMO), says, "I rarely get questions about market research from sponsors. In terms of sponsors asking us to conduct market research with consumers to understand what would motivate them to participate in specific clinical trials, this happens very rarely. Yet some sponsors are aware of the increased competition for patients to enroll, so I see more interest today in marketing for patient recruitment than I did in the late 1990s."

Table 6 **Case Study Showing Importance of Market Research to Enhance Patient Recruitment**

For a phase IIIb investigation of an asthma drug for a major pharmaceutical company, study coordinators were faced with a brief six-month recruitment window and narrowly written exclusion criteria. Potential patients who were recently diagnosed or were managing symptoms with other classes of drugs either were excluded, or were asked to terminate successful treatment with a bronchodilator and were required to be in treatment for at least six months. These requirements stymied enrollment, eliminating many potentially compliant patients

To jump start the recruitment process, a market research firm was brought in during the first month and introduced:

- A comprehensive local site support program, with one-on-one counseling for all sites and a comprehensive communications kit, which contained a broad range of public relations, advertising, marketing and community outreach materials.

- Materials for audiences of limited literacy. The IRB-approved language used to explain the study and inclusion/exclusion criteria was too technical for many prospective patients to grasp.

After consulting with clinical experts, the market research firm recommended modifying the inclusion criteria to accept subjects who had been on treatment for less than six months. Although this suggestion was not adopted, it does highlight the need for realistic inclusion/exclusion criteria.

A paid advertisement campaign was begun that could be modified site-by-site, and the enrollment eventually reached 70% of the target, which was 840 patients.

Source: Patients1st

It is worth exploring the reasons why relatively little market research is being conducted for patient recruitment by sponsors when those same companies spend $1.8 billion annually in direct-to-consumer advertising to promote marketed products.[9] Lewis of America's Doctor explains that this disconnect has its roots in the fact that for most sponsors, clinical research and development functions are totally separated from marketing activities. Cheryl Miller of Scirex says that historically, departments within pharmaceutical companies have always been very siloed, with power structures in place within each silo. Communication between silos is limited. She adds, "It's important to understand that these two functions have different goals. Research scientists want to answer scientific questions, and don't necessarily think about promoting the compounds they are developing."

Marchand of Patients1st agrees that R&D and marketing departments have different goals, yet both can be satisfied if marketing information is collected early on, including evaluation of the protocol. Once the data are analyzed, R&D scientists can share that information with selected outsourced partners responsible for developing strategies to fill later phase studies within designated timeframes. Marketing types can use the data to have a greater understanding of the targeted population, and can start crafting marketing messages. Marchand says that she sees R&D and marketing working together mostly for phase IV studies and late phase III studies, and that it is less typical in early phase III, and still more uncommon in phase II.

Barbara Kravitz, senior clinical scientist at SmithKline Beecham, explains that the disconnect between scientists and marketers can be addressed if the two groups interact early on during clinical development. "It's important to understand that the mindsets of the two groups are quite different, and they have very different training. We are seeing more interaction, but it could still happen earlier. As the drug progresses from phase II into phase III, the scientists become more aware of marketing than they were in phase I."

Kravitz says that SmithKline Beecham uses market research for patient recruitment efforts. The company has conducted focus groups with patients to collect information about the kinds of help they would like with their illness, and to talk about what the drug under discussion might or might not be able to do. Qualitative data generated by the research has proven helpful in writing protocols to facilitate the attracting and retaining of the right kinds of patients. She believes this approach is most effective when used upfront, as opposed to waiting until a rescue effort is needed.

Kravitz explains that sponsors can benefit from conducting research with patients because many have become more educated about their disease than was typical in the past. Patients have formed opinions and are more interested in taking an active decision-making role in their health. For example, Kravitz says, "In the case of women's health, we see the group of younger women much more involved in making medical decisions than their mothers were. The younger women are more likely to become their own advocates."

Soliciting input from patients is a relatively new tactic. Kravitz says that historically, sponsors sought opinions from clinical physicians about studies for new compounds, and in turn, the physicians would talk with their patients. While this approach is very much alive, garnering input from patients could prove to be a welcome addition as long as the market research efforts are not designed to be coercive.

WILL MARKET RESEARCH EVENTUALLY PLAY AN ACTIVE ROLE?

The pharmaceutical industry is renowned for its marketing prowess when it comes to promoting and positioning marketed or about-to-be marketed drugs. As evidence, the industry has been very successful in growing its business, with earnings per share rising at double-digit rates, year after year. Yet, it is not clear that this type of growth can be sustained as more trials than ever are underway, with many lagging in patient enrollment.

The tried and true formula of recruiting experienced investigators and opinion leaders with access to databases of specialized patient populations seems to be the method of choice for sponsors or CROs looking to enroll new studies. While this approach has yielded excellent results, and will probably continue to do so, it is critical to recognize that it is time to branch out beyond the tried and true.

A number of patient recruitment agencies have evolved that understand the many factors contributing to today's patient recruitment and enrollment dilemma. They are familiar with the growth in the number of trials, and see this increase complicated by the fact that difficult or even unrealistic inclusion/exclusion criteria in protocols are being written to answer specific scientific hypotheses. In addition, some studies require a particularly select population in an attempt to gain marketing advantage if the compound is successful.

All of these factors can make recruitment a daunting task, yet that is all the more reason for all parties involved in clinical development to explore new approaches. Sometimes, determining the best approach requires market research, because the best way to locate all of the required patients is not immediately apparent from the resources at hand. Market research, such as focus groups, one-on-one interviews, direct mail, Internet surveys, and other venues can be conducted to collect valuable information needed to design media campaigns most likely to attract the desired population. Multimedia efforts will probably be more effective and less costly if done early in the recruitment process, instead of waiting until a rescue effort is needed.

Technology today is allowing for the possibility of determining the feasibility of enrolling studies with particularly difficult inclusion/exclusion criteria. Making this determination might include researching vast databases, such as claims databases, which are being developed by some CROs. This effort allows the researchers to compute the likelihood of finding these patients. In addition, some market researchers might forward protocol summaries to a good number of experienced investigators who collectively can provide insight into a protocol's feasibility. The willingness to take these steps can spell the difference between failing to meet enrollment and meeting or exceeding the target in a timely fashion.

All of these tools are available, and they expand the options available for patient recruitment activities. The hope is that over time, clinical development partners will take advantage of these tools to accelerate the enrollment process.

REFERENCES

[1] CenterWatch, Boston, Massachusetts, May 2000.

[2] *Ibid.*, 1997.

[3] www.britannica.com/bcom/eb/article/5/0,5716,52265+1+51011,00.html, August, 2000.

[4] "Marketing Research and Information." The Portable MBA in Marketing. Alexander Hiam and Charles W. Schewe, John Wiley & Sons, Inc., 1992. p. 107.

[5] *Ibid.*, p. 97.

[6] "Marketing Research: Customers, Competitors, and Industries." Marketing for Dummies. Alexander Hiam. IDG Books Worldwide, Inc. 1997. p. 91.

[7] "Managing Market Information." Services/Marketing: Principles and Practice. Adrian Palmer and Catherine Cole. Prentice-Hall, Inc., 1995. p. 301.

[8] Pharmaceutical R&D Statistical Sourcebook 2000, Barnett International, p. 130.

[9] "Direct-to-Consumer Spending by Brand." MedAdNews. June 2000. p. 46.

CHAPTER 11

THE IMPORTANCE OF RETENTION AND PATIENT SATISFACTION IN CLINICAL TRIALS

Diana L. Anderson, Ph.D., Rheumatology Research International

Recruitment and retention of subjects are keys components of successful clinical research. The best protocols with the most innovative new drugs cannot move forward unless a sufficient number of subjects are recruited as well as retained.

Much of this book is dedicated to exploring issues and strategies leading to successful and timely patient recruitment, but patient retention is just as important. Data cannot be collected from an incomplete subject and if randomized subjects continue to drop out, those individuals either have to be replaced and/or study coordinators must identify reasons for the attrition. Both of these scenarios are time consuming and costly.

Closely linked to retention is patient satisfaction. Because each contact between the investigator site and the patient contributes to the possibility of continued participation or withdrawal, it is critical for sites to develop methods for retaining patients, and to see to it that patients are well-treated and satisfied with the care they are receiving. A review of the literature suggests that treating patients with respect and honesty from the very first contact, and throughout the trial, goes a long way toward creating satisfaction, leading to increased patient retention. Taking steps to keep individuals informed and involved can have a similar impact. Providing information about disease process, for example, can be empowering, and may increase the sense of buy-in to the research process. Offering onsite day care may facilitate a young mother's ability to keep an appointment for a study visit. Recognizing that older participants in an osteoporosis study may require round trip transportation may encourage them to remain in the study.

The literature contains many examples of observations and initiatives utilized to retain subjects in a wide variety of therapeutic areas. The literature also suggests that different approaches for retention are required in different therapeutic areas because the issues change depending upon the disease, age, sex, and possibly, ethnicity of the subject. Whether the focus is on retaining infants, asthmatic patients, people with HIV, or minorities in a hypertension study, the message is clear. Valuable resources are lost when enrolled participants fail to finish a study.[1] When significant attrition occurs, the resulting data may no longer be representative of the original population, significant bias may be introduced that affects study findings and generalizability to a larger population may not be possible.[2]

Table 1

Possible Predictors of People Predisposed to Drop Out of a Study

- Lower Income
- Lower Education Level
- Unstable or High Risk Physical Status
- Low Levels of Social Support
- An Ethnic or Socioeconomic Status Different from that of the Investigators

Source: "Factors Differentiating Dropouts from Completers in a Longitudinal, Multicenter Clinical Trial"

Dropout incidence is widely variable but rates of 15% to 40% are not uncommon, and even higher rates of participant loss have been reported.[3] Moser, Dracup and Doering focus on the high rate of participant loss in studies of infants at high risk for adverse events.[4] They comment on the lack of research conclusively identifying the factors that contribute to dropout, but their research suggests that some researchers hold opinions about characteristics that may be predictors of a subject predisposed to drop from a study. (Table One) Identification of factors associated with participant dropout from longitudinal research studies may help investigators plan future studies and anticipate dropouts.

Moser conducted a longitudinal multicenter study of 578 parents and other caretakers of infants at risk for cardiopulmonary arrest. Participants were recruited from five metropolitan area hospitals. The researchers investigated the psychosocial impact of teaching cardiopulmonary resuscitation training to parents and caretakers of high risk infants hospitalized in the neonatal intensive care unit after birth. Parents and caretakers also completed a packet of questionnaires at baseline, two weeks, three months and six months after baseline.

The purpose of the study was to determine the characteristics that differentiated those who completed versus those who dropped out of this multicenter clinical trial. In a secondary analysis, researchers reviewed the baseline sociodemographic, emotional, psychosocial and infant characteristics of those who quit the trial as compared to those who completed it.

Table 2

Caregivers Assignment to Random Groups for Analysis of Trial Completion

- CPR videotape only (63% completed study)
- Training from certified CPR instructor who was also an advanced practice nurse (59% completed study)
- Participation in a CPR support group in addition to training from a certified CPR instructor (55% completed study)
- Control group (usual care from the institution from which infants were discharged) (75% completed study)

Source: "Factors Differentiating Dropouts from Completers in a Longitudinal, Multicenter Clinical Trial"

Participants were randomized to one of four groups. (Table Two) The study was completed by 60%, or 347, of the participants. Those most likely to drop out were other caretakers or fathers (versus mothers) who were employed outside the home, spoke English; were assigned to an experimental group (versus a control group); had higher levels of depression, hostility and psychosocial distress related to the infant's illness; and held negative views about the effectiveness of health care for their baby.

In this study, reputed sources of retention difficulties, i.e., low income, less education, minority status, lack of social support or problems with family functioning, did not predict dropout. Also, the finding that the control group had the least amount of dropouts is contrary to the findings of other research.[5] Researchers can use this type of information to develop a profile of participants with a high likelihood of dropping out, and can plan strategies to maintain a study sample. It is important to mention, however, that providing continuing special attention or intervention in studies with a psychosocial and education component may possibly alter results by introducing confounding factors.[6]

Bender, Ikle, DuHamel and Tinkelman believe that patient attrition in clinical trials can significantly compromise study objectives, yet the topic receives little attention. This group reviewed the profiles of 362 patients, including adults and children, who had participated in a year-long, double-blind, placebo-controlled, randomized asthma trial.[7] Patients in the trial had been randomized either to beclomethasone diproprionate, theophylline or placebo. The purpose of the Bender et al study was to evaluate the medical, demographic and psychological characteristics of asthmatic adults and children who dropped out of this year long trial to determine if this group differed from those who completed it.

Table 3 Reasons for Patient Dropout From a Year-Long Asthma Study

Reason	%
Treatment Non-Compliance	17%
Treatment Adverse Effect	17%
Treatment Lack of Benefit	12%
Other Medical Condition	11%
Moved From Area	4%
Administrative Termination	22%
Other Reasons	17%

Source: Retention of asthmatic patients in a longitudinal clinical trial

Bender et al reported that initially 771 patients at thirty-one sites underwent a one-month prerandomization screening requiring several visits to document their asthma symptoms. In an effort to facilitate patient compliance and retention, patients who failed to complete these screening visits did not continue past the study baseline. Despite this careful planning, 24% of those who entered the study dropped out for various reasons, due mostly to noncompliance or treatment adverse effect. (Table Three) It is worth mentioning that patients may not always report the real reason for dropping out of a study. Citing inadequate symptom control may be a convenient way to quit a study, when the real reasons may be more complex or psychological in nature.[8]

Only eleven of the thirty-one participating centers had convenient access to a psychologist to conduct the psychological testing protocol designed to evaluate patient psychological characteristics and drug-specific psychological changes. The eleven centers represented 362 patients. Results from only those centers were included in the drop-out versus completers comparison.

All analyses were performed separately on the adult and pediatric study groups and on the subset of subjects that was present at baseline. A variety of statistical methods were used in the data analyses. (Table Four)

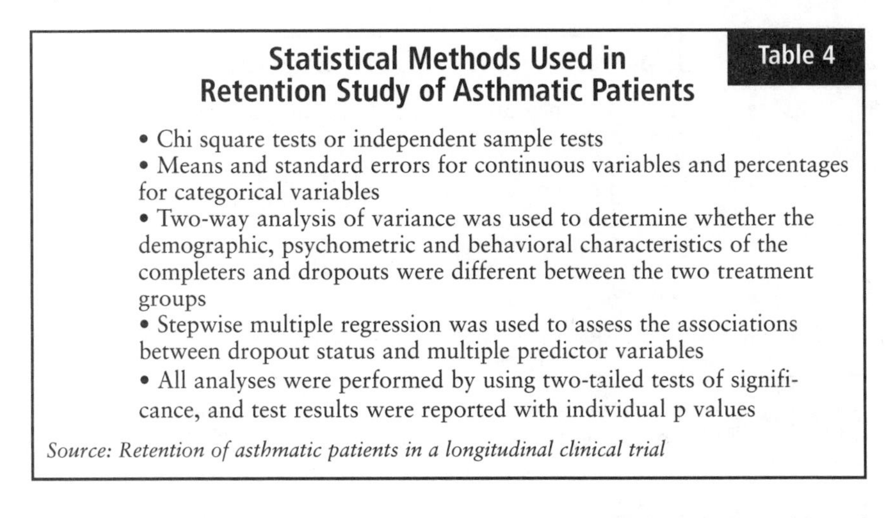

Table 4

Statistical Methods Used in Retention Study of Asthmatic Patients

- Chi square tests or independent sample tests
- Means and standard errors for continuous variables and percentages for categorical variables
- Two-way analysis of variance was used to determine whether the demographic, psychometric and behavioral characteristics of the completers and dropouts were different between the two treatment groups
- Stepwise multiple regression was used to assess the associations between dropout status and multiple predictor variables
- All analyses were performed by using two-tailed tests of significance, and test results were reported with individual p values

Source: Retention of asthmatic patients in a longitudinal clinical trial

Attrition rates were equal between adults and children, and profiles of adults who dropped out of the study were no different than those who completed. The pediatric evaluation, however, showed that those who dropped out were more likely to be female, have more reactive airways, have reduced scores on tests of intelligence and problem solving tests, and more likely to have increased behavioral problems.

Bender et al commented that when attrition includes a disproportionate representation of patients with more serious disease, medical and psychosocial study results may be biased. Specifically, it may be difficult to generalize medical results from completers to patients with more severe asthma.[9] Also, the fact that pediatric females with reduced scores on intelligence tests were more likely to drop out of this study suggests that data from the study were loaded with higher functioning patients, potentially biasing outcomes and hindering the study's generalizability of psychosocial and quality of life outcomes.

The authors make the point that a one month prescreen can shake out most candidates who are unlikely to keep appointments, submit incomplete or poorly complete diary cards, resist procedures or appear otherwise uncooperative. However, once the remaining patients are enrolled and randomized, patients must continue to experience satisfaction with their participation, otherwise they, too, could have greater drop-out potential. It is critical that staff be warm, friendly and personally interested in the patients. There are other important steps that can be taken to encourage retention. (Table Five)

Table 5 **Steps That Can Be Taken to Encourage Patient Retention**

- Offer convenient physical access and appointment times
- Send newsletters
- Provide written or telephone contact between visits
- Remember special occasionss, such as Christmas, birthdays
- Maintain contact with patient's primary care physician
- Assist with transportation
- Financial compensation (per IRB approval)
- Small gifts for pediatric patients

Source: Retention of asthmatic patients in a longitudinal clinical trial

Table 6 **Interventions That Can Be Used With Patients Likely to Drop Out of a Study**

- Increase communication
- Sympathize with problems
- Respond to complaints
- Consider decreasing the patient's workload by eliminating the daily diary cards or decreasing the number of required blood draws
- Reduce the frequency of study visits

Source: Retention of asthmatic patients in a longitudinal clinical trial

Despite these efforts, some patients will become disenchanted with the clinical trial and send out signals forecasting possible departure. Generally, these signals take the form of actions rather than words. Those who miss appointments, fail to return phone calls, complain about procedures, claim to be too busy to schedule a routine appointment or display a general lack of enthusiasm may be planning to drop out.[10] An effective dropout intervention strategy must include a system for early identification of these at-risk behaviors. A successful intervention strategy may involve negotiating a modified protocol to include those procedures that are essential to the study and within the patient's motivational reach.[11] (Table Six)

Retention is also an issue in studies targeting patients infected with HIV. Similar to what Bender et al had reported, Morse, Simon, Beach, and Walker noticed that issues of patient recruitment and retention are rarely addressed, yet the validity and reliability of data can be compromised if large numbers of patients drop out of studies.[12] Also, the ability to generalize results to broader populations is limited if the pool of randomized patients within a study continues to shrink.

In an article entitled, "Issues of Recruitment, Retention, and Compliance in Community-Based Clinical Trials with Traditionally Underserved Populations," Morse et al presented data from a survey of fourteen Community Programs for Clinical Research on AIDS (CPCRA). These programs were the result of a National Institutes of Health (NIH) initiative started in 1989. At that time, NIH dedicated funding for the establishment of eighteen CPCRAs to provide broader access to HIV clinical trials within community-based primary care settings.

The survey completed by the fourteen sites included information about the sociodemographic and lifestyle characteristics of the HIV-infected populations served (Table Seven), the structure and organization of the unit, patient services offered and successful and unsuccessful strategies used to address issues of recruitment, retention and compliance (RRC). The identified potential barriers to recruitment, retention and compliance were divided into client-centered and structural factors.

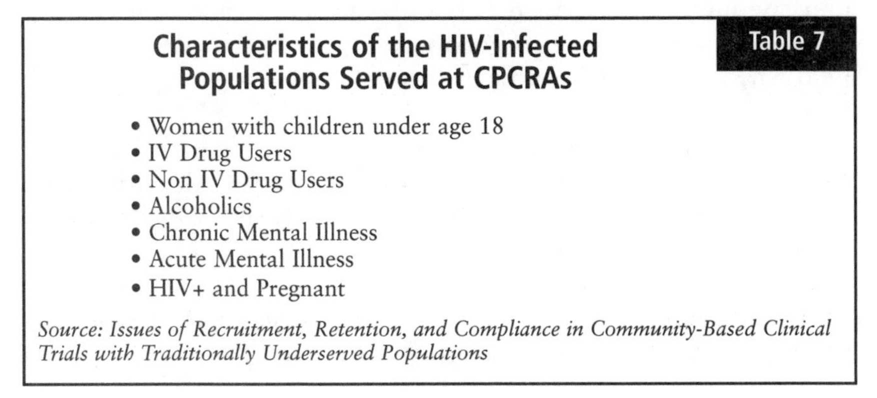

Characteristics of the HIV-Infected Populations Served at CPCRAs — Table 7

- Women with children under age 18
- IV Drug Users
- Non IV Drug Users
- Alcoholics
- Chronic Mental Illness
- Acute Mental Illness
- HIV+ and Pregnant

Source: Issues of Recruitment, Retention, and Compliance in Community-Based Clinical Trials with Traditionally Underserved Populations

Survey data were collected at two points in time; October 1990, and March 1991.

As seen in Table Eight, the client-centered factors affecting RCC remained fairly constant between the two time points with a few exceptions. The staff had little or no control over most of the client-centered factors, with the exception of fear of participation in clinical trials, negative staff attitudes and transportation difficulties.

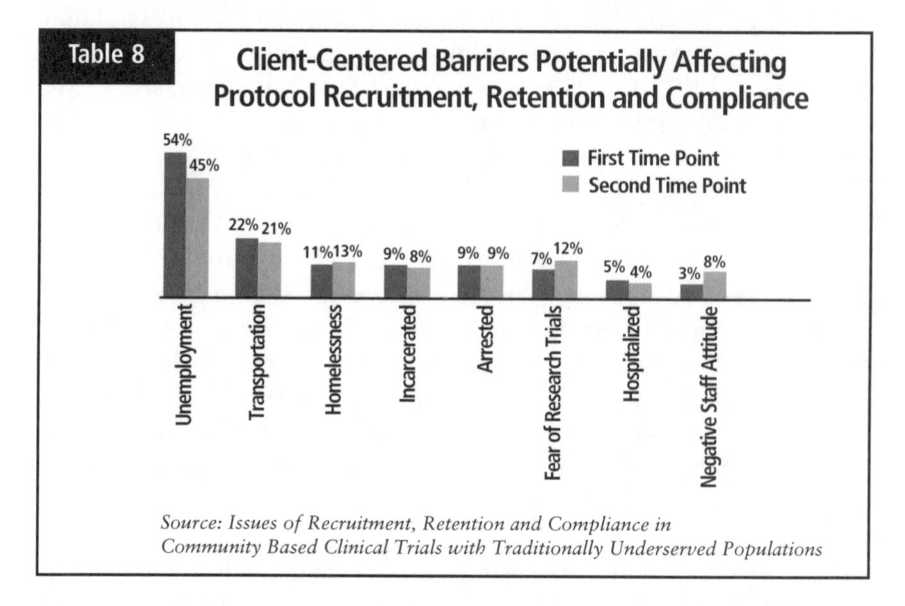

Table 8 **Client-Centered Barriers Potentially Affecting Protocol Recruitment, Retention and Compliance**

Source: Issues of Recruitment, Retention and Compliance in Community Based Clinical Trials with Traditionally Underserved Populations

Table Nine shows that between the first and second time points, the CPCRA staff recognized a dramatic change in the types of structural factors contributing to retention problems. For example, at the first time point, clinics identified lack of financial resources, clinic space and clinic staff as key barriers to recruitment and retention. However, after six months of experience, the sites named requirements of the protocols and the type of protocols available to their patients as the main barriers to RRC. Although this perception was not consistent across all participating CPCRA sites, there was a significant increase in appreciation of protocol-related issues as critical barriers to RRC. Part of this change may reflect the fact that most participating sites generally lacked background in clinical research, although they were experienced in delivering healthcare to special populations.

It is worth noting that sites with an awareness of potential protocol-based problems appeared to recruit participants more successfully than those that did not identify these same problems. Morse et al suggest that perhaps an awareness of the restrictive nature of protocols led to the development of ways to neutralize these barriers, resulting in greater patient accrual.[13]

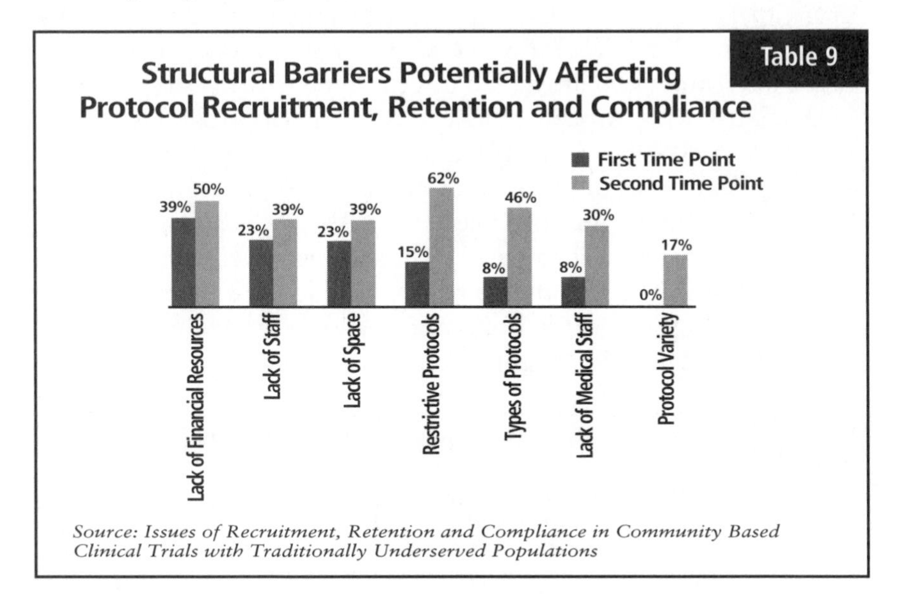

Source: Issues of Recruitment, Retention and Compliance in Community Based Clinical Trials with Traditionally Underserved Populations

Implications of this research suggest that nurses at the CPCRA clinical sites, who were experienced in working with underserved populations, had critical insight into the types of barriers that had to be overcome for successful recruiting. The more successful sites implemented clinic-based strategies such as flexible clinic hours, child care, and shelter and drug rehabilitation placement to enhance RRC efforts.

RECRUITING AND RETAINING MINORITIES

Results of large clinical trials are used to support decisions by physicians to treat broad populations of patients with similar therapeutic needs. If those clinical trials lacked sufficient patient diversity, it may not be in the best interest of the patient to assume that the results can be generalized to all or most ethnic groups. The literature suggests that researchers need to understand that studies sometimes include a less than ideal number of minorities, and that there are reasons contributing to this traditional under-representation and difficult retention of minorities in ethical clinical trials.

In "The Recruitment Triangle: Reasons Why African Americans Enroll, Refuse to Enroll, or Voluntarily Withdraw From a Clinical Trial,"[14] Gorelick, Harris, Burnett, and Bonecutter identify reasons why recruiting and retaining minorities, particularly African Americans, can be very challenging. Through use of an open-ended questionnaire (Table Ten), the researchers focused on one site of a multi-center study, and attempted to determine why the site's twenty-nine subjects in the African-American Antiplatelet Stroke Prevention Study (AAASPS) either remained in the study (nineteen subjects), voluntarily withdrew in the absence of an adverse event (four subjects), or refused to participate (six subjects). AAASPS was a double-blind, randomized clinical trial designed to determine the effectiveness and safety of aspirin and ticlopidine hydrochloride in the prevention of recurrent stroke, myocardial infarction, and vascular death among African-Americans with recent ischemic stroke.

Table 10 Open-ended Questionnaire for AAASPS Participants

- What were your reasons for participating, voluntarily withdrawing, or refusing to participate in the AAASPS?
- What circumstances or events may have influenced your decision to participate, withdraw, or refuse to participate in the AAASPS?
- Was the information regarding the study explained to you in words or terms that you could easily understand?
- Did the study coordinator treat you in a respectful manner?
- What was the opinion of your family members regarding your being asked to participate in the AAASPS?

Source: The Recruitment Triangle: Reasons Why African Americans Enroll, Refuse to Enroll, or Voluntarily Withdraw from a Clinical Trial

It has been widely publicized that in the past, African-Americans have been exploited by unethical medical experimentation, with the Tuskegee Syphilis Study being one of the most highly visible examples. Although few patients in the AAASPS made reference to the Tuskegee Study specifically, this backdrop may have contributed to recruitment difficulties because the study occurred during the high profile apology for these unfortunate studies issued by President Bill Clinton.

Of the nineteen patients who remained in the study, 84% responded that they had participated to reduce their risk of another stroke, and 32% to find a cure for stroke or to help others. Thirty-two percent were encouraged by their physicians to participate and 47% were encouraged by family or friends.

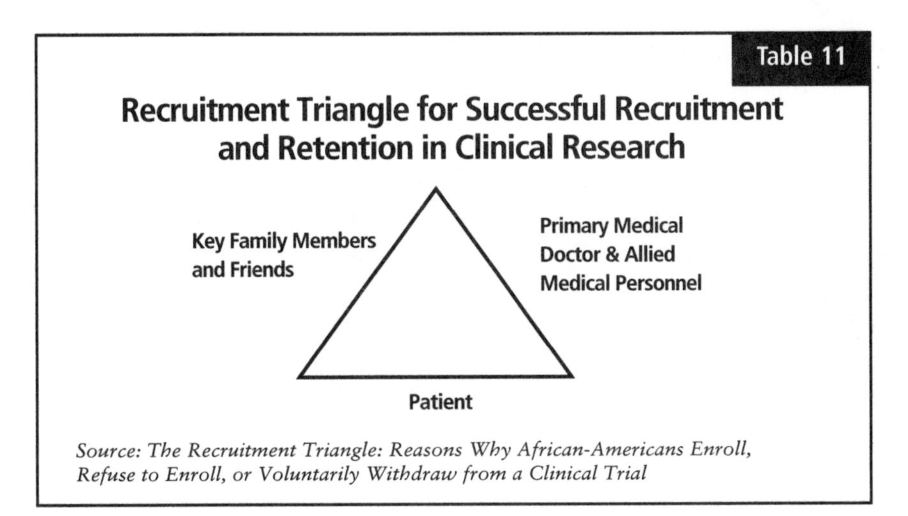

Of the four patients who withdrew, the key reason given was concern about being the subject of experimentation. When family and friends were consulted, they supported the decision to withdraw and expressed concern about government-sponsored research of African-Americans.

Of the six patients who refused to participate, half cited concerns about changing current stroke preventative medications or other life circumstances, and one-third referred the possibility of becoming a "guinea pig." When family or friends were consulted, 84% reinforced the patient's concern about medical experimentation.

According to Gorelick et al, these results suggest a "recruitment triangle" that is central to the enrollment and retention of patients in clinical trials.[15] The three walls of the triangle include the patient, key family members and friends, and the patient's primary medical doctor and other medical personnel. (Table Eleven) The walls are held together by social support, education about the nature of the research, and trust in study personnel and the overall program. Should one of the walls pull away from the triangle, the structure may collapse with resultant refusal to enroll, or subsequent dropout.

The results of the study are limited due to the small sample size, and because little demographic information was available on those who refused to participate in the study. The group of patients who remained in the study had more education and higher income than the small group of those who dropped out, but beyond these facts, there was insufficient demographic information available to draw conclusions about a demographic profile of a candidate more likely to remain in a study.

The Dietary Approaches to Stop Hypertension (DASH) Study was a multi-center trial sponsored by the National Heart, Lung and Blood Institute. Although DASH was open to a wide audience, aged 22 and older, there was a special effort to recruit and retain African-Americans, a group that suffers from hypertension disproportionately. Sixty percent of the 459 randomized participants were African-American[16], and the average age of African-American participants was 44.

The DASH Study was designed to compare the impact of three dietary patterns on blood pressure.[17] Patients were randomized to either a control diet relatively low in fruits, vegetables and dairy products with 36% of calories from fat; a diet rich in fruits and vegetables but otherwise similar to the control diet; or a combination diet that was rich in fruits, vegetables and low-fat dairy foods, and reduced in saturated fat, total fat and cholesterol. The feeding was controlled and obligated participants to eat (with the exception of some discretionary beverages) only those foods provided by the site. The trial demonstrated that a diet rich in fruits, vegetables and low-fat dairy foods, and reduced in saturated fat, total fat, and cholesterol, significantly reduces blood pressure independent of sodium reduction and weight loss.[18]

A variety of recruitment methods were used, but the most successful were bulk mailings to a broader audience that was weighted toward, but not limited to, minority participants. Generally, strategies targeting African-Americans exclusively were not productive. Each site had an ethnically diverse recruitment and clinical staff. At two of the sites, the principal investigator spoke at every recruitment presentation about the increased burden of hypertension in the African-American community, and the explicit goal of DASH to include two-thirds minorities so that the results could be extrapolated to minority populations. To encourage retention, sites reminded patients of their obligations to the study throughout the screening process, and they made efforts to identify and exclude those unwilling or unable to comply.

The DASH investigators received supplemental funding from the NIH Office of Research on Minority Health to assess factors affecting minority recruitment and retention in DASH.[19] As part of the supplement, each site requested its participants to complete a participation survey designed to explore their main reason, and up to two additional reasons why they decided to participate in DASH. Also, they were asked to state what they enjoyed most about the study and what factors made it most difficult for them to remain in the study. All questions were open-ended. The response rate to this participation survey

Table 12

Primary Reason for Participating in DASH Among Randomized African-American and White Respondents

Reason	African-American n=213	White n=132
Control blood pressure	46%	42%
Experience/gain weight	17%	18%
Healthy eating/weight control	20%	11%
Cash reimbursement/free food	6%	18%
Health monitoring	6%	2%
Other	4%	8%

Source: Recruitment and Retention of Minority Participants in the DASH Controlled Feeding Trial

Table 13

Most Difficult Aspect of Participating in DASH Cited by Randomized African-American and White Respondents

Reason	African-American n=208	White n=130
Time commitment/duration of study	5%	8%
Coming to clinical center each day	20%	12%
Eating only DASH foods	16%	28%
Lack of variety of DASH foods	13%	13%
Dislike some DASH foods	19%	14%
Study measurements	6%	9%
Large portion sizes	6%	5%
Scheduling problems	4%	6%
Other	2%	1%
No difficulties	8%	4%

Source: Recruitment and Retention of Minority Participants in the DASH Controlled Feeding Trial

Table 14 Most Enjoyable Aspect of DASH as Cited by Randomized African-American and White Respondents

Reason	African-American n=N/A	White n=N/A
Socialization with other study participants	57%	63%
DASH meals	11%	3%
Not having to buy/prepare food	8%	16%

Source: Recruitment and Retention of Minority Participants in the DASH Controlled Feeding Trial

was 81%. Data were presented for African-Americans and non-Hispanic White respondents. (Table Twelve, Thirteen, Fourteen)

Results of this research suggest that African-Americans and white participants were more similar than dissimilar to each other in their motivations for participating. Most were genuinely interested in the study and found few impediments to successful adherence. As evidence, the results shown in Table Twelve suggest that 83% of African-Americans and 71% of white participants cited positive, health-related factors that helped them comply rather than focusing on negative factors that hindered compliance.[20]

Vollmer et al point to a variety of factors for their success in recruiting and retaining minority participants. The nature of the study and the design were attractive. It dealt with food; the study lasted for only eight weeks following randomization; it was non-pharmacologic; and the ethnically diverse staff at the sites made diligent efforts to provide a caring, supportive and culturally sensitive environment. Also, the results were seen as directly benefiting African-Americans. More than three-quarters of the African-American respondents reported that the study was beneficial to them, and 88% reported that they would participate again in a similar study.

The authors were concerned about biased results because those who participated may have been systematically different than those who were ineligible or refused to participate. The African-American participants were mostly female (59%) generally well-educated, with 64% having attended at least some college, and 13% having attended graduate school. Seventeen percent reported an annual income exceeding $60,000. This may be the profile of groups more likely to participate in clinical trials as opposed to lower-income African-American men, a group that is particularly difficult to reach.[21]

Arean and Gallagher-Thompson report that older ethnic minorities are also difficult to recruit and retain.[22] Their psychosocial research indicates that recruiting and retaining older ethnic minorities becomes easier when methods are tailored to address the issues that prevent potential participants from engaging in clinical research.

According to Arean and Gallagher-Thompson, older white adults generally point to transportation problems to and from the site as a key reason for dropping out of a geropsychiatric study. Once the transportation is addressed, some researchers have found that older adults are far less likely to drop out than younger participants. The average dropout rate for geriatric studies is only 10%.[23]

Ethnic minorities have transportation issues too, but they also have more complex reasons having to do with cultural beliefs about mental illness and help-seeking behavior.[24] A common reason given is distrust of the goals and processes of research on older ethnic minority adults. According to the literature, attempting to recruit and retain an older ethnic minority person without involving the family may result in alienating the family and fueling distrust about research.[25] Others reasons are listed in Table Fifteen.

Table 15

Typical Reasons Cited by Older Ethnic Minorities for not Participating or Remaining in Psychosocial Clinical Studies

- Distrust of the goals and processes of research by older ethnic minority adults and their families
- Difficulties in transportation to research and clinic centers
- Lack of information about the disorder that is being investigated and negative cultural attitudes toward mental illness
- Lack of information about the kind of help that the participant or family can receive by participating
- Lack of culturally or racially compatible professional staff

Source: Issues and Recommendations for the Recruitment and Retention of Older Ethnic Minority Adults Into Clinical Research

A variety of retention methods are highlighted in the literature. Providing round trip transportation, offering flexibility in scheduling to allow for the fact that some ethnic seniors have custody of young grandchildren, calling patients to remind them of appointments, and providing some home visits to obtain follow-up data have resulted in retention rates of approximately 95%.[26] Home visits can be important for patients who do not want family or friends to know they are participating in a clinical study.

Arean and Gallagher-Thompson believe that cultural competence of the clinical staff is the most important factor to consider when researching an ethnic minority population. Unless the staff is culturally competent, the research project could fail. For various research projects seeking older patients, these researchers recruited staff who are Chinese, Hispanic and African-American. Using the approach of cultural competence among staff, retention of older African Americans rose from 60% to 98%.[27]

A LOOK AT PATIENT SATISFACTION

The news is encouraging. A review of the literature suggests that the majority of patients have very positive experiences in clinical trials. Although there have been stories in the main stream press heralding exploitative researchers and investigators, these examples are far from typical.

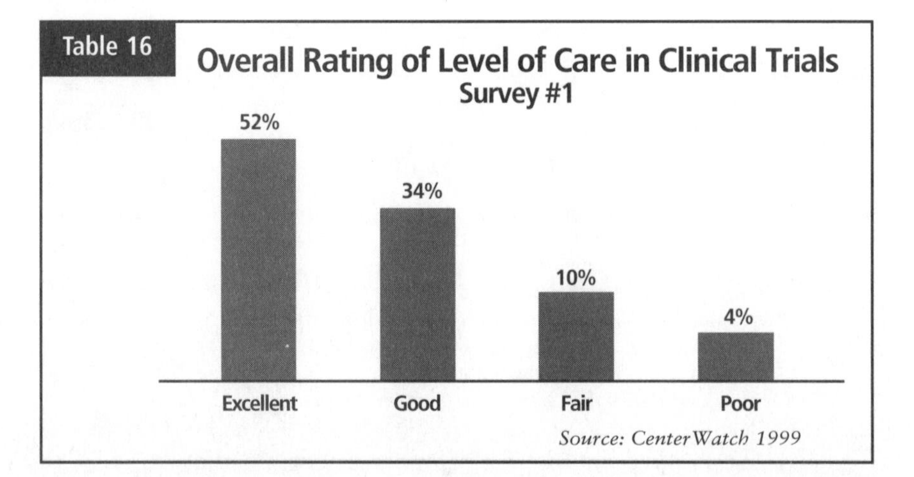

Source: CenterWatch 1999

CenterWatch has reported in two different surveys that more than half of the survey respondents rated their clinical studies experiences as excellent.[28,29] In the first report, CenterWatch surveyed 210 participants in 1999 across all therapeutic areas, with the largest percentage, 25%, having participated in oncology-related trials. Of the 210 respondents,

87% considered the quality of care received in the trial as either "excellent" or "good." (Table Sixteen) More than three-quarters (77%) stated they would definitely participate in another clinical trial. Forty-two percent rated the care they received in the trial as better than the care they receive from their own primary care physician.

Although these survey results were quite positive, one area of improvement cited by one-third of respondents was the desire to receive feedback and information about the study medication. For example, subjects wanted to know if the medication was found to be effective, and if it ever came to market.

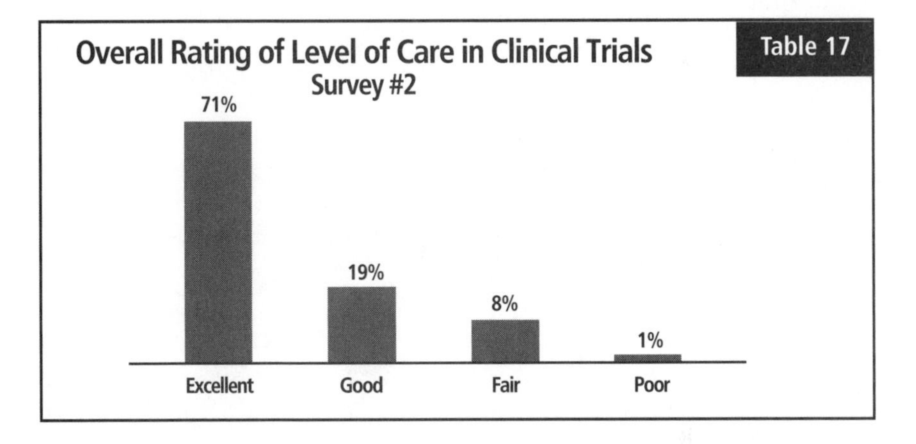

The second CenterWatch survey, conducted in 2000, included 1,050 people who had participated in clinical trials within the preceding year, and represented all therapeutic areas. As in the first study, this one yielded very positive ratings by study participants. Fully 71% rated the overall level of care in the clinical trial as excellent (Table Seventeen), and 75% reported that they would volunteer again for another clinical study. Forty-two percent rated the level of care received as better than the care they receive from their primary care physicians.

Areas of improvement identified by survey respondents included better de-briefing as the top request, similar to results in the first survey. They also cited several other areas as seen in Table Eighteen.

Information in the literature coincides with CenterWatch findings that many patients have good experiences while participating in clinical trials. Kennedy, Blair, Ready, Wolf, Steinhart, Carryer, and McLeod explored patients' perceptions of their participation in a

Table 18 Top Cited Areas to Improve by Clinical Trial Participants

Areas for Improvement	Percentage
Debrief and Post Study Follow-up	31%
Easier Communication with Staff	23%
Better Time Estimates	17%
Compliance Support	14%

Source: CenterWatch 2000

clinical trial for postoperative Crohn's disease by tallying results of a twenty-seven item questionnaire.[30] Sixteen items were specific statements about the trial and were framed in a positive manner. Patients evaluated the degree to which they disagreed or agreed using a five-point Likert scale. ("Strongly Disagree," "Disagree," "Neutral," "Agree," "Strongly Agree") Nine items were statements pertaining to improvements that could be made to the trial, and the two remaining items were questions regarding future participation in clinical trials.[31]

The survey instrument was mailed to all patients who had participated in a six year randomized controlled trial studying the effectiveness of mesalmine in preventing the recurrence of Crohn's disease postoperatively. The survey had an acceptable response rate of 66% (99 of 149).

Kennedy et al started with a commonly held belief that people who participate in clinical trials are inherently different from those who do not, yet there is little information documenting these differences. Also, there are few data about patient perceptions. Although the survey sought to explore patients' perceptions about various aspects of this trial for postoperative Crohn's disease patients, the key objective was for subjects to identify aspects of the trial that could be improved. The goal of the research was to use the survey results for developing strategies leading to increased enrollment and decreased attrition in future trials.

Participants generally held positive views about the trial. (Table Nineteen) In fact, 91% stated they would be willing to participate in another trial, and only 6% reported that time commitment for the study interfered with personal life. A large majority (80%) enjoyed the altruistic purpose of their participation possibly helping others. There was still room for improvement, however. Forty-six percent of the respondents either agreed or strongly agreed with the statement, "I would have preferred more information about the trial prior to its commencement." Seventy-five percent agreed or strongly agreed with the statement, "I would have preferred more information about the trial while it was in progress." Sixty-two percent agreed or strongly agreed with the statement, "More education about my disease should have been incorporated into the trial." Strategies to provide patients with better education about their disease may result in patients feeling they benefited from participation.[32]

Kennedy et al point to the fact that the study had only a 66% response rate as a limiting factor. Because it is likely that the responders and the nonresponders had different perceptions of the trial, the results must be interpreted with caution.[33] Despite this limitation, the results of the survey still provide information about what some patients perceived as positive and negative. At the end of a trial, patients who enjoyed participating may suddenly feel let down, so sites may consider developing newsletters, or groups. These tools may serve to encourage patients to participate in future studies, as there is a perception that patients who have previously participated in clinical research are more likely to do so again. For this reason, it is important to remain in contact with patients, and not "abandon" them after the close of a trial.

Table 19 Participant Response to a Post-Operative Crohn's Disease Clinical Trial (n=99)

Benefits to Participation	Percentage
Received better medical care than they would have otherwise	55%
An excellent opportunity to receive medicine and/or tests	63%
Improved awareness of their disease	48%
More control over the disease	41%

Source: Patients' perceptions of their participation in a clinical trial for postoperative Crohn's Disease

The Systolic Hypertension in the Elderly Program (SHEP) was another trial followed by a patient satisfaction survey. SHEP was a randomized, double-blind, placebo-controlled multicenter study of 4,281 men and women, aged 60 and older, with a primary endpoint of fatal and nonfatal stroke. Average follow-up lasted for four and one half years. Schron, Wassertheil-Smoller and Pressel developed a ten item satisfaction/attitude questionnaire designed to evaluate the personal benefits that participants expected from the SHEP trial, motivation for joining, and satisfaction with the clinic staff and operations.[34] Schron et al made the survey available to all SHEP participants at the last clinic follow-up visit. The goal of the research was to develop data that could be useful in the planning and carrying out of clinical trials in older and minority populations.

Table 20 Summary of Areas of Satisfaction and Problems for SHEP Patients

Area of Satisfaction or Problem	Percentage Who Agree
Staff were friendly	99.8%
Staff provided good care	99.4%
SHEP will provide important information	99.2%
I didn't mind taking SHEP medication	94.2%
Transportation was a problem	15.6%
Too many visits	7.8%

Source: Clinical Trial Participant Satisfaction: Survey of SHEP Enrollees

Of the 4,281 participants, 88% (3510) responded to the survey. Responses were high among all groups, but higher among those who were younger, white, more educated, and did not have a myocardial infarction (MI) or stroke during the trial. Level of satisfaction was high across all groups as evidenced by the fact that 93% stated that they would volunteer for the SHEP again based on their experience in the study. As seen in Table 20, there was a sharp division between the positive and negative areas of comment. For example, 99.4% of the respondents reported that the staff provided good care, yet a mere 7.8% said the study required too many visits. Transportation was problematic for 15.6% of respondents, particularly for those who were older, African-American, female, less educated and experienced a nonfatal MI or stroke during the study.

The research showed that the most important reasons for joining SHEP were altruistic, and this result varied little by age, race, gender, whether respondents had been in the placebo or active group, or whether they had had a non-fatal MI or stroke. The desire to contribute to science, and ultimately, to improve the health of others

(Table Twenty-One) indicates the key reasons for participation. African-American participants were considerably more likely to state that free medical care was important to them as compared to whites and others. (85% for African-Americans versus 62% for whites and others.) Also African-Americans were nearly twice as likely to consider someone to talk with as an important reason for joining SHEP. (60% for African-Americans versus 32% of whites and others.) Those with less than a high school education stated having someone to talk with as important nearly twice as often as those with at least a high school education or more. (51% vs. 28%)

Schron et al conclude that participants were overwhelmingly satisfied with their experience in SHEP, however there were some differences in needs and expectations by age, race and gender. Findings of patient satisfaction from this study coincide with those from other long term national trials, such as the Beta-Blocker Heart Attack Trial, and the Aspirin Myocardial Infarction Study.[35]

Reasons Why Participants Joined SHEP — Table 21

Reasons for Participation	% important or very important
Contribute to science	96%
Inprove health of others	96%
Improve my health	93%
Free medical care	65%
Someone to talk to	35%
Some place to go	19%

Source: Clinical Trial Participant Satisfaction: Survey of SHEP Enrollees

RETENTION AND PATIENT SATISFACTION— A FINAL THOUGHT

Pipelines are filled with many promising therapeutics. The number of clinical studies for these new products continues to grow, and studies are becoming more complex. The number of patients per new drug application (NDA) is approximately 4000, and expanding 7% annually.[36] Reaching the targeted figure of enrollees can be especially daunting if many participants drop out along the way.

A review of the literature suggests that retention of study subjects, while long a neglected topic, has attracted the attention of a number of forward-thinking researchers. When studies have drop out rates ranging from 15% to 40%, this is certainly a call to action for investigators charged with reaching enrollment and randomization targets.

The natural tendency of researchers interested in boosting retention may be to develop protocols with a pre-randomization screening period that can identify subjects unlikely or unable to keep appointments, or comply with protocol demands. Another approach is to create inclusion/exclusion criteria that would result in attracting patients who are likely to comply, remain and benefit from the study.[37] Unfortunately, stacking the deck this way is generally considered to lead to biased results that may not be generalizable to a larger, more realistic population. This realization encourages researchers to develop strategies that allow them to meet their research goals while including patients that resemble a general population.

A common theme for retention is treating all patients with respect. Beyond this basic premise of ethical research with human subjects, strategies for retention vary from therapeutic to therapeutic area. Retaining a young single mother who works full time may require different approaches than retaining a retiree who is skeptical of medical research and lives far away from the clinical research site. These types of issues can be addressed by an experienced staff that offer flexible appointment hours, day care and transportation.

Retention also seems to increase if the staff composition is somewhat ethnically diverse at sites interested in conducting trials that attract ethnic minority participants. This factor seems to be particularly important for older participants.

As sites make greater efforts to retain patients, they tend to find that patients who are retained are often satisfied. People want to have a satisfactory experience because they generally participate in a study to seek relief from a troubling condition. Some may also enjoy the altruistic aspect of their participation possibly leading to the helping of others with similar conditions. When sites recognize these motivating factors, and then treat volunteers with respect, offer a knowledgeable caring staff, and possibly relief, this is a prescription for a satisfied patient. Recent data from CenterWatch showed that 71% of participants in clinical trials rated their level of care as excellent. Three-quarters reported a willingness to participate in additional studies.

Although participants in clinical trials may inherently be different than those who do not participate, the number of participants in studies may grow as they are attracted by the treatment possibilities, and then retained by a caring, well-trained staff.

REFERENCES

[1] "Factors Differentiating Dropouts from Completers in a Longitudinal, Multicenter Clinical Trial." Nursing Research. Debra K. Moser, Kathleen Dracup, Lynn V. Doering. March/April 2000, Vol. 49, No. 2. p. 110.

[2] "Subject Loss in Infancy Research: How Biasing is it?" Infant Behavior and Development. G.A. Richardson, & K.A. McCluskey. K.A, 6, 1983. p. 235-239.

[3] *Op. cit.*, Moser, Dracup, Doering. p. 109.

[4] "Factors Differentiating Dropouts from Completers in a Longitudinal, Multicenter Clinical Trial." Nursing Research. Moser, et al. pp. 109-116.

[5] "Reduction of Patient Attrition from Experimental Behavioral Interventions: Nursing Research." C.W. Given, B.A. Given, & B.W. Coyle. 1985, 34. pp. 293-298.

[6] "Factors Differentiating Dropouts from Completers in a Longitudinal, Multicenter Clinical Trial." Nursing Research. Debra K. Moser, Kathleen Dracup, Lynn V. Doering. March/April 2000, Vol 49, No. 2. p. 114-115.

[7] "Retention of Asthmatic Patients in a Longitudinal Clinical Trial." Journal of Allergy and Clinical Immunology. Bruce G. Bender, Ph.D.; David N. Ikle, Ph.D.; Thomas DuHamel, Ph.D.; and David Tinkelman, M.D. 1997; Vol 99, Number 2. pp. 197-203.

[8] *Ibid.*, p. 198.

[9] *Ibid.*, p. 200.

[10] *Ibid.*, p. 202.

[11] "Adherence and its Management in Clinical Trials: Implications for Arthritis Treatment Trials." Arthritis Care and Research. J.L. Probstfield. 1989. 2:S48-S57.

[12] "Issues of Recruitment, Retention and Compliance in Community-Based Clinical Trials with Traditionally Underserved Populations." Applied Nursing Research. Edward V. Morse, Patricia M. Simon, C. Lynn Beach, and Janice Walker. February 1995, Vol. 8, No. 1. p. 9.

[13] *Ibid.*, p. 13.

[14] "The Recruitment Triangle: Reasons Why African-Americans Enroll, Refuse to Enroll, or Voluntarily Withdraw from a Clinical Trial." National of the National Medical Association. Philip B. Gorelick, M.D., MPH; Yvonne Harris, MPA; Barbara Burnett, MSW; and Faith J. Bonecutter, MSW. 1998. Vol. 90, No.3. pp. 141-145.

[15] *Ibid.*, p. 143, 144.

[16] "Recruitment and Retention of Minority Participants in the DASH Controlled Feeding Trial." Ethnicity & Disease. William M. Vollmer, Ph.D.; Laura P. Svetkey, M.D., MHS; Lawrence J. Appel, M.D., MPH; Eva Obarzanek, Ph.D., MPH; Patrice Reams, BS; Betty Kennedy, MA; Kathy Aicher; Jeanne Charleston, RN, MSN; Paul R. Conlin, M.D.; Marguerite Evans, MS, RD; David Harsha, Ph.D.; and Stephanie Hertert, M.Ed. Vol. 8, Spring 1998. pp. 199-208.

[17] "Rationale and Design of the Dietary Approaches to Stop Hypertension Trial (DASH)." Annals of Epidemiology, F.M. Sacks; E. Obarzanek; M.M. Windhauser; L.P. Svetkey; W.M. Vollmer; M. McCullough, et al. 1995. 5: 108-118.

[18] Dash Collaborative Research Group. New England Journal of Medicine. L.J. Appel; T.J. Moore; E. Obarzanek; W.M. Vollmer; L.P. Svetkey; F.M. Sacks, et al. 1997; 336: 1117-1124.

[19] "Recruitment and Retention of Minority Participants in the DASH Controlled Feeding Trial." Ethnicity & Disease. Vollmer, et al, p. 201.

[20] *Ibid.*, p. 206.

[21] *Ibid.*, p. 205.

[22] "Issues and Recommendations for the Recruitment and Retention of Older Ethnic Minority Adults into Clinical Research." Journal of Consulting and Clinical Psychology. Patricia A. Arean, Dolores Gallagher-Thompson. Vol. 64, No. 5, 1996. pp. 875-880.

[23] "Participation of Older Adults in Health Programs and Research: A Critical Review of the Literature." The Gerontologist. W.B. Carter, K. Elward; J. Malmgren; M. L. Martin; & E. Larson. 1991, 31, 584-592.

[24] *Op.cit.*, Patricia A. Arean, Dolores Gallagher-Thompson, p. 876.

[25] "Caring Roles of Grandparents and Chronic Illness in Black Families." Presented 1994, P. Dilworth-Anderson & Anderson.

[26] "A Comparison of Outreach Strategies for Hispanic Caregivers of Alzheimer's Victims." Clinical Gerontologist. D. Gallagher-Thompson, R.S. Moorehead; T.M. Polich; D. Arguello; C. Johnson; V. Rodriguez, & M. Meyer. 1994, 15, 57-63.

[27] "Issues and Recommendations for the Recruitment and Retention of Older Ethnic Minority Adults into Clinical Research." Journal of Consulting and Clinical Psychology. Patricia A. Arean, Dolores Gallagher-Thompson. Vol. 64, No. 5, 1996. p. 878.

[28] "A Word From Clinical Trial Volunteers." CenterWatch. Editorial Staff. June 1999, Vol. 6, Issue 6. p. 9.

[29] "Patient Experiences in Industry-Sponsored Clinical Trials." Research Roundtable. Ken Getz. September 2000.

[30] "Patients' Perceptions of their Participation in a Clinical Trial for Postoperative Crohn's Disease." Canadian Journal of Gastroenterology. E.D. Kennedy, M.D.; J.D. Blair, RN; R. Ready; B.G. Wolff, M.D.; A.H. Steinhart, M.D.; P.W. Carryer, M.D., R.S. McLeod, M.D. Vol. 12, No. 4, May/June 1998. pp. 287-291.

[31] *Ibid.*, pp. 288-289.

[32] *Ibid.*, p. 291.

[33] *Ibid.*, p. 290.

[34] "Clinical Trial Participant Satisfaction: Survey of SHEP Enrollees." Journal of the American Geriatric Society. Eleanor B. Schron, Sylvia Wassertheil-Smoller, Ph.D., and Sara Pressel. 1997, 45. pp. 934-938.

[35] "Participation in a Clinical Trial: The Patients' Point of View." Controlled Clinical Trials. M.E. Mattson; D.J. Curb; R. McArdle.; and the AMIS and BHAT Research Groups. 1985:6. pp. 156-157.

[36] DataEdge LLC. Fort Washington, PA. October 1998.

[37] *Énhancing Retention in Clinical Trials of Psychosocial Treatments: Practical Strategies.* Kathleen M. Carroll. Yale University; Department of Psychiatry. p. 4.

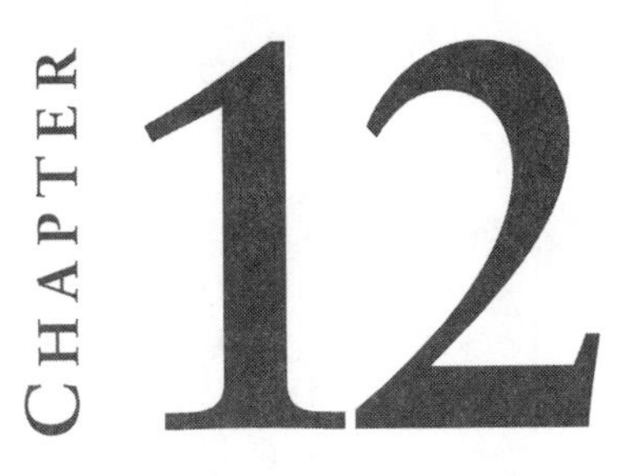

The Investigator Site Perspective: Patient Recruitment Considerations and Issues Facing Site Personnel

Terry Reece, Melynda Geurts and Diana L. Anderson, Ph.D.,
Rheumatology Research International

In today's market, speed is of the essence in recruiting study subjects. Recruiting and enrolling subjects for clinical trials is increasingly becoming more of a challenge for individual investigator sites. As more compounds are entering the developmental pipeline, pharmaceutical companies and Contract Research Organizations (CROs) are focusing on working with sites that can enroll subjects quickly and efficiently as well as produce quality work.

In many instances, sites must consider having a patient recruitment plan in place prior to study start-up in order to meet their enrollment commitments. While centralized recruitment is effective in accelerating patient enrollment, the site must also continue to recruit subjects locally through various patient recruitment venues. If the site does not have a recruitment or marketing department, then it is the responsibility of the research team not only to identify potential subjects, but also to provide methods to help retain these study subjects.

This chapter will focus on methods used to facilitate timely and efficient enrollment by staff at the site level. A variety of recruitment methods (both internal and external) that can be developed by site personnel will be discussed. In addition, obstacles that may be encountered during the course of the study will be presented.

RECRUITMENT AND THE RESEARCH TEAM

Effective recruitment at the site level begins with the principal investigator and the study coordinator. Together, they comprise the core of the research team. The team consists of the principal investigator, study coordinator, and other research staff such as the receptionist, lab and x-ray personnel. It is imperative that the research team work together to complete enrollment within the designated enrollment period.

Throughout the course of the study, each team member plays an integral role in recruiting subjects for a study. For example, the principal investigator can serve as a recruiting asset in the community. By participating in speaking engagements at educational forums and support groups, the principal investigator can generate interest in the study and help establish name recognition for the site.

Like the principal investigator, the study coordinator is also responsible for patient recruitment. The role the study coordinator plays is crucial in developing a close relationship with the patient. Not only does the study coordinator collect data and dispense medication, but also they can serve as a mentor and encourage the patients to remain in the study. According to David Ginsberg, "There is an oft repeated truism in the clinical trial industry, that the most important individual at the investigative site is not the investigator, but the study coordinator."[1] Without a dedicated, knowledgeable study coordinator, a site cannot conduct a successful clinical trial.

Finally, it is important to remember that all staff members have an impact on the performance of the study. The service patients receive from the time they enter the research center can determine if they stay in the study or return to participate in future studies. Therefore, it is important for the site to build team involvement to facilitate enrollment. This can be accomplished by conducting a group meeting with the research team prior to study initiation. The purpose of this meeting is to help the staff understand the complexities of the protocol and study as well as be cognizant of enrollment goals and deadlines. At the site level, it must be recognized that not just one person is responsible for patient recruitment. In fact, the entire research team must compliment each other throughout the study in order to yield successful trial enrollment.

BUDGETING FOR AND TRACKING ENROLLMENT

Funds allocated for recruitment initiatives can vary significantly depending on the study design. Table One is an example of a single site recruitment budget for a contraceptive study. This table illustrates a simple tracking form that can be implemented by site personnel. In this example, the initial recruitment budget was for $2,000.00. During the course of the study, the site realized that they would need additional funding to maintain the enrollment momentum. They received an additional $4,700.00, yielding a total recruitment budget of $6,700.00. Within this budget, each recruitment strategy was itemized. This enabled the research team to identify the actual cost of each venue. Additionally, they were able to track invoicing and payments to and from the sponsor.

However, recruitment funds are not always allocated to support enrollment. In this instance, sites must look to other resources such as community outreach, discussed specifically in this chapter. However, sites that have recruitment tracking processes in place, which illustrate the results of specific strategies (number of calls,

Table 1

Patient Recruitment Budget

Contraceptive	
$2,000.00	Recruitment Budget
$4,700.00	Additional Funding
$6,700.00	Total Budget Available

Venue	Expenses	Remaining Balance	Sponsor Billed	Invoice Date	Pay't Rec'd
Ad/Flyer Design	$23274	$6,467.26	Y	6/26/00	Y
College Student Paper	$189.00	$6,278.26	Y	6/26/00	Y
Brookhaven Community College	$120.00	$6,158.26	Y	6/26/00	Y
Young Country Radio	$2,100.00	$4,058.26	Y	6/26/00	Y
The Edge Radio	$1,610.00	$2,448.26	Y	6/26/00	Y
Young Country Radio	$2,300.00	$144.26	N		N
Ad Design	$75.00	$73.26	N		N

advertising cost, number of randomized subjects per venue), can help the site in securing recruitment budgets for future studies.

Given the competitive nature of clinical trials, clinical research sites can also begin to differentiate themselves in the market by collecting historical metrics related to recruitment initiatives. Sites can begin tracking these metrics by implementing the use of a recruitment report as illustrated in Table Two. This particular recruitment report tracks response rates from ten different recruitment methods across six studies. Additionally, it tracks the number of scheduled subjects and those that did not qualify. Collecting this particular information in conjunction with cost per venue is helpful in determining cost per subject for a specific study. Moreover, it provides the site with a forecasting tool when developing a recruitment plan. Sites that are

Table 2

Recruitment Report for a Six-Month Period for a Large Multispecialty Investigator Site

Study	Chol	HTN	RA	OA	IBS	OP
TV	134	1	38	465	12	
Radio						
Newspaper	105	50		130		35
Letter						98
Database	88	1	9	40	114	3
Seminar	5	4	14	23		8
Previous Ads		66	58	68	1	22
Health Fairs		33		90		68
Flyer	10	5	2	2	4	
Other	100	12	5	5	3	
Total Calls	442	172	126	823	134	234
Scheduled	162	26	46	135	8	
DNQ Declined	39	71	29	112	6	

Chol=Cholesterol; HTN=Hypertension; RA=Rheumatoid Arthritis; OA=Osteoarthritis; IBS=Irritable Bowel Syndrome; OP=Osteoporosis

Source: Rheumatology Research International, 1998

able to provide sponsors with this historical data are in a better position to secure advertising monies for a study otherwise not granted.

INTERNAL VERSUS EXTERNAL ADVERTISING METHODS

No one advertising method can be successful in recruiting subjects.[2] Therefore, a multi-faceted approach obviously will reach a broader network of potential subjects as well as yield higher response rates. In terms of the research site, these approaches may be comprised of "internal as well as external" advertising strategies.

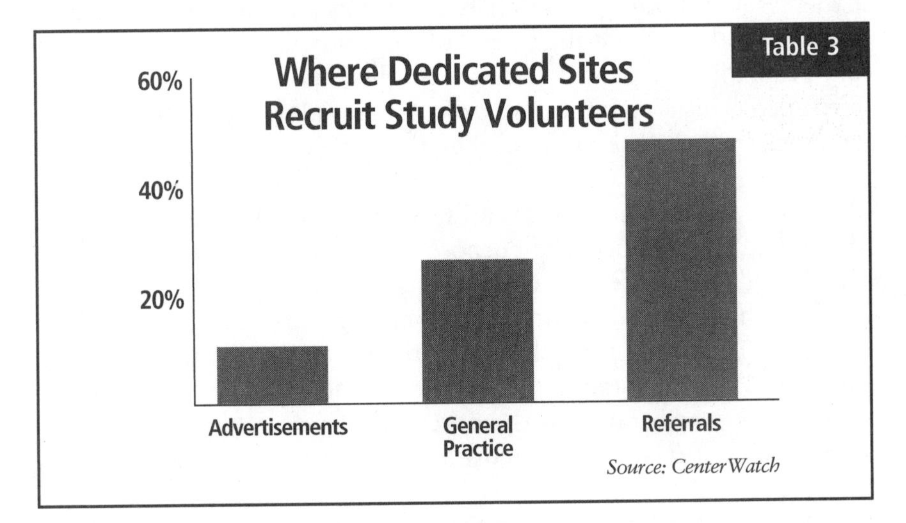

Table Three depicts what vehicles dedicated sites used to recruit study volunteers. Based on this data, 55% of volunteers are recruited through external methods, 35% through internal methods and 5% through physician referrals.[3] Hence, a combination of both types of advertising strategies can aid the sites in developing a complete and comprehensive recruitment plan for recruitment of subjects.

To ensure the success of the recruitment plan, it is essential that the research team supports the plan and has an understanding of the study criteria. However, the research team must also have a fundamental understanding of these types of advertising strategies before recruitment practices can be employed.

Internal Advertising Methods

The first stage in developing a recruitment plan is to evaluate internal resources. First, the research team should define the target audience for a particular study based on the study criteria. Once the target audience is defined, a recruitment plan can be developed that will assist in completing the study within the appropriate timeframe.

There are several internal advertising options that a site may elect to employ such as performing database searches, conducting open forums and building and maintaining site awareness. First, the site should look within their own patient population to identify potential patients. A review of the database as well as patient charts should be researched throughout the course of the study. Maintaining an ongoing evaluation of patient charts will allow potential subjects to be identified. This is an important process especially when there has been an amendment to the protocol that alters the conduct of the trial.

Another type of strategy that can serve as a recruitment tactic is conducting group forums. The purpose of holding a group session is to further educate potential participants about clinical trials and the study at hand. The benefits of holding a group orientation include decreasing people's fears, lowering their skepticism and increasing their level of understanding about clinical trials. Another advantage to the group orientation is the potential of new referrals a site may receive with a relatively low cost and minimum investment of time.

Finally, investigative sites can implement strategies, which consistently remind the research staff of the ongoing clinical trials. This can be accomplished through weekly meetings, reminders on the patient charts, distributing study specific information cards, posting fliers and/or posters in each exam room and sending e-mail reminders to all of the principal investigators, sub-investigators and study coordinators.

External Advertising Methods

This leads to the second stage in developing a recruitment plan, the evaluation of external resources. Some of these resources may include media and community resources, the Internet and the utilization of media buyers. Additionally, utilizing these resources in conjunction with internal resources can further support the recruitment plan.

Media Resources

Researching the market is imperative in reaching the target audience through local advertising, which may include radio, newspaper and television. It is important to note that depending on the study and geographical location of the site, call responses can vary across different venues. Newspaper advertising can be an effective recruitment method. Depending on a site's geographic location, advertising in the main or metro section of the newspaper may generate a large call response rate. Again, it all depends on the target audience a site is trying to reach. Case example: A rheumatoid arthritis study was conducted in Oklahoma City, Oklahoma, utilizing radio and newspaper advertisements. Four calls were received from the print ad, none of which qualified for the study. However, the radio commercial did extremely well. Twenty-one calls were received and four subjects were randomized into the study. Clearly, radio was the best advertising venue for this market. The site must know its target market to be successful. In this example, print advertising for a more obscure disease such as rheumatoid arthritis (2.5 million people in the U.S. with this disease) is not a good use of the allocated recruitment dollars.

Television can also be used effectively in recruiting subjects, but in most markets it is expensive to advertise. However, television advertising is an effective way of reaching a broad range of potential subjects. If you are working within the confines of a limited budget, advertising on local cable stations as opposed to national stations may lower costs, although the reach is not as great.

Finally, before implementing any type of advertising campaign, the sponsor and the Institutional Review Board (IRB) must review and approve all recruitment materials used to recruit study volunteers. The first step is to develop the recruitment materials and submit them to the sponsor for approval. Once the sponsor has approved the material, the next step is to forward the materials to the IRB. It is important to note that IRBs have different approval processes. For example, one IRB may need to approve the radio script and listen to the actual commercial before it is aired, while another IRB will only need to approve the radio script. It is imperative that the research team understands this approval process when implementing a recruitment plan. Table Four shows the approval process of patient recruitment materials beginning with the sponsor.

External Mailings

Another type of external advertising is the utilization of external

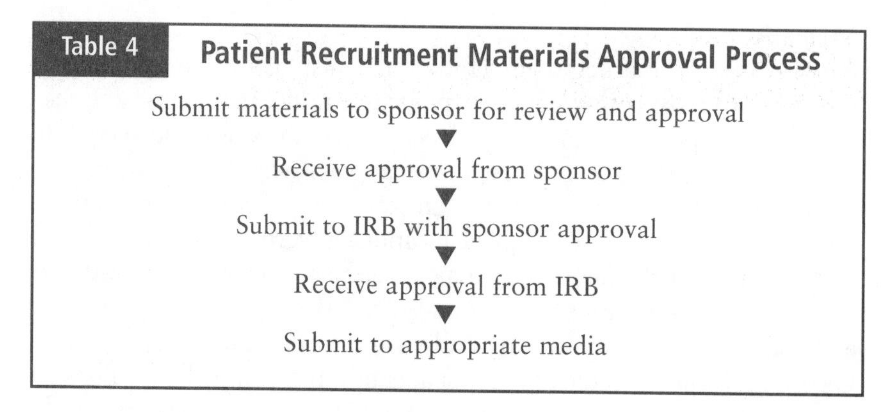

Table 4 **Patient Recruitment Materials Approval Process**

Submit materials to sponsor for review and approval
▼
Receive approval from sponsor
▼
Submit to IRB with sponsor approval
▼
Receive approval from IRB
▼
Submit to appropriate media

mailings. Direct mail, physician-to-patient letters and physician-to-physician letters are examples of external mailings. The physician-to-patient letter, shown in the Appendix One, is an efficient method in notifying a site's patient population about a new study that may potentially benefit them if they choose to participate in the study. Likewise, the physician-to-physician letter (Appendix Two) is way of informing other physicians about the conduct of a trial and the availability to their patients. This letter is used primarily to generate referrals from area physicians.

Furthermore, conducting a direct mail campaign is similar to the physician-to-patient mailing. In comparison to the physician-to-patient mailing, the direct mail piece is typically a postcard mailer as opposed to a letter. (Table Five) This postcard can be mailed to both internal and external databases. There are various clearinghouses that maintain health specific databases that allows for a more targeted mailing to occur.

When creating these external mailings, it is crucial that the information be study specific. The message must convey the therapeutic area being addressed, study criteria, and what potential benefits may be received by participating in the study.

Internet

The Internet is another advertising medium that began impacting patient recruitment in the late 1990's. On the World Wide Web today, more than 10,000 websites focus on health and medical topics, and the wealth of information continues to expand rapidly. In this age of technology, the number of people "surfing the net" is huge.[4] As seen in Table Six, it is projected that approximately 77

Table 5

ATTENTION

DIABETES?

ABC Research Center is conducting a clinical research study for individuals with Diabetes. To be eligible, you must be male/female, 30-60 years of age, with a diagnosis of Diabetes and presently on oral medication or insulin. Participants must be willing to eat an individualized diet aimed at maintenance of current weight. Those who qualify will receive a complete physical exam, eye exam, laboratory assessments and a glucometer at no cost. Upon completion of the study, participants will receive $135.00 honorarium.

Please call ABC Research Center at (123) 456-7890

ABC Research Center is located at 123 Town Street, Anywhere, USA 12345

million people (80%) will be using the Internet by the year 2001. This represents a 75% growth in Internet users since 1997.

As patients are becoming more educated about their disease process, traditional approaches such as fliers, physician referrals, and direct mailings need to be integrated with new methods of advertising. Compared to other media formats, (i.e., newspaper and radio) advertising on the Internet is relatively inexpensive. However, while cost per subject obtained is low, the up-front cost can be high. Most websites require a minimum of $2,000.00 to advertise on their site.

Sponsors and CROs are taking advantage of the Internet's resources by posting clinical trials on various websites including CenterWatch, which maintains one of the most comprehensive websites posting industry sponsored clinical trials. On the average, the Sponsor and/or CRO will post the study on the Internet for about ten months to one year and this listing generally includes an average of nineteen geographic sites.[5] Investigative sites can also take advantage of this medium by creating their own website. By developing a comment or request box for users to complete when visiting the website, a site may gain exposure to potential participants which they might not have reached through traditional advertising as well as increase their patient recruitment database.

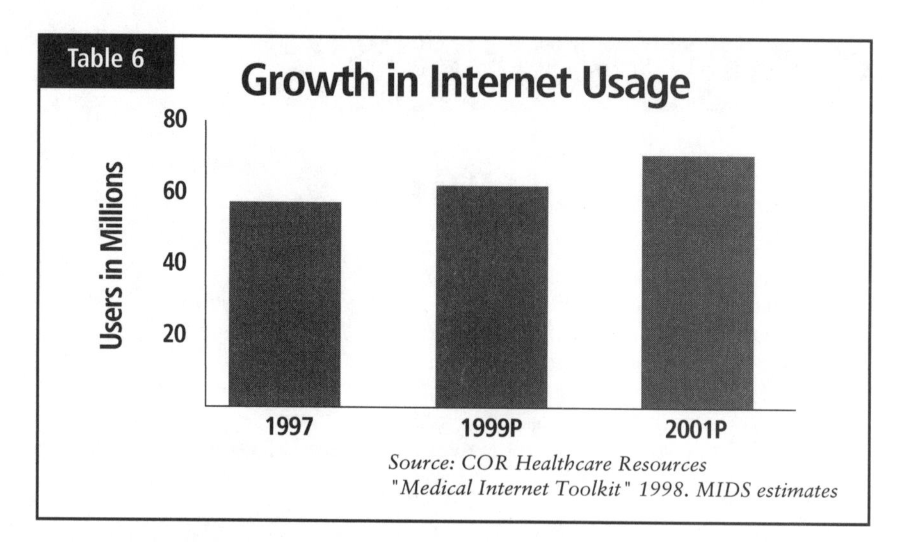

Media Buyers

Oftentimes, sites do not have the time or resources to research the market nor place advertising based on experience or knowledge. This is where the services of a media buyer can be utilized. If a site does not have a marketing or recruitment department, the media buyer will research the market, recommend which course of advertising would yield a greater response for the study, and place the advertisement for the site. Typically, there are no up-front costs for the site to pay. The commission a media buyer receives is usually from the newspaper, radio or television station. It is important to note that when utilizing a media buyer, the site should use a media buying company that specializes in healthcare, specifically clinical trials if possible.

ADDITIONAL CHALLENGES

The failure to recruit subjects accounts for almost one out of every four delays occurring in the development phase. Among the reasons for low participation is poor protocol design, negative public perceptions and lack of patient's trust in the healthcare providers.[6] Patient's attitudes have changed. Sites must be open and flexible to their demands, such as extending office hours. For example, if sites can extend office hours to evenings and weekends, more patients may take advantage of participating in a research study. In addition, providing ample parking and scheduling visits when traffic times are slower can be advantageous to the site. This can be especially important if seniors are participating in a study. Other barriers to overcome are protocol amendments, patients' lack of understanding about the study, and potential side effects compared to their current regimen. One way to alleviate this concern is to let the subject read in the Physicians' Desk Reference, the side effects profile of the medications currently being taken versus the study drug.[7]

As discussed throughout this chapter, the success of each recruitment method varies based upon multiple factors such as target market, geographic site location, type of study. Table Seven reveals survey findings conducted by Rheumatology Research International (June 2000) of over 100 clinical research sites and offers insights into why certain recruitment tactics are more successful than others.[8] Interestingly, the majority of sites who responded to the survey

Table 7

Results of Patient Recruitment Methods of Over 100 Research Sites

I.	75% of sites use advertising for patient recruitment
II.	Sites have a higher ratio of recruiting subjects in the spring and fall versus the summer when individuals are taking vacation and in the winter during the holiday season
III.	81% receive an advertising budget for individual studies
IV.	31% of sites feel that funds are not adequate
V.	Fliers and physician-to-patient letters rank high on materials most useful in recruiting subjects. Followed by posters, print ads, brochures, quick study reference cards and physician-to-physician letters
VI.	Other materials helpful in recruiting subjects: direct mail, prepaid postcards to send to potential patients for response to studies, toll-free number for patients to call to discuss study
VII.	88% of sites have the capabilities to respond to calls generated through an advertising campaign
VIII.	56% of sites would utilize a centralized toll-free number to prescreen patients
IX.	38% said the experience with utilizing a toll-free number was fair. Others felt a patient would be more compliant if drawn from their own database or another physician that has a history on the patient as well as calling a local number for personal health issues
X.	81% of sites used letters as their primary form of internal communication followed by direct mail and fliers (38%) and posters (19%)

received monies for recruitment and were actively advertising for the studies. However, they felt the funds received were not adequate for recruiting new subjects.

Finally, it is important to try to predict potential recruitment challenges when developing a recruitment plan. Through identifying possible recruitment obstacles for a study, the site will be better prepared to establish processes to minimize and/or eliminate these obstacles so to not negatively impact site enrollment.

CONCLUSION

Sponsors and CROS are consistently looking for sites that can perform studies efficiently. Sites who initially identify the major obstacles in recruiting for a particular study and develop a recruitment plan of how to enroll and retain potential subjects are typically more successful in securing patients. As the study progresses, recruitment initiatives will need to be evaluated on an on-going basis to ensure effectiveness.

Whether a site decides to utilize internal or external recruitment methods, the advertising methods discussed in this chapter can serve as guidelines to facilitate patient recruitment at the site. It is important to remember that the success of the trial is greatly dependent upon the professionalism and dedication of the research team.

REFERENCES

[1] "The Investigator's Guide to Clinical Research." CenterWatch, Inc. Dr. David Ginsberg. Boston, MA. 2nd edition, 1999. p. 89, 138.

[2] Rheumatology Research International. Market Research Findings, 1999.

[3] CenterWatch, Inc. 1998.

[4] COR Healthcare Resources. "Medical Internet Toolkit." 1998, MIDS estimates.

[5] "Surf's Up—An Update on Recruiting Subjects via the Internet." Applied Clinical Trials. Kenneth Getz and Ann Kennon. Volume 7,

Number 5, May 1998. p. 58-59.

[6] "The Investigator's Guide to Clinical Research." CenterWatch, Inc. Dr. David Ginsberg. Boston, MA. 2nd edition, 1999. p. 89,138.

[7] *Ibid.*

[8] Rheumatology Research International. Clinical Research Site Survey, June 2000.

AUTHOR BIOGRAPHY

Terry Reece is the Site Recruitment and Relations Coordinator for Rheumatology Research International (RRI). Ms. Reece serves as the patient recruitment liaison to research centers (sites) participating in various rheumatology studies. She is responsible for assessing each sites patient recruitment needs and conducts ongoing advertising analysis throughout the course of the individual studies.

Ms. Reece has over 12 years of healthcare experience and was previously employed by Integris Health in Oklahoma City, Oklahoma where she worked in the ProHealth Marketing department assisting with physician marketing and recruitment.

A graduate of the University of Oklahoma, Ms. Reece holds a B.A. in Advertising and is a public education committee member for the North Texas Arthritis Foundation chapter.

Sample Physician-to-Patient Letter

September 29, 2000

Jane Doe
123 Town Street
Anywhere, USA 12345

Dear Ms. Doe:

ABC Research Center is participating in a clinical research study to test the safety and effectiveness of an investigational medication for the treatment of Erosive Esophagitis.

The 8-week study consists of 3 endoscopies. The first one will be at the start of the study, the second at week four and the third at week eight. Qualified participants will receive up to $150.00 for their participation.

If you qualify, you will also receive study medication, study related laboratory tests and study related examinations at no charge.

For more information about this study, please call ABC Research Center at (123) 456-7890.

Sincerely,

John Doe, M.D.

Sample Physician-to-Physician Letter

September 29, 2000

Jane Doe, M.D.
123 Town Street
Anywhere, USA 12345

Dear Dr. Doe:

We are currently conducting a clinical research trial with an investigational medication and are looking for patients who may be eligible to participate. The purpose of this letter is to ask you to take an active role in helping us to find suitable patients by considering whether any of your own patients may be eligible to take part. Based on preclinical information, this investigational product has the potential to reduce joint deterioration caused by rheumatoid arthritis.

To qualify for this study, the patient must be 18 years of age or older, have been diagnosed with rheumatoid arthritis for at least 6 months, and currently taking methotrexate.

All study-related procedures including physician, laboratory and x-ray exams, as well as study medication, will be provided at no cost to the patient. The study lasts three years. **We would of course follow your patient only for study-related treatment and will keep you fully informed of the patient's progress.**

If you have patients who you think may want to take part, please send the enclosed sample physician-to-patient letter to those individuals. If the patient is interested, he/she is asked to call ABC Research Center at (123) 456-7890 to obtain information about the study. In addition, if you would like to have further information about this study, please call Study Coordinator Doe at (123) 456-7890.

Rheumatoid arthritis is still a devastating disease. Clinical drug studies such as this may allow us to offer more effective treatments to our patients. Thank you for your help.

Sincerely yours,

John Doe, M.D.

CHAPTER 13

A Practical Approach to the Development of Community Resources to Fulfill Recruitment Goals and Commitments

Margo Whitley, Radiant Research, Dallas

"Goodwill is the one and only asset that competition cannot undersell or destroy." –Marshall Field, Retail Entrepreneur

The success of any business depends largely on its ability to establish a good, solid reputation among the audience it serves. Common sense dictates that smart advertising, name branding, excellent service and a good product are crucial to a company's survival, clinical research being no exception.

However, the most commonly overlooked variable in promoting a research site is quite possibly the most obvious and least expensive, community involvement. The purpose of a business is to create and keep a customer. To do that, it is important to do those things that will make people want to do business with a company.

Almost everyone is acquainted with how a new business first strives to involve themselves in the community by joining the Chamber of Commerce, Rotary Club, Lions Club and other civic organizations. Other examples include involvement in sponsoring Little League,

PTA, County Fairs and similar events of significance to the community. The smart and savvy businessperson soon learns it's not always what you know, but who you know and who knows you.

Companies all over the world spend billions annually on advertising, celebrity endorsements, sponsorships and promotion. For building trust and capitalizing on the targeted audience, there is no substitute for community outreach. In terms of an investigator research site, this often means the ability of an entire staff to represent the business (the site) in a positive and favorable light by supporting and serving those organizations/events that are important to the patient population. Research shows that giving back to the community can increase a firm's reputation for social responsibility and for being known as a well-run business, factors that can enhance a company's overall market value.

Patient recruitment involves far more than creating clever ads and gathering demographics. A patient population must become as familiar as your own family, know their likes, dislikes, where they congregate, what their hobbies are and what their favorite radio and television programs are. A site cannot expect to thrive if it ignores the surrounding community.

Acquiring this information requires resourcefulness, tenacity and consistency. Developing and maintaining a high profile in the community allows sites to recruit informed, quality, study participants.

I LIVE IN LITTLEVILLE/LARGVILLE—HOW DO I GET INVOLVED?

"The purpose of a business is to create and keep a customer."
–Theodore Leavitt, Editor, Harvard Business Review

An investigator site can be located in a small town in Kansas or in a sprawling urban city like Chicago, but the formula for "getting involved" remains the same.

Join, Join, Join...Support, Support, Support...An offer to provide juice and doughnuts for an upcoming 5K run to "Save the Whales" might be just the entree to mix and mingle with a segment of the population heretofore untapped. In another case scenario there might be a Board of Director position open within a non-profit organization and staff could be allotted time to volunteer for a few hours a week. With little effort and expense, the site's mission and need for recruitment resources are made apparent to another segment of the population. The message is clear. The Chamber of Commerce has "business mixers" for a reason and the key word here is "NETWORKING." (Table One) Part of networking is realizing what can be done for others, and it is quite possibly the most effective way of creating contacts.

Table 1

How can your time and talent benefit your community?

Attend the ***Get On Board!*** *Fair, a unique opportunity to meet a variety of area nonprofit organizations that need qualified board members who represent our diverse community.*

This is your chance to make a difference!

Join us

Thursday, October 5

4:30–7:30 p.m.

Center for Community Cooperation

2900 Live Oak, Dallas

It's Free!

Call 214-826-3470

Visit *www.cnmdallas.org* to register

Premier Sponsor
BANK ONE

Sponsors:
Alcatel, SBC Foundation, JC Penney, Jenkens & Gilchrist, P.C. and The Dallas Morning News

Present by
CENTER FOR NONPROFIT MANAGEMENT

In partnership with
Asian American Chamber of Commerce, American Indian Chamber of Commerce of Texas, AMAP (Association of Mexican American Professionals), Dallas Black Chamber of Commerce, National Pan-Hellenic Council—Dallas, City of Dallas Economic Development Department, Greater Dallas Chamber—Leadership Development, Greater Dallas Hispanic Chamber of Commerce, Hispanic Women's Network of Texas, Junior League of Dallas, YMCA of Metropolitan Dallas and United Way of Metropolitan Dallas

PROFIT FROM NONPROFIT

"Success is measured by the degree that one helps and enriches others, even if he helps himself at the same time."
–John Marks Templeton, World's Greatest Investor

Establishing a good working relationship with nonprofit organizations is a "win-win" situation, one that benefits a company in countless ways. Participating in public service can help a company as much as it does the nonprofit organization they are helping. Success comes in finding a need and filling it at the same time.

Take for instance the case of a site involved primarily in arthritis studies. Joining up with the local chapter of the National Arthritis Foundation provides a perfect vehicle for offering clinical research to a population searching for relief and/or a cure for arthritis. Becoming involved with nonprofit organizations can be achieved on several levels. Employees can serve on a board, volunteer to fundraise, or have physicians and staff offer a forum on what's on the horizon in new treatments for a specific disease. No matter what your area of expertise in any given therapeutic area, partnering with a nonprofit organization is a giant step towards integrating into the community.

Becoming a viable member and supporter of one or more of these nonprofit organizations can be both valuable to a business and rewarding for staff. Businesses that encourage their employees to volunteer and contribute benefit if they themselves have a reputation for public service. Many a fledgling business has bolstered revenues and customer base through public service. If this tried and true formula works for major companies like Johnson & Johnson, General Motors and AT&T, it certainly merits serious consideration by clinical research sites around the country.

THE MEDIA, A DOUBLE-EDGED SWORD

"Advertising is the genie which is transforming America into a place of comfort, luxury and ease for millions."
–William Allen White, Owner of the Emporia Gazette

The media may seem as elusive and difficult to access as the bald eagle, but it is surprising how often they are eager for a story.

Approach the media with press releases on every novel study that comes down the pike. If it is Breast Cancer Awareness Month and there is a study that ties in, present it to the local newspapers, radio and television stations. The more the press is exposed to a company name, the better chance the site stands of acquiring additional press coverage. Once a relationship is established with the media, follow up with a thank you note for the coverage and an invitation to have them return. Even the most seasoned reporter appreciates being treated with civility and courtesy. Fostering an ongoing relationship with the press is good business, which helps serve the goals of recruitment.

RADIO—MAN'S CONSTANT COMPANION

"The business that considers itself immune to the necessity for advertising sooner or later finds itself immune to business."

–Derby Brown, Entrepreneur

Advertising via radio is one of the most effective means of reaching an audience. The radio keeps America company in the home, office, car and points in between. Branding a research site name and advertising for study participants is achieved by studying the demographics and reach of the radio stations in a geographic area.

Common sense dictates that placing a commercial on a hip-hop station to attract age fifty plus participants makes as little sense as contracting with a conservative talk show format for teens and young adults.

If two radio stations have the same demographics, reach, plus are in the same price range, consider telling the station rep that advertising dollars will go to the competitor who can arrange a "perk" for the site. Perks can range from interviewing a medical director to exhibiting in an event planned for the station. Whatever the extra edge offered by the station make it work for the site. Sales representatives are in a position to make deals, so it is not necessary to be shy about negotiating. "Marketing" is giving the site a favorable position in the market, it's up to those responsible for patient recruitment to find that niche.

TELEVISION—THE UNFORGIVING MEDIUM

"You can have brilliant ideas, but if you can't get them across, your ideas won't get you anywhere."

–Lee Iacocca, CEO Chrysler Corporation

Many budgets do not allow for the extravagance of producing a study-specific commercial for television; if there's the opportunity to produce a commercial spot, make it as professional and as direct as possible. Costs can run from $500 to $500,000 depending on a number of factors.

A site may choose to use a local production company to create a generic or study-specific commercial that can be used on multiple stations. It is a good idea to request a sampling of the production company's previous work before signing on the dotted line. A reputable firm will also be willing to supply references upon request. The number of "fly-by-night" video services is multiplying, so caution should be exercised when making a selection. Remember too that cable stations make television affordable for the small business owner and having the ability to target geographic areas makes cable all the more attractive for recruitment purposes.

Whether a site chooses to employ professional actors or use members of its staff for a commercial, the targeted audience should be the first consideration. A receptionist might be a dead-ringer for Madonna, but it would make little sense to use her as the main character in a commercial targeting volunteers for a male-pattern baldness or post-menopausal study. Miscasting can "turn-off" the very audience that one is trying to "turn-on."

Some television stations have a "Medical Reporter" on staff that covers items of interest in the medical arena. Like all employees, medical reporters exhibit varying degrees of expertise, interest and overall talent when it comes to doing their job. If approached for an interview about the clinical research trial occurring at the site, be prepared for what a "medical segment" entails. First, clear with the sponsor and assuage any fears or questions they might have concerning the integrity of the segment. Believe it or not, most sponsors are probably not acquainted with the wide world of medical reporting and have to be convinced that agreeing to allow this type of exposure almost always translates into a new source of potential subjects. Traditionally, IRBs are not involved in a medical segment since the sponsor or drug name are not mentioned. There is no hard and fast rule regarding IRB approval of a medical segment[2], but it is always prudent to contact the IRB and advise them of the upcoming segment.

Preparing for the actual filming of the medical segment usually requires providing an overview of the study, a study participant(s), a physician and auxiliary staff. If television can make an actor appear 10 pounds heavier, it can exaggerate other flaws as well. Personnel should be reminded that it's possible the spot will be seen by thousands of viewers; attention to grooming and professional garb is essential. Be prepared to do some housekeeping, and refurbishing in the area being filmed.

All parties involved in the filming must sign a consent form for release of subject matter (Appendix One). It is also essential to provide the medical reporter with a telephone number that viewers can call to obtain more information on the segment. Interest generated by a segment of this nature usually results in a large number of calls; telephones need to be adequately staffed to obtain optimum results. A well-done medical segment is advertising that money can't buy—all bases must be covered.

HEALTH FAIRS

"More business is lost every year through neglect than any other cause." –Jim Cathcart, Professional Speaker & Motivator

In today's health conscious society, there is a constant clamoring for more information about health and wellness. Thus, springs up the catchall term "Health Fair." Hospitals, nonprofit organizations, corporations, municipalities, schools and universities, put these events on with regularity and are always seeking quality exhibitors to help inform the public about the ever-changing medical field.

This venue can be the time to offer the public a look at what an investigator site does and how it operates. It's always good idea to have printed materials in the form of brochures and flyers. Materials should identify a site's capabilities, personnel and studies being offered. Always keep in mind that the company's name is being branded into the public's subconscious at these events, logos and credentials need to be boldly featured whenever possible.

Health fairs are usually annual events and chances of being selected for inclusion are enhanced by offering a service, such as blood pressure testing, cholesterol screening or bone density readings. Give-aways are always popular with the attendees and are another means of advertising the site. Providing a give-away without including a phone number and company name is akin to throwing money out the window.

Employees representing the site at these public events should be friendly, neatly groomed and equipped with a name badge that identifies their position and company's name. An exhibitor who is uninformed and does not interact with the public during the event might as well stay home. Remember the axiom, *you never get a second chance to make a good first impression.* These exhibitors should represent the site in a professional and courteous manner.

AN INFORMED PUBLIC

"In business the competition will bite you if you keep running, if you stand still, they will swallow you."

–William Knudsen, Presidential Advisor

Do not confuse health forums with health fairs. Health forums are usually conducted by a physician and geared toward an invited audience. Most successful forums target a specific disease category and are addressed by a specialist in that field. Events of this nature take careful planning, because without adequate preparation, the event is a disaster with five or six people in attendance and a disgruntled speaker who feels that their time has been wasted.

There are no set rules for putting on a forum, however, the following guideline is helpful:

- Identify a speaker and check availability.
- Saturday's traditionally yield the best attendance. Avoid holidays and months when the weather is severe.
- Mail invitations (Table Two) to a targeted audience, advertise through public service announcements, newspapers and flyers. Always include an invitation to the press.
- Reserve a location in advance. Hospitals and municipal centers make excellent venues and are rarely expensive.
- Decide on the format of the event. Will refreshments, door

prizes and screenings be provided? Never forget for a moment that "food" is the universal language and can prove an enticement for people to attend.

- Questionnaires, give-aways, and flyers on enrolling and upcoming studies should be made available.

- Funding for the event is available from several sources. Partnering with nonprofit organizations, pharmaceutical sponsors and other exhibitors provides opportunities to share expenses. Sites can also factor these events into the annual budget under patient recruitment expenses.

- Capture names and addresses of those who attend these events and send a follow up thank you letter with a list of upcoming studies that you think might be of interest to them.

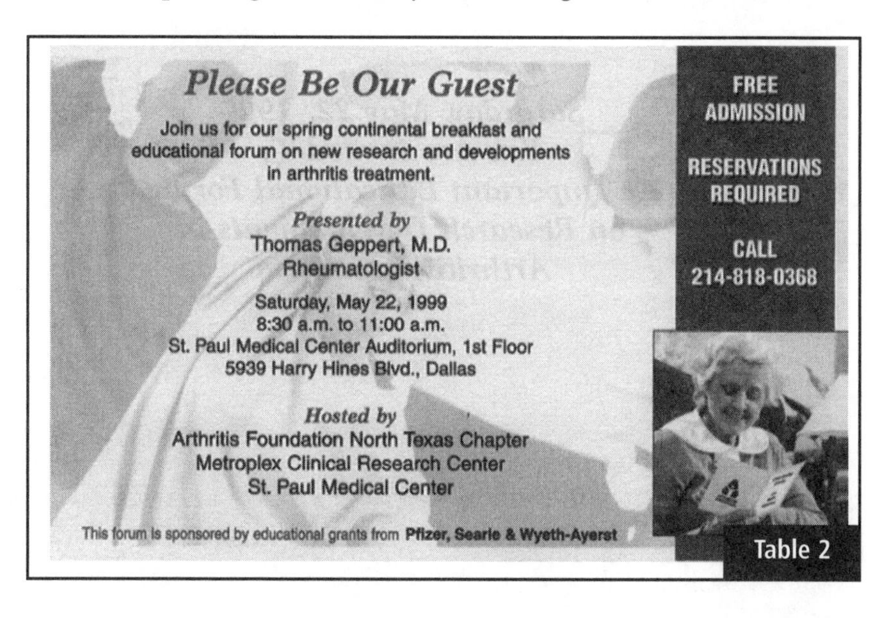

Please Be Our Guest
Join us for our spring continental breakfast and educational forum on new research and developments in arthritis treatment.
Presented by
Thomas Geppert, M.D.
Rheumatologist
Saturday, May 22, 1999
8:30 a.m. to 11:00 a.m.
St. Paul Medical Center Auditorium, 1st Floor
5939 Harry Hines Blvd., Dallas
Hosted by
Arthritis Foundation North Texas Chapter
Metroplex Clinical Research Center
St. Paul Medical Center
This forum is sponsored by educational grants from Pfizer, Searle & Wyeth-Ayerst
FREE ADMISSION
RESERVATIONS REQUIRED
CALL
214-818-0368
Table 2

Notify the speaker that there will probably be a "question and answer" session immediately following the presentation. It is also helpful to provide a list of enrolling and upcoming studies to the presenter prior to the speech. It is beneficial to keep metrics of the attendees who are recruited for clinical research studies as a result of attending the event.

THE WRITTEN WORD

"Advertising is like learning—a little is a dangerous thing."
–P.T. Barnum, Circus Owner

It's said "if you read it in the newspaper, it has to be true." Don't underestimate the power of the printed word, particularly when it appears in the local newspaper. The cost of print advertising varies from region to region, city to city, but traditionally, advertising in the local newspaper is the best return for an investment. Placement, frequency and subject matter play an important part in how successful an advertising campaign will be and control must be exerted over all three components.

Again, fostering a relationship with an advertising representative allows a site to request and receive preferential placement. Saying, "Place the ad beneath the two sisters, on the crease and away from all of the 'fad ads'" translates into "Place the ad under Dear Abby or Ann Landers, aligned at the crease and grouped with more stable, trusted advertising." A rep familiar with particular likes and dislikes

Table 3

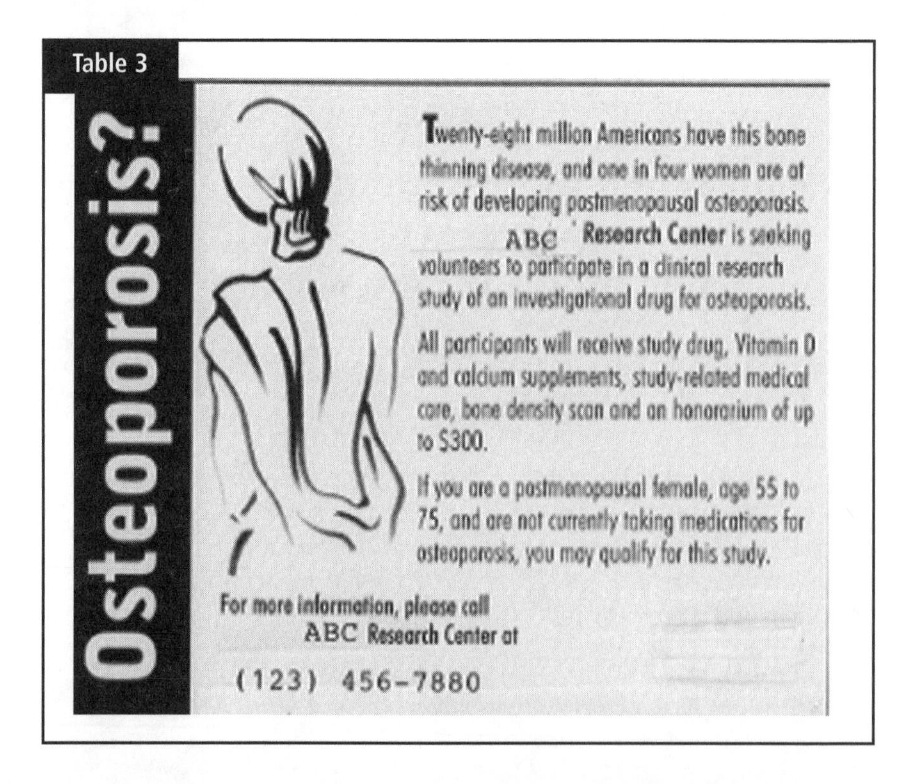

makes placement much easier, with less explanation necessary. Placing one ad at a time on an infrequent basis rarely garners the number of participants it requires to meet enrollment. A contract negotiated with the newspaper for multiple runs is a better deal in the long run.

The physical look of an advertisement requires the assistance of a professional designer to establish a "look" that identifies the site. The site logo, name, location and phone number should be readable and strategically placed. Graphics and clip art are handy tools when used effectively, but they should not overpower the message. (Table Three) Shy away from cartoon figures, typically this type of message is not one traditionally partnered with clinical research. Sensitivity to the ethnic and religious make up of the readership is essential when using artwork. A study designed for Asian Americans or American Indians would hardly be served by an ad featuring a picture of someone with blonde hair and blue eyes. The nuances of attracting a certain population and age group should be factored into the design for each study.

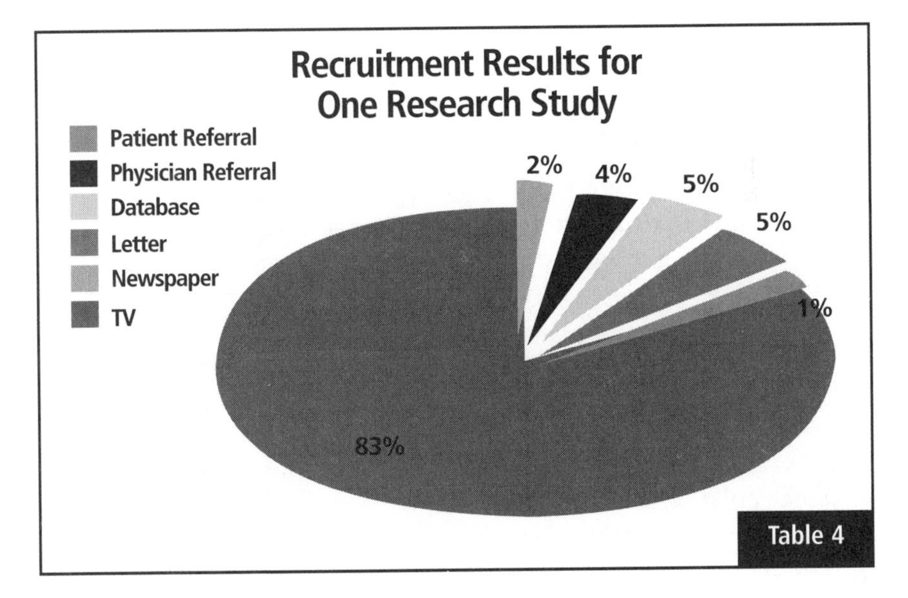

Table 4

Last, but certainly not least, results should be tracked after placement of each ad. How many calls were received after each placement? How many subjects were scheduled, did not qualify, and were not interested? These metrics will show where the patient population is located and how successfully they were accessed. When it comes to convincing a sponsor that a site has the patient population for their particular study these statistics are invaluable. (Table Four)

INSTITUTIONAL REVIEW BOARDS

"A man would do nothing if he waited until he could do it so well that no one could find fault with it."
–Cardinal John Henry Newman, Man of Letter

Just a note of caution when going forth with such enthusiasm into the community, don't do it with wild abandon. Always consider the guidelines of the ruling IRB when presenting study-specific press releases and ads. All print ads, press releases, radio and television commercials should be submitted to the sponsor for approval prior to IRB submission. Allow plenty of time to complete this process because the turnaround time for both sponsors and IRB's vary. Failing to produce advertising for review in a timely manner may result in the study closing before advertising can be implemented. Once the IRB approves advertising (with or without changes), placement and distribution can begin immediately.

SUMMING IT UP

"It takes more than capital to swing business. You've got to have the A.I.D. degree to get by...Advertising, Initiative and Dynamics."
–Ken Mulford Jr., Businessman

Trust, name recognition, involvement, dependability are a few of the words that come to mind when venturing out to establish a site's standing in the community. Every employee in the company is an ambassador for the site and should project an image in the community that bolsters their name and reputation. Employees who work like they own the company will also put their best foot forward in the community to get the message out that their site is the best place for clinical research.

It is in the best interest of every company to include their staff during the decision-making and poll them for their opinions about what they think will work and what won't. Team spirit is what gives companies an edge over their competitors, and the achievements of any successful organization are the combined efforts of each individual. Statistics prove that employees treat customers the way their employer treats them.

It will be up to the individual site to sift through all of the suggestions and come up with a plan that best suits its needs. Whatever the outcome of the search for the best way to involve a site in the community, remember that opportunity dances with those who are ready on the dance floor. Be prepared, be proactive and success will follow.

REFERENCES

[1] Recruitment Results, Radiant Research. Dallas, Texas. March 2000.

[2] "Recruiting Study Subjects." Food and Drug Administration Office of Health Affairs. Information Sheets, Guidance for Institutional Review Boards and Clinical Investigators. September 1998.

AUTHOR BIOGRAPHY

Margo Whitley is Director of Marketing and Patient Recruitment at Radiant Research in Dallas, Texas. Radiant Dallas is a multi-specialty investigator site dedicated to performing quality clinical research, phases II–IV. Radiant Research opened its doors in 1984 as Metroplex Clinical Research Center (MCRC). In 1999, MCRC joined Radiant Site Management Organization. Radiant Dallas conducts 65 to 70 clinical trials annually and all advertising/recruitment initiatives are under the direction of Ms. Whitley. A database of over 10,000 study patients and a strong recruitment team are hallmarks of her efforts to build a strong recruitment and retention program. She has developed novel approaches to both meeting enrollment and retaining study participants. Ms. Whitley has an extensive public relations background and serves on the boards of several local organizations.

Appendix 1

Release, Authorization and Consent for Media

I hereby authorize Research Center ABC to use and record on photographic film, motion picture film, videotape, audiotape or other medium my name, voice, likeness and performance, and I acknowledge that the recording is the sole and exclusive property of Research Center ABC in perpetuity.

I authorize in perpetuity any display, exhibition, sale, rental, publication and/or broadcast of said recording in all media now known or hereafter devised and throughout the universe irrespective of whether a fee, admission, rental, payment or other charge is required, and in doing, waive all rights that I may have for any claims to payments or royalties in connection therewith.

I hereby consent to the use of my name, likeness and biographical information for publicizing and promoting such distribution or use. I acknowledge that I have no right to compel my name, likeness, voice or performance to be included in any display, exhibition, sale, rental, publication and/or broadcast.

I warrant that I am free to enter into this license and that this agreement does not conflict with any existing contracts or agreements to which I am a party. I hereby release Research Center ABC, it's agents, employees, assigns, or distribution parties from any claims and any liability arising from the taking or subsequent distribution of the recording.

This authorization and release shall be for the benefit of Research Center ABC, and it's agents, employees, assigns and distributing parties and is binding an my heirs, executors and assigns.

Signature ______________________________

Printed Name ______________________________

Address ______________________________

City/State ______________________________

Date ______________________________

For Research Center ABC
AGREED & ACCEPTED BY: ____________________

CHAPTER 14

WOMEN AND MINORITIES: ELIMINATING BARRIERS FOR CLINICAL TRIAL PARTICIPATION

Marilyn North-Arnold, The Arnold Group

"In the past, medical research has focused on males and all too frequently, women have been included as an afterthought. Eliminating these barriers is the right thing to do."

–David Kessler, M.D., Former FDA Commissioner

Regulatory policy changes in the early 1990's lifted the barriers that prevented women, especially women of childbearing potential, from participating in clinical trials.[1, 2, 3] Women are no longer excluded from research studies that hold the promise to improve their health status and save lives. Today, the drug development pipeline contains more than 348 drugs focused on a variety of women's health issues: cardiovascular disease, muscoloskeletal disease, immune disorders, endocrine disease, urological disorders, psychiatric disorders, and cancer.[4]

The same 1993 NIH Revitalization Act also addressed the inclusion of minorities in clinical trial participation. Although no specific FDA guidance exists addressing minority participation in clinical trials, the FDA 1993 Gender Guideline clearly elucidates the FDA's expectation that all appropriate demographic subgroups be included in the drug development process.

These regulatory changes brought new challenges to the patient recruitment and retention process, requiring new and specific strategies to reach these expanded patient populations. The purpose of this chapter is to provide the reader with an easy to use guide, which highlights the basic issues and presents practical strategies in the recruitment and retention of women and minority populations. (This chapter offers the reader an examination of the basic issues and presents practical strategies for the recruitment and retention of both women and minorities in clinical trials.)

WHY INCLUSION?

The safety and efficacy of new drug treatments has traditionally been tested in the white male population, with results extrapolated to women. Because women have been excluded from the clinical trial process, alarming gaps in knowledge, including the effects of hormonal fluctuations and potential harm to a fetus, exist about many women's health conditions, thus negatively impacting their diagnosis, treatment and prevention.

The exclusion of women makes little sense, not only from a health perspective but also from a numbers perspective, since women compose 52% of the population[5], make 61% of physician visits, purchase 59% of prescription drugs, and make 75% of the health care decisions in U.S. households.[6]

Just as women have been excluded from clinical trial participation, so have minority populations. (Minority populations include African Americans, American Indians, Alaska Natives, Asians, Native Hawaiians or other Pacific Islanders and Hispanics in the U.S.)[7] Minorities suffer disproportionately from many diseases, exhibit higher rates of premature death and experience a poorer heath status during all stages of their lives. For example, lupus erythematosus occurs more often in Hispanic and African-American women than in White women and Puerto Rican and African-American men bear an increased incidence of prostate cancer.

These inequities extend into the research realm where under representation of minority populations are the norm. Only when these populations are included in numbers adequate to permit valid analyses of differences in treatment interventions can society at large gain equitably from the advances in new treatments and interventions.

PATIENT PERCEPTIONS

As with any outreach endeavor, an understanding of how the target customer thinks is critical to developing the appropriate recruitment and retention strategy. It is critical to understand the underlying attitudes and beliefs that influence their actions. For example, many women distrust the research process because of past negative events such as DES and thalidomide.[8] Others harbor resentment toward a male-dominated medical establishment that has for so long ignored their needs. Yet others readily participate, fervently believing that they are helping future generations through their participation. This attitude is so prevalent among women participants that a term has been coined to describe it: the construct of altruism.[9]

Minority groups generally harbor mistrust and suspicion about an establishment where there is so little common ground. Among the African-American groups mistrust of research exists because of abuses such as the Tuskegee experiment.[10] African-Americans are often unwilling to be "guinea pigs." In Hispanic groups where the patriarchal male dominates, women are often not permitted to participate in clinical trials.

Beliefs about the nature and prognosis of illness vary greatly among racial and ethnic groups. In addition the manner in which various cultural groups define symptoms and how and when they seek help, either through the formal health system or by utilizing folk medicines, varies enormously. These differences are largely unrecognized by health care providers. (Appendix One)

Strategies

Changes in potential patient perception are most readily achieved through the creation of three types of relationships: (1) between the research group and community groups, (2) between the study staff and potential study participant, and (3) between former study participants and current or potential patients. These relationships provide education about the clinical research process and a source of reliable and trusted information.

For each specific population, it is necessary to gather and analyze information such as: what community group(s) is most trusted by that population? Is it a church-based group? A low-income clinic? A daycare center? A rural community group? Who are the community leaders? Such an analysis provides a valuable framework for the development of subsequent patient recruitment and retention plans.

Clinical research staffs should reflect the composition of the target population and be familiar with and able to address their issues and concerns. Efforts need to be made to increase the numbers of women and minority investigators as well as well-trained research staff.

The development of "ambassador" programs linking former study participants with potential or current participants provides an invaluable resource. A well-known breast and cervical cancer screening program, "A Su Salud," targeted Hispanic women, informing them about the importance of screening as well as how and where to obtain services.[11] The success of the program resided in the use of role models providing personal testimonials to the target population. Creation of such relationships based on mutual trust and respect can begin to create positive attitudes among potential research participants and increase the patient pool.

ACCESS TO RESOURCES AND SERVICES

The ability to access resources and services is related to a person's socioeconomic status. Because women and minorities compose the majority of lower socioeconomic groups, an understanding of their lifestyle needs is critical to patient recruitment and retention success. Barriers to participation include childcare costs, transportation access and cost, food costs and the inability to take time away from a job.

Access can also be impeded by responsibilities inherent in the role of caregiver. Women are most frequently the caregivers to children, parents and spouses, leaving little time for clinical research participation. (Appendix Two)

Strategies

Strategies that address the constraints of limited time and financial resources are critical to successful recruitment and retention. Programs designed to increase access to clinical sites and services, bringing the service to the consumer, are effective. On-site solutions include providing flexible and extended clinic hours, childcare and transportation services. In addition mobile services, such as vans equipped with mammography and other screening technologies, increase patient protocol compliance. Financial remuneration for dependent care and transportation costs should be provided when not available at the site. Utilization of patient stipends that does not create coercion or a sense of undue influence is also appropriate.

COMMUNICATION AND OUTREACH EDUCATION PROGRAMS

Language and cultural barriers present one of the greatest challenges in minority patient recruitment and retention efforts. Low literacy levels and/or limited knowledge of English can impede understanding of critical information. In addition lack of understanding about the clinical trials process and specific health issues also prevent trial participation. For example, confusion about the issues of patient confidentiality is of primary concern among women.

Many women and minorities, especially those in low-income and low literacy levels, need to be better informed about health issues in order to change unhealthy lifestyle behaviors. However the groups at highest risk for not receiving understandable health information are often the most difficult to reach. Outreach programs designed with messages that are tailored to the particular cultural, social and economic circumstances of the target population provide excellent opportunities to include information about the clinical trials process and current trial opportunities. (Appendix Three)

Strategies

Plans to utilize the primary language of the target population in all aspects of clinical trial conduct is crucial, from outreach efforts through the informed consent process and beyond. Targeted media channels, ethnically appropriate messaging, low literacy materials and minority spokespersons are key components to a successful communication strategy. Additionally utilization of appropriately written patient education materials that explain the clinical trials process and information about specific health issues can help eliminate barriers to participation.

Identification of large-scale prevention campaigns, funded by the government and implemented at the community level, often provide venues for offering information about specific health related issues and an opportunity to inform patients about ongoing or future clinical trial opportunities. Private sector efforts, utilizing the resources of local businesses and the cooperation of non-profit organizations, are also effective in educating target populations.

Delivery of the message can be accomplished through a variety of communication methods and physical settings including health fairs, newsletters, "campaign" buttons, posters, TV and radio announcements, billboards, door-to-door canvassing, bus advertising, schools, work-site programs, grocery stores and educational programs in churches, workplaces and community centers.

Community partnerships and alliances with patient advocacy groups can provide a strong bond between research sites and potential patients. Often times a significant disconnect exists between minority groups and the medical establishment, including research sites. Partnerships within the community can create understanding and shared goals. Alliances with patient advocacy groups can provide culturally appropriate materials about specific disease states and health issues, as well as ideas on how to effectively reach the target population.

All members of a clinical research staff need appropriate training in the nuances of recruiting and retaining members of specific patient populations. The knowledge, enthusiasm, sensitivity and commitment displayed by staff when discussing a clinical trial can directly affect a patient's perception about clinical trial participation.

Patient referrals by community physicians can be another source of potential patients. A recent survey conducted by the Society for the Advancement of Women's Health Research indicates that women rely on their primary care physician as a primary source of clinical trial information.[12] Outreach education and increased awareness of clinical trial conduct to these physicians within the medical community can be a valuable resource to investigative sites.

OTHER ISSUES

Most of the strategies discussed above involve the design, implementation and evaluation of specific patient recruitment and retention strategies. Important related considerations include:

- Recognition of gender, cultural and ethnic issues related to patient recruitment and retention by the sponsor in the very early planning and design of a clinical trial. This includes protocol design, resource planning, and informed consent design and site selection.
- Allocation of sufficient resources to patient recruitment budgets to allow for the customization of patient recruitment strategies and support materials.
- Acknowledgement by clinical research sties that additional resources, such as increased staff time for training and outreach efforts, may be required to access particular patient populations.
- Enforcement of guideline and regulatory requirements that encourage and mandate the inclusion of a balanced and diverse study population.

THE INTERNET

Internet technology holds the promise to transform the clinical trial process, including patient recruitment and retention effort, especially those directed toward women. A recent national survey of women, ages 25 to 49, conducted by Georgetown University Medical School Department of Obstetrics and Gynecology found that 73% of women use the Internet to find health related information.[13]

Although still in its infancy, potential barriers exist to patient recruitment efforts. Issues such as effective screening processes, patient confidentiality, conversion of screened to enrolled patients, matching potential patients to participating sites and access to the Internet by lower socioeconomic groups need to be addressed.

EVALUATION

No strategy is complete without an evaluation or metrics component. A method must be established to capture, analyze and evaluate information on techniques employed. This provides valuable information for mid-course corrections, if needed, and future patient recruitment and retention plans.

SUMMARY

If recruitment and retention strategies are to be effective, education and outreach programs must involve the target patient population, including "subgroups" such as women and minorities, related community networks and clinical research providers. For any study that is to include these subgroups, sponsors and investigators need to make a substantial commitment to address the issues discussed in this chapter in every aspect of study design and conduct.

Broader issues include patient perceptions that are the result of societal and cultural practices, access to services, communication and linguistic issues, community networks and outreach education.

Successful patient recruitment and retention is about people developing relationships. Patients give a "gift" of themselves when participating in clinical research. Adherence to Good Clinical Practices provides protection, research ethics provides respect for persons, but relationships developed at the sites supply the element of trust and caring. There is no media or technology that can be substituted for these valuable relationships.

"Medical research volunteers are modern day heroes (heroines). Without these pioneers we wouldn't have many of our modern day advances."
–David McCall, M.D., American Heart Association spokesperson

REFERENCES

[1] NIH. Revitalization Act, 1993.

[2] Food and Drug Administration. "Guidelines for the Study and Evaluation of Gender Differences in Clinical Evaluation of Drugs." 1993.

[3] FDAMA. Section 115, 1997.

[4] PhRMA. Survey 1999.

[5] U.S. Census Bureau data, 1996.

[6] Smith Barney Research. "Women's Healthcare." April 1977.

[7] Office of Research on Minority Health, NIH.

[8] Ragavan. "Drug Development and Women." John Wiley and Sons, Inc., 1998.

[9] Women and Health Research, Volume I. National Academy Press, 1994.

[10] Des Jarlais. Am J Public Health 1991; 81(11): 1393-94.

[11] Vellozi et al., Women's Health Issues 6 (March/April), 1996.

[12] Society for the Advancement of Women's Health Research, Survey Results, 1999.

[13] Newsedge Work Groups.com, July 13, 2000.

AUTHOR BIOGRAPHY

Marilyn North Arnold is the President and founder of The Arnold Group, a professional practice consulting group, providing clinical trial and medical communications services to the pharmaceutical, biotechnology and device industries. An expert in the area of business start-ups and "greenfield"site deployment, Ms. Arnold founded the first Site Management Organizations devoted solely to conducting women's health clinical trials.

A long-standing women's health advocate, Ms. Arnold is professionally and personally committed to improving the standard of women's health care in the U.S. Her membership activities include: Past Chair of the Corporate Advisory Committee of the Society for the Advancement of Women's Health Research; member of the Board of Directors of the American Medical Association Foundation; AMWA's committee on the Advanced Women's Health

Curriculum; the Task Force of the National Academy of Women's Health Medical Education; the Steering Committee of AMA's Women's Health Summit; and the Steering Committee of the Association of Reproductive Health Professional's National Adolescent Reproductive Health Initiative.

Ms. Arnold also serves as a member of the Drug Information Association's journal editorial board and is a PhD candidate in the field of bioethics.

Barriers and Strategies in Recruiting Women and Minority Volunteers—Patient Perceptions

Barrier	Strategy
Mistrust, suspicion and lack of understanding about the clinical research process.	Identify the specific concerns of the target population. Train the clinical trial staff about sensitive racial, cultural or gender issues. Create culturally appropriate education material which address the clinical research process. Educate patients about the regulatory requirements, including the informed consent process, which protect human subjects. Identify community, business and/or religious leaders who can help to create community partnerships and common goals and act in an advisory capacity. Establish, develop relationships between: Community groups and the research group; Research staff and prospective study participants; Former and prospective study participants ("ambassador" program); Employ clinical research staff that reflect the composition of the target population; Stress the importance of one-to-one relationships between research staff members and study participants.
Denial and fear surrounding a suspected illness or health condition may preclude participation.	Development of specific health related programs and support groups which provide information and supportive group dynamics.

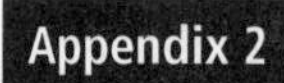

Appendix 2

Barriers and Strategies in Recruiting Women and Minority Volunteers—Limited Access to Resources and Services

Barrier	Strategy
Time constraints imposed by role as caregiver prevents clinical research participation.	Establish flexible and/or extended clinical hours Provide child care or home care services or reimbursement for same Develop alternative sources of service delivery (mobile mammography services, in-home examinations)
Transportation to research site is unavailable or too expensive for lower socioeconomic groups.	Provide transportation or cover the cost of travel
Financial constraints that prevent clinical research participation (such as the inability to pay for meals and child care).	Provide patient stipends that cover out of pocket costs

Appendix 3

Barriers and Strategies in Recruiting Women and Minority Volunteers—Communication and Education

Barrier	Strategy
Language barriers	Plan to use primary language of the target population in all aspects of the clinical trial. Use of minority spokespersons/community leaders. Employ research staff who speak the language of the target population.
Lack of low literacy and culturally sensitive health information	Design ethnically appropriate low literacy materials. Create community partnerships that provide a link between research sites and potential patient subgroups. Develop alliances with patient advocacy groups.

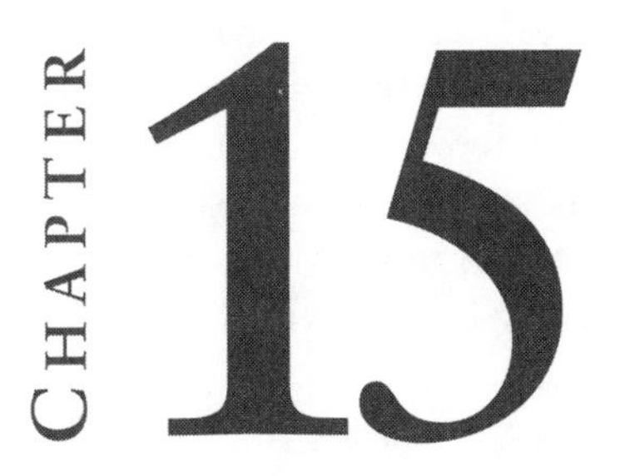

Issues in the Recruitment of Pediatric Subjects: New Challenges and Possibilities

Molly Matthews, Matthews Media Group, Inc.

For parents of children confronting serious illness, a pediatric clinical trial may be a life-giving antidote for despair, the hope that at least some measure of relief, if not an actual cure for a child's suffering, is within their grasp. Depending on the nature of the disease itself, a clinical research study may be a more questionable opportunity, where the experiment's risk tends to outweigh potential benefits for a given child or children in general. For other parents a study may simply represent the only means for their uninsured child to receive the sophisticated medical care that can make a difference and, as such, represents a purely economic decision.

Children and adolescents are not merely "little adults" in physiological or biochemical terms any more than they are in psychological terms, and prescribing medications that are only weight-dosed could (and often does) carry unforeseen consequences. Children metabolize certain drugs differently than adults, making formulaic weight-extrapolated dosing problematic. In addition, pediatric physiology, certainly through puberty and into early adolescence, is a work in progress, and the effects of medications on these developing systems, both short- and long-term, can be markedly different from the effects on mature adults.

Clinical research is required to support and further medical advances. However, Americans now stand in the troubled light of a number of well-publicized ethical lapses in the conduct of research. This same light casts shadows across the purview of watchful federal regulators who are charged with protecting the public interest as they maintain a special vigilance around research involving children.

For pharmaceutical companies, pediatric trials offer the means to expand a medication's approved indications, bringing valuable therapies to a needy population while simultaneously protecting and enhancing formidable opportunities in an increasingly competitive marketplace.

Children themselves might carry different perspectives about clinical research participation. Being a patient in a trial can create a sense of pride for a young person who values the significant fulfillment in being selected to support research that will benefit many others with the same illness. To another child in that same study, trial participation is not a badge of honor but a burden, a reminder and further reinforcement that they are different because of an illness.

Many other competing or conflicting issues at play, flavored by a mix of players whose goals and concerns are frequently at odds, recruitment for pediatric clinical trials presents a unique set of challenges. Successful patient recruitment for pediatric trials demands a multifaceted understanding of the motivations and expectations of patients, parents, siblings, physicians and other health care providers, regulators, researchers and sponsors, along with both experience and skill in communicating directly and effectively with each of these groups. As discussed throughout this text, these challenges are complicated by the fact that the current climate for medical research places premiums on accelerated recruitment, requiring rapid response to a study protocol's need, with little time for reflection.

OVERLOOKED AND UNDER STUDIED

Until recently, pediatric clinical trials drew little attention because children, like minorities and women, represented an essentially under-studied segment of the human community when it came to drug research. As a result, medications prescribed for children for illnesses shared with adults (e.g., diabetes, asthma, bipolar disorder) were rarely tested specifically on a pediatric population, and dosage recommendations were simply weight-based recalculations of approved adult dosages. The term "therapeutic orphans" has been historically used to describe the state of neglect attended to children in pharmaceutical research, a situation that extended well into the waning years of the twentieth century. A 1990 report of the American Academy of Pediatrics noted that 80% of new molecular entities approved from 1984 to 1989 had no information on pediatric use.[1] Four years later a survey conducted for the Food and Drug Administration reported the ten medications most often prescribed for children and adolescents on an outpatient basis (accounting for 5 million prescriptions annually) contained either inadequate information regarding pediatric use in their labeling, or none at all.[2]

THE FDAMA KICK-START

The Federal Government has, since the late 1970s, sought increasingly greater data from pharmaceutical companies regarding the effect of medications prescribed in pediatric populations. Those initiatives have culminated in legislation and regulations that provide "carrot and stick" incentives for pharmaceutical companies to include children and adolescents in clinical research.

The Pediatric Rule of 1997 (codified in 21CFR201.23, 314.55, 601.27) is the stick: it requires sponsors to conduct pediatric studies of certain new and marketed drugs that have pediatric indications; moreover, after December 2, 2000, all new drug applications (NDAs) for pharmaceuticals used to treat, diagnose, or prevent illnesses that occur in both adult and pediatric populations will have to demonstrate safety and efficacy through clinical trials conducted specifically in a pediatric population.[3]

If the Pediatric Rule is the stick, Section 505(A) of the Federal Drug Administration Modernization Act (FDAMA), signed into law on November 21, 1997, holds forth the proverbial carrot. It extends six-months of additional patent exclusivity for a number of currently approved and new medications if those drugs, in response to a written request from the FDA, are tested for their specific effects on children and adolescents.

As of February 10, 2000, the FDA had issued requests for pediatric studies on 115 medications currently prescribed for children.[4]

Seventeen of these drugs have, after fulfilling the stipulations of the FDA requests, received 6-month patent extensions. The additional protection periods extend to all uses of a drug, not just its pediatric applications. For a blockbuster drug, an additional 6-months of patent protection could mean staggering revenues.

To qualify for extended patent protection, sponsors face a sundown date of January 1, 2002. After that date, the FDA can grant the additional 6-month exclusivity only under special circumstances. That, in turn, places pressure on sponsors to accelerate pediatric recruiting efforts for trials.

Therapeutic orphans no more, children and adolescents have now been thrust front and center into the world of clinical research. Those involved in that recruitment, sponsors, investigators and outsourcing agencies, have had to focus on the problems and particulars of finding, enrolling and maintaining patients in pediatric trials, some of which are described below.

A LOOK AT THE CHILDREN

What criteria define a pediatric patient? The answer might seem obvious, but criteria and definition are basic to recruitment for pediatric clinical trials. Toddlers are definitely pediatric patients, but so too, according to FDA guidelines, are 16-year-olds. On the other hand, 17-year-olds may not be. The enormous disparities in physical development between a first-grader and a teenager raise certain flags and will obviously affect study design. In selected pediatric studies being conducted under FDAMA guidelines that have broad age inclusion, i.e., 6 years-old to 16, the FDA has requested that sponsors make efforts to ensure that their study population be stratified by age and balanced by cohort. For example, a certain percentage of the study cohort must be grouped between ages 6 and 10, with an equal percentage aged 11 to 16. This stratification is intended to capture data on any differences in the drug's efficacy and utilization that occur across varying stages of physical development. Similarly, the developmental differences between girls and boys suggest, for certain compounds, the need to assure a representative sample of both sexes in the study. Requiring representative numbers of participants from different age groups and both genders carries, in turn, impacts on recruitment strategies and methods.

Coupled with these factors are the even greater disparities in social development. Younger children are likely to listen to their parents and take medications when told; teenagers decidedly less so. Teenagers may have the ability to read and understand an informed consent document, but no elementary school age child can. Moreover, the soaring sense of self and power that accompanies adolescence may make teenagers unwilling even to admit they are ill. To do so, and to further acknowledge illness by participating in a clinical trial, amounts to an acceptance of their own limitations, a dent in their belief in their own invincibility. That belief resonates with particular strength among certain ethnic teenagers, who place great emphasis on the virtues of strength and stoicism associated with adulthood.

For those attempting to recruit for pediatric trials, these social differences will affect the kinds of messages crafted and the media in which they appear. Who is the proper spokesperson, Barney or Madonna? Big Bird or a cast member from *Dawson's Creek* or *Buffy*? What's a better retention item, a CD carrying case or a coloring book? Is advertising placed on radio stations that attract teen listeners, or focus only on the stations that appeal to their parents, who in the end will have to make the ultimate decision about their child's participation?

Our experience has revealed techniques and approaches that address the variations in recruiting for pediatric clinical trials. For young people who have already expressed pride in volunteering and participating, recognition of their efforts can be as simple as a well-designed certificate of appreciation, or include a variety of retention items, such as hats, T-shirts, or water bottles bearing a study's logo and name. A comic book that used a superhero-based narrative line to explain a study, its goals, and the altruistic aspects of participation proved to be a compelling, highly effective, and "kid-friendly" communication tool.

Extensive planning was invested to assure that the comic book's language and underlying message was not coercive and presented a balanced view of trial participation, emphasizing the significance of language and word choice in attracting young people to a research study. Just as the dramatic but tailored story line of a comic book proved to be a successful recruitment tool, a shopping mall screening table drew far more children (and parents) on behalf of a juvenile diabetes study with a banner asking "Does Diabetes Run In Your Family?" rather than simply stating "Free Diabetes Screening."

Altruism and community welfare are meaningful concepts to children, more than many adults realize. Young people take pride in highly-developed social values, and advertising messages that invoke or echo these values are inevitably more successful than straightforward announcements of medical research efforts. The mainstream logic of public relations would hold that use of the word "free" is always the best attractor, but we learned that speaking to altruism was, in fact, a greater attractor. This observation underscores a pivotal concept in recruiting children to clinical trials: children and adolescents respond to advertising and calls to action that are not only communicative, succint and easy to remember, but invoke a sense of family care, concern and social responsibility.

RECRUITING CHILDREN—AND THEIR PARENTS

The key role parents must play in pediatric recruiting underscores the fact that recruitment among children focuses only partially on the child who may happen to have the specific medical condition that meets a drug protocol's inclusion criteria. It is the parent or guardian, after all, who provides legal authorization for a child to participate in a clinical trial. It is the parent/guardian who will struggle with issues of benefit and risk. It is the parent/guardian, in addition to the child, with whom study coordinators and investigators will discuss the rights and responsibilities of a study subject, informed consent and the importance of placebo. It is therefore the entire family who is the communications target audience for clinical trials involving children.

But the role of parent/guardian of a child in a pediatric trial transcends the clinical and legal requirements for participation. When recruiting for pediatric clinical trials, especially studies that require newly or non-diagnosed patients or those not receiving medication, it is the parent's or guardian's antennae that must be activated. A child may not want to go to school or play with friends, but it is a parent or guardian who must first question whether these behaviors reflect an emotional or personality disorder. Parents face these quandaries all the time—when, for example, can a teenager's problem with weight be reclassified as obesity? And if so reclassified, how much medical attention is justified or appropriate? How or should this child enter a weight-reduction or hypertension study?

A similar line of questioning has surrounded the efficacy of the stimulant methylphenidate (Ritalin). At what point is an ebullient and energetic child, in fact, dysfunctionally hyperactive, and in need of intervention? Are clinical screening instruments for hyperactivity and attention-deficit disorders accurate? What do we really know about the effects of amphetamine-based stimulants in children? This debate, with its swamp of troubling, and unanswered, questions, illustrates the ambiguity that exists for medical providers, researchers and parents when faced with making rational and humane decisions about what constitutes normal childhood behavior, and what demands medical intervention.

In the course of navigating such difficult ethical terrain, the very act of acknowledging a child's illness or susceptibility to illness, the usual *sine qua non* of clinical research, may be viewed as an indictment of parenting ability. In the case of the obese child sought for a hypertension study, for example, many parents might be reluctant to admit their overweight children are in fact obese, an often pejorative label that could imply they did not provide proper nutrition or are unable to control their child's impulses. Recruiting children for trials involving mood disorders or mental illness raises similar challenges as parents' wonder why they cannot ease their child's anxieties or fears, and at what level of severity these fears constitute a "diagnosis" that infers a parenting failure.

Equally important as familial attitudes toward illness are cultural perspectives exhibited by different ethnic groups. Shyness has recently been identified as a behavioral diagnosis, and trials are already being designed to test certain drugs that may offer symptomatic relief. In families of Middle-Eastern origin, where custom limits a child's exposure to social situations, extraordinary shyness, clinically diagnosable shyness, will go unrecognized. Similarly, in contrast to the American fascination with waif-like thinness as a mark of beauty, South Asian tradition places a premium on fullness. Recruitment for childhood obesity trials might fall on deaf ears in that population. Expressions of pain or discomfort is discouraged among many African-American or Hispanic boys, in keeping with the general dictates of their cultures, a factor that could limit their willingness (or familial interest) in participating in studies investigating analgesics.

While some parents are reluctant to identify their children as potentially eligible candidates for clinical research for either cultural or attitudinal reasons, others find clinical trials a route to otherwise unavailable medical care for their children. A clinical trial may be the last and only avenue to the level of physician care that offers true hope for impoverished children and families, bringing a child access to specialist physicians denied under managed care or insurance-based programs.

Whatever the route that opens the way for a parental decision, be it economic need or overcoming philosophical or sociocultural objections, recognizing that a child might qualify for a clinical trial is only the first step that demands parental and familial involvement. Once a child is accepted into a study, compliance becomes a family activity. Someone has to accompany the child on every visit to the research study center, which may be located far from the neighborhood. A parent must take time away from work; brothers and sisters miss school. In-laws may be called upon to help with transportation, or stay with younger children at home during study visits. Medication must be taken on time, diets may have to change, study diaries maintained, all of which have an impact on a family's regular activities. Invariably, the fact that every family has a unique set of interdependencies will one way or another be reflected in a child's enrollment and participation in a pediatric clinical trial.

Familial relationships also affect a child's participation in clinical research in other subtler ways. If a child senses that the family deems it important to continue in a study, the child may experience (even if it is never overtly stated) a quiet pressure to remain in the study. This, in turn, can lead a study participant to withhold information when not feeling well in order not to disappoint, or to hide or misstate symptoms to avoid rebuke for not being a "good patient." The desire to accommodate expectations typically extends to the relationship a child develops with the research team as well. The possibility that a child may subvert his or her personal experience in order to please an adult authority figure, parent or otherwise, needs to be considered when crafting and explaining informed consent materials. This issue becomes even more stark when monetary reimbursement is provided for participation: imagine the pressure on a child from a family of little means whose honest answer to the questions "Is everything okay?" or "Any problems since you started taking the new medicine?" could cost the family dollars.

SITES AT THE READY

If the psychological and cultural issues impacting pediatric clinical trials are formidable, other equally difficult logistical concerns affect pediatric recruitment. The choice of principal investigator (PI), site location and amenities, and study support with communication and outreach tools might seem elementary, the ordinary nuts and bolts of running a study. Still, these points often escape those involved in structuring and executing recruitment for trials.

Sponsors of clinical research routinely look to a PIs past and current patient panels as rich sources for trial patients. At times the specific nature of a physician's practice, patient catchment and demographics, or the economic indicators driving medical care choices in the physician's area are either superficially assessed or not included in an overall assessment of any given physician's suitability as a principal investigator. When recruiting for an unusual genetic disorder or pediatric cancer trials, signing pediatric specialists and sub-specialists as PIs would logically be the best route for research sponsors, since children with these conditions are nearly always referred for specialty care. On the other hand, pediatric rheumatologists may not be the most successful recruiters/investigators for a chronic fatigue study that seeks children as yet undiagnosed and untreated. Those patients are more likely to be identified initially by their primary care pediatricians or family practice teams, including physicians, physician assistants and nurse practitioners.

Office hours are another consideration. The standard 9-to-5 regimen doesn't lend itself to optimal participation for pediatric trials. During most of those hours children are in school, and many parents are reluctant to have them miss more class time than they normally would. It also means that working parents, who would have to accompany their children for the office visits required by the study, must miss work, a luxury many simply cannot afford. Solutions seem simple, later hours, weekend appointments, but too often researchers and their staffs are unwilling to revise schedules to accommodate their pediatric trial participants' needs.

Basic amenities at a research site matter to children and their parents or guardians. Waiting rooms should have play areas, children's books and art that appeals to pediatric patients. Such factors go a long way toward taking the sting out of a child's office visit, offering activities to occupy them during the often long or unexpected waits that invariably occur, and helping to take their minds off what may be an uncomfortable and fearful experience.

These practical issues are compounded by sharp and steady growth in the number of independent research centers aligned with private practice physicians, as opposed to the academic medical centers where much of the nation's clinical research has previously been conducted. With incomes squeezed by managed care, many physicians with relatively little research experience seek to augment their revenues by serving as principal investigators for clinical trials. At many of these sites, unfortunately, inexperience shows: the proper infrastructure may be lacking, there may not be enough qualified research staff, and no real emphasis is placed on active recruitment or targeted outreach. The PIs and their study coordinators often lack an established network of referring physicians or ongoing relationships with intermediary and support groups who can be invaluable sources of recruits for clinical trials. And while these issues certainly affect recruitment for all studies, they carry particularly significant impact for pediatric trials where so many other critical variables, cultural, psychosocial, economic, and logistical, are also in play.

LESSONS LEARNED

Despite daunting challenges, recruitment for pediatric and adolescent clinical trials can succeed provided those involved in recruitment are aware of the challenges and take carefully planned steps to meet them. Based on our experiences recruiting for pediatric clinical trials on behalf of both government and industry sponsors, a group of useful guidelines for pediatric recruitment initiatives have emerged that are both illustrative of recruiting needs and applicable across a variety of clinical research objectives.

Motivate Mothers

Promotional materials and advertising placements for pediatric trials need to target parents more than children. In most families this means mothers, since decisions about health care, especially a child's health care, are made by mothers. Advertising campaigns must target mothers listening and reading habits. As mothers respond to concerns raised by other mothers, testimonial-type advertising is also quite effective.

When distributing materials, a corner beauty salon where women get their hair done is a better location for a poster seeking kids for an asthma study than the local video arcade where asthmatic children may spend much of their free time. The "easy listening," oldies, or soft rock stations that appeal to adult listeners are more appropriate for radio advertising than the hard rock and rap stations adolescents favor. Daytime television targeted to women (talk shows, Oprah, daytime dramas) offer sensible points for airing TV commercials in support of pediatric trials, as opposed to Saturday morning children's programming, or Monday Night Football.

Motivate Children

The idea that a clinical trial may provide a remedy for a child's health-related problem could be a powerful incentive for a parent. It may not, on the other hand, be such a potent motivator for the child who must take a medication, give up Saturday mornings, or have blood drawn on a regular basis. To offset the obvious misgivings a child might experience when faced with these options, an attempt must be made to instill a sense of uniqueness and significance in clinical trial participation. It works far better, from a young person's perspective, if a study is memorable in the way other child-focused products are, with bright color schemes, a memorable name, an easy acronym, a well-defined logo and individualized graphics.

Incentive items can underscore a study's recognition factor with participants, creating a further resonance with consistent and clearly-designed graphic elements on study materials such as posters and brochures. One successful incentive example is a recognition book that tracks each visit and specifically thanks children for their efforts on behalf of a study. After each visit a child can redeem a visit recognition certificate for an appreciation item. Conveying uniqueness, offering a degree of pleasure and reward, and underscoring a child's sense of pride in making a valued contribution are all methods of both "branding" a study and offering an opportunity to enhance and maximize communication between children and their parents, as well as between participating families, PIs, and site personnel.

Access Intermediary Groups

Parents rely on trusted individuals, organizations and institutions for information like; advocacy groups, their churches, their children's schools, their pediatricians and clinics. Outreach to these organizations, at both the local and national levels, can provide valuable allies in raising awareness among parents about their children's health and their options for treatment, including clinical trials. Specific advocacy or intermediary-based outreach techniques that have proven successful in bringing patients to clinical trials include:

- disease-specific screenings held at churches or in community clinics ("Does Diabetes Run In Your Family?")
- informational seminars at churches, libraries, or community centers that present, discuss, and answer questions about a trial and its objectives
- direct mailings from established advocacy groups on behalf of a trial, with contact points for more information
- articles placed in advocacy newsletters or content on advocacy web sites about a clinical trial with contact points for more information about sites and screening criteria partnerships between advocacy groups and research sites to share resources and optimize access to and for potential participants
- support to advocacy groups and/or sites with professionally created graphics and communications solutions

It's a Family Affair

Remembering that children cannot elect to enroll themselves in clinical trials is critical in the implementation of strategies aimed at successful and large-scale recruitment of children. Families must be the focus and target of virtually all marketing and communication outreach efforts, and various points of timing and placement become important in reaching children...and their parents. If random intercepts or off-site screenings are an important element in recruitment, choose sites and times when children will actually be accompanying their parents. Rather than schedule an event at a local mall for Saturday, when kids go there to be with their friends and to get away from their parents, think about a back-to-school sale day when the family is shopping together. Include the family when designing incentive packages and retention programs: a dinner for four, a trip to the movies, or a day at the ballpark are all ways to effectively say thanks for the efforts of children and their families on behalf of that all too often go unrewarded.

PEDIATRIC CLINICAL TRIALS AT A CROSSROADS

For the first time in the history of modern medicine and pharmaceutical development, regulatory and legislative mandates fuel substantive research initiatives on behalf of children's health. Despite this fresh national energy supporting improved and comprehensive pediatric trials. The challenges remain significant, not the least of which involve complex ethical issues surrounding familial beliefs about health and medicine, children's expectable hesitancy about being subjects of research, and various institutional and industry needs to maximize recruiting goals.

For far too long children shared with the elderly the problem of being at a nearly invisible edge of the social continuum: out of the way and off the economic chart. Yet the welfare of children lies at the heart of our most valuable cultural and spiritual imperatives, and with that holds a definitive social and scientific importance for all of us. Successful pediatric clinical trial recruitment demands vigorous, eclectic and innovative approaches to the array of issues, concerns, needs and individuals involved in the multi-tiered business of clinical trials. The vital thread that has proven consistently effective in linking strategies to children, parents and investigators rests in keeping all recruiting efforts participant-centered, and always remembering the fundamental concern at stake, the health of children everywhere.

REFERENCES

[1] "Regulations Requiring Manufacturers to Assess the Safety and Effectiveness of New Drugs and Biological Products in Pediatric Patients, Proposed Rule." Department of Health and Human Services, Food and Drug Administration, 21CFR 201, 312, 314, 601. *Federal Register*. August 15, 1997. Vol. 62, p.43900.

[2] *Ibid.*

[3] "Regulations Requiring Manufacturers to Assess the Safety and Effectiveness of New Drugs and Biological Products in Pediatric Patients, Proposed Rule." Department of Health and Human Services, Food and Drug Administration, 21CFR 201, 312, 314, 601. *Federal Register*. December 2, 1998. Vol. 63, p.66631.

[4] Pediatric Exclusivity Statistics. U.S. Food and Drug Administration, Center for Drug Evaluation and Research. www.fda.gov/cder/pediatric/wrstats.htm. May 18, 2000.

AUTHOR BIOGRAPHY

Molly Mahoney Matthews is the founder, president and chief executive officer of Matthews Media Group, Inc. (MMG), a full-service health communications and public relations firm in Rockville, Maryland. Recognized by the Washington Business Journal as the fourth largest public relations firm in the Washington, D.C. area in 1999, MMG is known for its award-winning public education and patient recruitment campaigns, graphic solutions, web sites and videos.

MMG's government clients include many of the institutes at the National Institutes of Health (NIH), including the National Cancer Institute and the National Institute of Allergy and Infectious Diseases; the Department of Health and Human Services Office on Women's Health; and the Centers for Disease Control and Prevention. Private pharmaceutical relationships include Bristol-Myers Squibb, Eli Lilly, Glaxo Wellcome, Janssen Pharmaceutica, and SmithKline Beecham.

Ms. Matthews has developed a participant-centered focus in providing patient recruitment services to NIH and the pharmaceutical industry, a unique recruitment model that includes working closely with community-based clinics, partnering with intermediary organizations and utilizing local and national media strategies.

Ms. Matthews was selected for the Leadership Washington class of 2000. She sits on the board of directors for KidSave International, whose mission is dedicated to ending the neglect of institutionalized children and to providing nurturing home solutions for them. Ms. Matthews is also a member of the national board for Operation Smile, a charity that provides free reconstructive surgery to children with facial deformities.

CHAPTER 16

Multinational Guidelines and Obstacles to Patient Recruitment

Diana L. Anderson, Ph.D., Rheumatology Research International

Clinical trials are truly a global concern as 60% of studies now contain a global component.[1] Successful patient recruiting means understanding and respecting the idiosyncrasies inherent in recruiting worldwide. Prospective patients around the world have varying levels of awareness of clinical trials, and governments have vastly different degrees of openness and acceptance of the conduct of clinical research.

Table 1

Four Key Factors Influencing International Patient Recruitment Practices

- National Laws
- Ethics Committees
- Investigators and their Perceptions
- The Patients Themselves

Source: CenterWatch

Approaches deemed appropriate for patient recruitment reflect a country's culture, history, regulatory environment, ethical concerns, general awareness of clinical trials and the nature of its healthcare delivery system. Table One identifies four key factors that influence the type of patient recruitment initiatives practiced in different countries.[2]

Although the types of patient recruitment activities vary from country to country, there are global principles that serve as the underpinnings for all recruitment efforts. Most of these principles are ethical standards adopted by clinical investigators around the world in an effort to protect research subjects from unreasonable risks and to treat them with respect. How these principles are interpreted around the globe leads to today's diversity in recruitment practices.

THE EVOLUTION OF PATIENT RECRUITMENT PRACTICES

Clinical trials have been in existence for centuries, but the modern randomized double-blind, placebo-controlled multi-center study is largely a product of the twentieth century. Going into the twenty-first century, the conduct of trials that are increasingly complex and global highlights the need for standardization of protocol adherence, data collection, data cleaning and data submission. Some of the international guidelines address these issues. Methods of patient recruitment, however, are far from standardized. They vary tremendously across the globe, despite the fact that the practices tend to spring from the same sets of universal clinical practice standards. This is a reflection of diverse cultural norms and the fact that the international guiding principles do not state specifically what recruitment materials can say or are appropriate. Ethics Committees

Table 2 **First Principle of the Nuremburg Code**

The voluntary consent of the human subject is absolutely essential. This means that the person involved should have legal capacity to give consent, should be so situated as to be able to exercise free power of choice, without intervention of any element of force, fraud, deceit, duress, overreaching or ulterior form of constraint or coercion; and should have sufficient knowledge and comprehension of the elements of the subject mater involved as to enable him to make an understanding and enlightened decision. This latter element requires that before the acceptance of an affirmative decision by the experimental subject there should be made known to him the nature, duration and purpose of the experiment; the method and means by which it is to be conducted; all inconveniences and hazards reasonably to be expected; and the effects upon his health or person which may possibly come from his participation in the experiment.

The duty and responsibility for ascertaining the quality of the consent rests upon each individual who initiates, directs or engages in the experiment. It is the personal duty and responsibility, which may not be delegated to another with impunity.

Source: Nuremburg Code

are charged with reviewing the wording and presentation of recruitment materials, and because there are thousands of Ethics Committees around the globe, it is possible to have thousands of interpretations of "acceptable" recruitment approaches.

This multinational diversity may have its roots in the Nuremberg Code of 1947, which is one of the first collections of global principles guiding clinical trials and was part of the judgement handed down by the war tribunal following atrocities committed in World War II, including human experimentation.[3] This code contained ten principles, the first of which established that informed consent must be given freely, without coercion, by prospective subjects. (Table Two) The other principles in the code speak to the taking of precautions to prevent unnecessary mental and physical suffering by subjects, and state that research should be conducted by scientifically qualified staff.

Table 3

Efficacy Topics from the International Conference on Harmonization

- Standards for Dose Response Studies
- Standards for Carcinogenicity Testing in Subjects
- Good Clinical Practice
- Clinical Safety Data Management

Source: ICH Guidelines

The Declaration of Helsinki was first adopted in 1964 by the World Medical Association (WMA) and has been revised several times, most recently in 1996.[4] A revised draft was presented to the WMA in 1999, but was rejected. This declaration is widely regarded as the definitive set of ethical standards for the conduct of biomedical research using humans. Since 1964, the declaration has evolved from a relatively broad set of ethical principles to a more defined, prescriptive set of guidelines addressing numerous subject protections and investigator guidelines. It is difficult to obtain global consensus on interpretations of the declaration because perceptions of ethical standards are not universal. As an example, vague terms such as "acceptable risk" can be interpreted in an infinite number of ways.

The International Conference on Harmonization (ICH), initiated in 1990, is a joint initiative involving both regulators and industry as equal partners in the scientific and technical discussions of worldwide testing procedures. ICH brings together the regulatory authorities of Europe, Japan and the United States and experts from the pharmaceutical industry in these regions to discuss scientific and technical aspects of product registration for new drugs. ICH has several categories including Quality Topics, Safety Topics, Efficacy Topics and Multidisciplinary Topics. Efficacy Topics address standards for conducting clinical studies in human subjects, including Good Clinical Practice (GCP). (Table Three)

The topic of GCP refers to an international ethical and scientific quality standard for designing, conducting, recording and reporting trials involving the participation of human subjects. The objective of GCP guidelines is to provide a unified standard for the European Union, Japan and the United States to facilitate the mutual acceptance of clinical data by the regulatory authorities in these jurisdictions. The guidelines were developed with consideration of the current good clinical practices of the European Union, Japan, the United States, Australia, Canada, the Nordic countries and the World Health Organization.[5]

The GCP guidelines define responsibilities of institutional review boards or ethics committees, and in section 3.1.2 there is mention of patient recruitment. Because of this guideline, patient recruitment activities are considered to fall under the auspices of the ICH. (Table Four).

Table 4 **Guideline 3.1.2 of the Guideline for Good Clinical Practice**

The IRB/IEC should obtain the following documents:

Trial protocol(s)/amendment(s), written informed consent form(s) and consent form updates that the investigator proposes for use in the trial, **subject recruitment procedures (e.g. advertisements)**, written information to be provided to subjects, Investigator's Brochure (IB), available safety information, information about payments and **compensation available to subjects**, the investigator's current curriculum vitae and/or other documentation evidencing qualifications and any other documents that the IRB/IEC may need to fulfill its responsibilities.

Source: ICH Harmonised Tripartite Guideline: Guideline for Good Clinical Practice

Although these international principles are in place and widely recognized, it is critical to reiterate that they do not specifically address standards or specific approaches to be adopted for patient recruitment initiatives. For example, the first principle of the Nuremberg Code focuses on a subject being able to give informed consent freely, but a subject cannot give informed consent until he or she is first recruited. The code does not discuss patient recruitment initiatives perhaps because at the time that it was written, its purpose was to establish humane standards for clinical research; not the reaching of enrollment targets for industry-sponsored trials. This gap in international standards leaves countries free to develop their own recruitment regulations based on the customs and practices of each country. With this setting as a backdrop, it is not surprising that the definition of acceptable patient recruitment initiatives is highly variable around the globe.

A LOOK AT THE UNITED STATES

As the number of clinical trials continues to increase, along with the emphasis on timeline acceleration, American companies involved in study conduct have evolved toward a highly aggressive approach to patient recruitment to reach enrollment targets. Advertisements for clinical trials that appear in print, on radio, television, various Internet sites as well as direct mail from databases are permissible and acceptable in the United States as long as they are acceptable to the studies designated Institutional Review Boards (IRBs) and to the sponsor companies. Subjects who enroll and participate often receive remuneration, plus reimbursement for travel expenses. The amount of compensation paid to those who complete the trial is often mentioned in recruitment advertisements.

These open, assertive approaches reflect the entrepreneurial style of the American clinical trials industry and may follow the lead of direct-to-consumer advertising that is becoming more commonplace for marketed drugs. In 1999, pharmaceutical companies spent in excess of $1.8 billion on direct-to-consumer advertising.[6] At the same time, annual patient recruitment expenditures in the U.S. are estimated to be in the $200 million to $250 million range.[7]

It is obvious from the allowable tactics in the United States that the guiding principles, namely the Nuremberg Code, Declaration of Helsinki, the International Conference on Harmonization, and the succession of U.S. policies known as the Common Rule* are interpreted to permit a vast array of multi-media recruitment methods. Perhaps the current thinking is driven by the fact that 78% of today's clinical trials fail to meet patient enrollment deadlines[8], so many and varied ethical means are being explored. This philosophy works hand-in-hand with the fact that some Americans actively seek information about clinical trials instead of taking the traditional route of relying on their trusted physicians as the sole information source. The growing popularity of Web-based clinical trials and healthcare sites is further evidence that consumers want ready access to this media-based healthcare information as it fuels a greater sense of empowerment and control over their own health.

As discussed in Chapter One, however, American patient recruitment initiatives have sometimes become too aggressive, especially when investigators are enticed by handsome compensation for meeting or exceeding recruitment goals within negotiated timelines. Stories of coercion, enrollment of patients who do not qualify and investigator conflicts of interest have been reported over the past few years, attracting the attention of the Food and Drug Administration (FDA), the Office of Inspector General (OIG) of the Department of Health and Human Services and the U.S. Congress.

Following investigations into questionable recruitment practices and inadequate oversight by IRBs, the OIG issued a series of reports detailing their findings. The first of the documents, *Institutional Review Boards: A Time for Reform*[9], was released in June 1998, and was followed by several others, all highlighting purported problems in the patient recruitment process, ranging from an erosion of informed consent to the critical need for IRB members and investi-

Table 5 Documents from the OIG that Address Serious Problems with the Patient Recruitment Process

Date	Title	Report #
June 1998	Institutional Review Boards: A Time for Reform	OEI-07-97-00193
April 2000	Protecting Human Research Subjects—Status of Recommendations	OEI-01-97-00197
June 2000	Recruiting Human Subjects—Pressures in Industry-Sponsored Clinical Research	OEI-01-97-00195
June 2000	Recruiting Human Subjects—Sample Guidelines for Practice	OEI-01-97-00196

Source: Office of Inspector General

gators to be properly educated about human subject protections. (Table Five)

In terms of patient recruitment specifically, the June 2000 report, "Recruiting Human Subjects—Pressures in Industry-Sponsored Clinical Research"[10], recommends that industry and the research communities determine appropriate recruiting practices that would be helpful to all parties involved in clinical research. The report recommends that parties explore the following questions:

- Is it acceptable for sponsors to offer bonuses to investigators for successfully recruiting subjects?
- Should physicians be allowed to receive fees for referring their patients as potential subjects for a clinical trial?
- Should the financial arrangements between sponsors and investigators be disclosed to potential subjects?
- Does searching medical records for potential subjects constitute a breach of confidentiality?

The companion piece, "Recruiting Human Subjects—Sample Guidelines for Practice"[11], focuses more on guidance for IRBs. The report's key recommendation is for the Department of Health and Human Services (HHS) to provide IRBs with direction regarding oversight of recruitment practices. It calls for HHS to clarify that IRBs have the authority to review certain recruiting practices based on existing Federal regulation and to disseminate guidance on what IRBs can address in their review of recruitment practices. The goal of the report is to foster the development of a "level playing field" in which sponsors and investigators adhere to common standards in recruiting human subjects. Issues such as recruitment incentives, dual investigator-physician role and the confidentiality of medical records are discussed in this report.

It is clear that the subject of patient recruitment guidelines is garnering lots of attention in the United States. How the OIG reports ultimately influence or change recruiting practices remains to be seen, but it appears that an entrepreneurial style of direct-to-consumer advertising will continue, although there may be some changes with regard to investigator incentives, referral fees and other issues that could be interpreted as coercive, leading to conflict of interest or to erosion of informed consent. The Department of Health and Human Services issued a fact sheet announcing that it will pursue legislation to enable FDA to levy civil monetary penalties for violation of informed consent and other important research practices of up to $250,000 per clinical investigator and up to $1 million per research institution.[12] In the meantime, aggressive multimedia patient recruitment campaigns continue, perhaps with a more cautious eye. Also, repercussions caused by this governmental scrutiny may impact proactive recruitment strategies happening in Europe as site management organizations (SMO) proliferate.

CHANGE IS AFOOT IN THE UNITED KINGDOM

Conventional wisdom held that patient recruitment campaigns were neither allowed nor culturally acceptable in the United Kingdom. However, with a new set of recruitment guidelines launched by the Association of the British Pharmaceutical Industry (ABPI) in late 2000, and changing cultural norms, there is a greater openness in recruitment initiatives than in the recent past. Today, limited radio, newspaper and magazine advertisements are permitted. Television advertising is extremely rare due to the prohibitive cost, the small number of stations and a general lack of acceptance of this approach by consumers and clinical trials ethics committees.

Table 6 The Type of Clinical Trial Information Contained in the UK Web Site, www.controlled-trials.com

- The design and methodology of the study.
- Details of the number of patients included in a trial, including which groups of patients have been included and which excluded.
- Details of the length of the trial, including the start and finish dates.
- Contact details for further information about the clinical trials.

Source: Association of the British Pharmaceutical Industry

A new recruitment avenue is opening in early 2001.** At that time, the new web-based listing service of clinical trials is to be launched, sponsored partly by industry and by ABPI. The web site, *www.controlled-trials.com*, is to provide details of clinical trials for investigational compounds within three months of their having been registered in any major world market and involving UK citizens. The type of trial information appearing on the web site is listed in Table Six.

In July 2000, the National Health Service published "Changes in the Relationship Between the NHS and the Private Sector."[13] That report states that the development of a deeper partnership between industry, the National Health Service (NHS) and Government is in the best interest of the United Kingdom. As mentioned in that report, by April 2001 the NHS plans to streamline the work of research ethics committees, including making patient recruitment more effective. (Table Seven)

Table 7

Changes in the Relationship Between the NHS and the Private Sector

By April 2001 we will have developed ways of streamlining the work of research ethics committees whilst preserving all the necessary safeguards. This will allow faster and more effective recruitment of patients into clinical trials, enabling new medicines to be brought on stream more quickly.

Source: NHS, July 2000

Despite this new openness, the types of recruitment campaigns that are undertaken in the United Kingdom remain quite conservative by American standards. Paul Evans, Ph.D., and COO of Synexus, a U.K.-based site management organization (SMO), says, "There are strict limitations on what can be said and where the ads can be placed. What is allowed is basically fairly dull advertising, because anything that would attract more attention could be considered coercive. Similarly, patients cannot be compensated because that, too, could be construed as coercion. Also, doctors in the United Kingdom generally don't consider advertising to recruit patients to be ethical."

This attitude is rooted in the fact that the medical establishment is very conservative and government run. Due to the socialized healthcare delivery system, studies are conducted largely at hospitals or at the offices of government-based general practitioners as opposed to private sites that are commonplace in the United States. SMOs are relatively new in the United Kingdom, and they generally conduct their studies in hospital-based facilities.

The doctor-patient relationship is strong in the United Kingdom, and patients have a high degree of trust in their General Practitioners (GP). For these reasons, a patient considering participation in a trial would generally prefer using his own practitioner and would resist going to another doctor. Evans explains that because of this high level of trust and the fact the more GPs are organizing themselves into networks and securing more research grants, the GP-investigator is a good source of patients. "A GP can tell his or her patients about a study either during patient visits or by sending a letter to his or her patients on letterhead. This approach is very acceptable," he says. It is also acceptable to inform associations, such as those for diabetes, cancer or heart disease of upcoming trials and to send direct mail*** to patients known to suffer from various diseases.

GP interest in recruiting patients may expand as more of them negotiate directly with sponsors, bypassing the hospital. It has been reported that a growing percentage of industry-sponsored clinical grants in the United Kingdom are going directly to physicians.[14] This set-up is more economical for sponsors as their cost for underwriting a trial conducted at hospitals, particularly academic medical centers, exceeds the cost of having it operated by a network of office-based GPs (Table Eight). With these incentives growing, it is possible to speculate that at least some GPs may be looking to take a more pro-active patient recruitment stance.

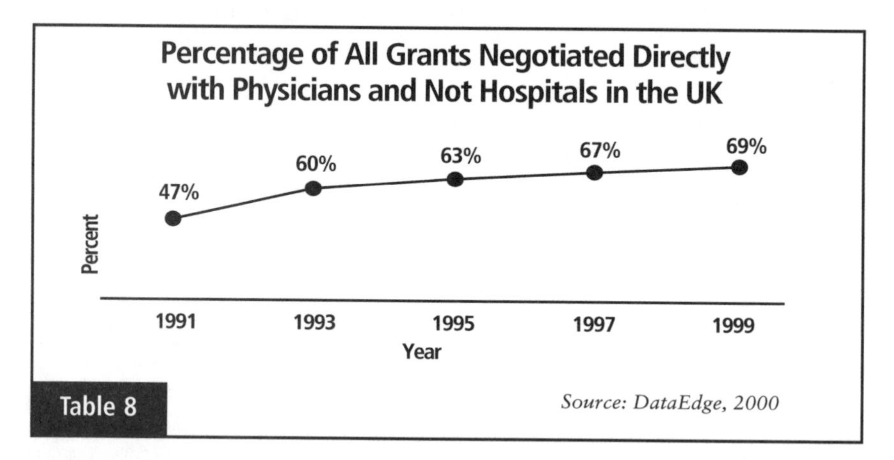

Table 8

Source: DataEdge, 2000

Expanding patient recruitment efforts beyond the limited amount of permissible advertising is bound to be challenging because the United Kingdom has a deeply entrenched government system of Local Research Ethics Committees (LRECs) that function similarly to American IRBs. Historically, LRECs had a reputation for not allowing advertisements, and although this has been changing with the new ABPI guidelines, LRECs maintain a general distaste for it. Each regional health district has its own LREC, translating into more than 300 of them in the United Kingdom, each functioning autonomously.

To make matters more complex, the National Health Service introduced another bureaucratic layer in the fall of 1997. At that time, a system of multicenter research ethics committees (MRECs) were established regionally in response to a growing concern that administrative and ethical problems as well as time delays were being encountered when large numbers of LRECs were involved in reviewing the documents associated with clinical studies. The MREC in each region is charged with reviewing proposals for studies taking place within the boundaries of five or more LRECs. Approval given by an MREC is to be binding in the whole United Kingdom. LRECs are to consider studies only with respect to issues that may affect acceptability locally.

There are numerous cases, however, of the system not functioning as intended. One published study of a clinical trial involving 125 LRECs and one MREC showed that only 40% of the LRECs reviewed the trial documents in accordance with the National Health Service directive and that 67% of the changes requested by LRECS addressed issues that were not local in nature.[15]

Evans says, "The subject of LRECs versus MRECs is very contentious in England. The LRECs are generally more conservative and have basically been accountable to no one. They were simply part of the regional health authority. The MRECs are more forward thinking in terms of contributing to the change in attitude toward advertising for clinical trials. If they determine that advertising is acceptable for certain studies, the LRECs have to accept it. MRECs are answerable to the Department of Health, and the MREC Chairmen meet on a regular basis to discuss ethical issues. These regular meetings will encourage more continuity in decisions about patient recruitment strategies."

The MRECs were also created as a result of new directives on Good Clinical Practice coming from the European Union designed to achieve uniformity in activities of study conduct across sixteen European countries. One of the directives is that each country is to have a national ethics committee. LRECs were not empowered with national clout so Britain's response was the MREC.

As this book goes to press, the new ABPI guidelines for patient recruitment are in final form, and they have been endorsed by the General Medical Council, the British Medical Association, the Royal College of General Practitioners, the Royal College of Physicians and the Chairmen of several MRECs. Richard Tiner,

Medical Director of ABPI, says, "The guidelines will be implemented as soon as the final draft is printed and distributed." Several of the guidelines appear in Table Nine. The complete set of guidelines appears on the association's web site at *www.abpi.org.uk*. Exactly how these recruitment guidelines will coincide with GCP directives coming from the European Union is not known at this time.

Table 9 Guidelines for Patient Recruitment Issued by the Association of the British Pharmaceutical Industry

Research Ethics Committees would be invited to review all materials used to recruit subjects for all phases of clinical trials, including, but not limited to:
- Television and radio advertisements
- Letters, posters, newsletters
- Newspaper advertisements
- Internet web sites

Essential Information for an Advertisement:
- A statement indicating that the study involves research
- A contact name and phone number for the subject to contact
- Some of the eligibility criteria
- The likely duration of the subject's participation for a specific study
- That the advertisement has been approved by an ethics committee
- That your general practitioner will be informed that you are taking part in the clinical trial

Additional Permitted Consent:
- The purpose of the research may be described
- The location of the research
- The company or institution involved may be named if appropriate

Statements that Should Not be Used:
- Implied or express claims of safety or efficacy
- Undue emphasis on reimbursement
- Any express or implied claim that the research is FDA or MCA approved
- Use of the term 'new' unless qualified, i.e., 'new research medicine,' 'new investigational medicine'
- The compound's name
- Care should be taken to ensure that advertisements are in no way promotional for the medicine concerned

Source: Association of the British Pharmaceutical Industry

RECRUITING FRENCH STYLE

In France, the system of oversight for protection of subjects in clinical trials is based on the Huriet Law which was implemented in December 1988. The Huriet Law distinguishes between two types of clinical trials—*avec ou sans bénéfice individuel direct*—which translates as trials with individual direct therapeutic benefit or those without it. Michel Wurm, M.D., an independent consultant to the clinical research industry, explains that the distinction between these two types of trials has a direct impact on the way that patients can be recruited. "Advertising using any medium is authorized for trials deemed to be without individual direct benefit, provided the advertising is approved by an ethics committee. Patients can receive remuneration up to a restricted amount per year. In contrast, for trials with individual direct therapeutic benefit, patients cannot be remunerated, and advertising, while not actually forbidden, is tough to organize and get approved," says Wurm.

Studies with or without individual direct therapeutic benefit are best defined by the location where the studies occur. Those trials without individual direct benefit can only be conducted at clinical pharmacology centers, which, by definition, do not treat patients. (Table Ten) Studies with individual direct benefit can only be carried out in public or private healthcare facilities, including hospitals and private medical practices.

Definition of a Clinical Pharmacology Center — Table 10

- Resuscitation Nearby
- Clinical Pharmacologist on Staff
- Accreditation from the Ministry of Health

Source: Michel Wurm, M.D.

According to Dr. Wurm, because of the restrictions placed on trials with therapeutic benefit, more pharmaceutical companies are trying to have their studies registered as being without individual direct benefit. He comments, "I've seen studies as late as Phase IIb being carried out under the definition of being without individual direct benefit so they can advertise for patients. The definitions of with or without therapeutic benefit have become so ambiguous that I doubt that you could find specific definitions anywhere." Phase III studies, however, are considered to be with therapeutic benefit.

Wurm continues, "Approximately 1000 of the 1300 trials carried out annually in France are with therapeutic benefit. In France, you cannot have access to patients for these trials without the involvement of those patients' physicians. At this time, there is no place in the market for private, professional sites because they fall within a gap in the law. Private sites do not fall within the definition of a clinical pharmacology center, nor within the definition of a hospital or private medical practice. If a patient were to be attracted to a private site offering a study with therapeutic benefit, you would be sued by that patient's doctor for diverting the patient away from that doctor's practice. Doctors are opposed to the idea of study sites because they get paid per patient, so if they lose the patient temporarily, they won't get paid for that patient. Therefore, there are not many ways to recruit for studies with therapeutic benefit without the involvement of the private practitioner. It is not so problematic for studies taking place at clinical pharmacology centers because by definition, they do not offer therapeutic benefit."

In France, two recruitment trends may be underway. One involves pharmaceutical sponsors continuing to work toward having trials registered as being without therapeutic benefit to take advantage of the advertising that is allowed, and the lack of reprisal by private physicians. The other trend is exploring the creation of Internet-based trials listings specific for Europe, listed country by country. Wurm estimates that there are approximately five million to eight million regular Internet users in France, which translates into 13% of the population. This is a fairly low usage rate, which is reasonably expected to increase. Patients with serious or terminal conditions such as HIV/AIDS, cancer or painful arthritis might want to know about ongoing clinical trials, so the Internet could become a welcomed source of information for those health problems. Additionally, web sites could be extended to include information on studies in France for other types of chronic medical conditions.

For non-life threatening illnesses, French patients who choose to participate in clinical trials generally do so either at the suggestion of their physicians or in response to advertising to gain access to a promising new treatment or for the more altruistic reason of wanting to participate in an experiment that could lead to less suffering in the future. There are no other objective reasons for patients to participate because in France, as in Western Europe, patients generally have access to free medical care. This is unlike the scenario in the United States in which patients with more limited access to health care may be attracted to the free care offered by a trial and the associated compensation.

AUSTRALIA—A LOOK DOWN UNDER

In this continent of twenty million people, hundreds of clinical trials are underway. From July 1, 1999 through June 30, 2000, approximately 430 clinical trials notifications were received each quarter by the Therapeutic Goods Administration (TGA), the Australian equivalent of the Food and Drug Administration. Most notifications are for Phases III and IV studies, and most, 310 to 320 of the 430 notifications, are for multicenter studies. When a sponsor plans to conduct a clinical trial in Australia, that company submits the protocol and other essential documents to an appropriate investigator who then submits the package to his or her ethics committee for consideration. If the ethics committee approves the protocol, the company then submits a clinical trials notification to the TGA. According to the TGA, approximately 60% of the trials notified under the clinical trial notification scheme are industry-sponsored. The remaining 40% include trials conducted by government, individual doctors, hospitals and universities.[17]

Denise Clarke-Hundley, Clinical Research Manager for a major pharmaceutical company, comments that the clinical trials notification is just that, a notification of intentions to start a trial. "The onus for approving the conduct of the trial lies solely with the Human Research Ethics Committee (HREC), not with the TGA," she explains.

Clarke-Hundley says that in Australia, each academic institution has its own HREC, and there are also independent ethics committees that function outside of the hospital system, mostly on a regional level. Regardless of the location of the ethics committee, the sponsor submits the protocol package to the principal investigator who then submits it to the appropriate HRECs. Most studies are conducted in hospital settings, although some are being conducted in the offices of General Practitioners. The regional Ethics Committee may cover a specific geographic region of GP-based practices.

Ethics committees are charged with reviewing patient recruitment materials and making decisions to approve or reject them. According to Clarke-Hundley, a wide range of media advertising is allowed, such as in newspaper, magazines and radio, but television advertisements would be unusual.

In Australia, however, patients are generally not compensated for participating in phases II, III and IV clinical trials. Patients may be reimbursed by the Investigator for transportation costs to protocol-specified site visits. Compensation for participation in phase I trials is acceptable.

Table 11 Section 4.8—Informed Consent of Trial Subjects

4.8.10 Both the informed consent discussion and the written informed consent form and any other written information to be provided to subjects should include explanations of the following:
(k) The anticipated prorated payment, if any, to the subject for participating in the trial.
(l) The anticipated expenses, if any, to the subject for participating in the trial.

Source: Note for Guidance on Good Clinical Practice, July 2000

The basis for compensation of research subjects is found in the CPMP/International Conference on Harmonization/135/95, in section 4.8 which is entitled "The Note for Guidance on Good Clinical Practice." Section 4.8 refers to informed consent of trial subjects. (Table Eleven) In Australia, however, Section 4.8 requires further explanation beyond "The Note for Guidance on Good Clinical Practice" to include input from local regulatory requirements. The fact that this section continues to be under review in Australia may explain why subjects in that country are generally not compensated.

Table 12 Ethical Guidelines from the National Health and Medical Research Council

Year	Document
1966	Statement on Human Experimentation
Various	Supplementary Notes
1992	National Statement on Ethical Conduct in Research Involving Humans (the 'Act')
June 1999	Latest Revisions to the National Statement on Ethical Conduct in Research Involving Humans

Source: National Statement on Ethical Conduct in Research Involving Humans

Australia has been proactive in developing standards for the conduct of ethical research based on the Declaration of Helsinki and ICH principles. In 1966, the National Health and Medical Research Council (NHMRC) issued its first "Statement on Human Experimentation," and over time added various supplementary notes to turn the original document into a widely used standard for ethical review. This statement was followed by the "National Statement on Ethical Conduct in Research Involving Humans," which consists of a series of guidelines made in accordance with the NHMRC Act 1992 (the "Act"). This Act established the NHMRC as a statutory entity to pursue and foster issues relating to public health, and specifically requires the NHMRC to issue guidelines for the conduct of medical research and ethical matters relating to health. Table Twelve lists dates for various revisions to ethical guidelines. The latest revision to the national statement, released in June 1999, identifies the ethical principles and values that should govern research involving humans. It provides an expanded guidance for researchers, ethics committees, institutions, organizations and the public on how such research should be designed and conducted to conform to the ethical principles.

Section 12 of this 1999 revision is entitled "Clinical Trials"[18] and mentions specifically that a Human Research Ethics Committee must consider all aspects of the design of a clinical trial and be satisfied that the trial's methodology provides:

- A rationale for the selection of appropriate participants.
- An appropriate method of patient recruitment.
- Adequate, understandable information for the purpose of obtaining participant consent.
- A clear description of the intervention and observation to be conducted.
- A sample size adequate to demonstrate clinically and statistically significant effects.

The complete document is available at the NHMRC Web site, *www.nhmrc.health.health.gov/au/publicat/pdfe35.pdf.*

Although Australia allows diverse approaches to patient recruitment, one last horizon will be use of the Internet for web-based listings of clinical trials. At the time of this writing, Australia does not yet have an Internet listings service. A spokesperson for the NHMRC stated in October 2000 that the NHMRC currently has no position about the ethics of a clinical trials web site as it does not yet exist.

NETHERLANDS

Advertising as a patient recruitment tool has been an accepted practice in the Netherlands for a number of years, as long as there is

Ethics Committee approval. Phil Davies, Director, Clinical Pharmacology Unit of Kendle International B. V. in the Netherlands, says that newspapers, magazines and the Internet are commonly used, as is sharing information about trials with patient support groups. He adds that there are no guidelines or regulations specifically governing types of allowable patient recruitment activities. "The accepted recruitment methods depend on the patient categories to be studied, and the final decision is always according to the opinion of the responsible Ethics Committee," says Davies.

Recruitment via the treating physician is accepted in all cases, and depending on the severity of disease, this may be either at the GP level or via specialists. Davies explains that there is diverse opinion among the medical establishment in terms of their acceptance of advertising for patients to reach enrollment targets. "Some physicians disapprove of more active recruitment, such as through advertising, but others use this strategy themselves for research they have initiated. In terms of society at large, people seem to accept advertising because they can make a choice about participating in a study. If however a study were to interfere with treatment already prescribed by a physician, such as involving a wash-out period, patients can usually only participate in those trials with the approval of their own physician." According to recently initiated changes in the laws covering clinical trials in the Netherlands, an independent physician should also be available to subjects to give advice about their participation in a clinical trial.

According to Davies, Kendle has been allowed to advertise for patients from many therapeutic areas including studies for incontinence, benign prostate hyperplasia, migraine and dysmenorrhea. "So far, we have not been allowed to advertise for diabetes patients, and we have had mixed experience with asthma studies. Our policy is to discuss upfront with an ethics committee what its current opinion is. We believe that greater acceptance will come in the near future and that there will be more opportunity to use advertisements. It will continue to be important to involve the patient's own physician in the final decision of including individual patients in a specific trial," Davies says.

In December 1999, a new law, the "Medical Research Involving Human Subjects Act" (WMO–Dutch initials), was implemented by the Central Committee on Research Involving Human Subjects (CCMO–Dutch initials). WMO specifically controls the activities of ethics committees, whereby only committees approved or recognized by CCMO can make judgement for clinical trials accepted to be performed in the Netherlands. Davies comments, "Some view this law as having made the business of performing clinical trials somewhat more cumbersome. However, from a Kendle perspective, and particularly for clinical pharmacology studies, the new law has increased our flexibility to initiate phase I and IIa studies more quickly than was previously the case."

The following comments are related to Clinical Pharmacology studies which are in the majority of cases single site studies. By co-operating with more than one of the recognized committees we are able to ensure that the timeline from submission to receipt of a final opinion of the ethics committee is reduced compared to the previous instance. We are now free to select the committee we apply to provided that their own constitution allows review of external protocols. Earlier feedback from the ethics committee implies that we are able to initiate advertising campaigns sooner. This significantly enhances the recruitment rates. If there are some clarifications required to a study submission but in principle there is an intent to approve the protocol, then we are able to already initiate advertisements (which are part of the ethics committee submission). In the near future we also anticipate being able to run pre-approved advertisements for general information purposes, something we do not currently undertake. This will however only be initiated after completion of ongoing discussions with the appropriate ethics committees that we are working with.

MEXICO EMERGES

Mexico, with a population of 100 million, is an emerging market for clinical trials. Cristina Torres, M.D., General Manager of Quintiles Mexico, says that some very limited advertising is allowed and must be approved by an ethics committee. She explains, "Advertising is done in a very discrete way. Some institutions may place a small announcement in a newspaper stating that a clinical trial is underway for patients with specific characteristics, but the actual indication is not mentioned. A telephone number is provided. We don't see ad campaigns including newspapers, magazines, radio and direct mail."

According to Torres, patients are not compensated for participating in trials. She also says that she is not aware of any Internet-based clinical trials listing service for Mexico, nor of any plans to develop one in the near future.

Regulations addressing patient recruitment activities in Mexico can be found at *www.ssa.gob.mx*, and then searching for "Ley General de Salud, Chapter on Investigacion and on Reglamento de la Ley General de Salud en material de Investigacion para la Salud." Torres says that Mexican guidelines and the Helsinki Declaration are used for determination of ethical practices, but there is a movement toward integration of ICH guidelines.

VARIABILITY IS HERE TO STAY

A compound under development needs to be tested in various countries for several reasons. First, different subpopulations may react differently to the same compound, so only through clinical research in diverse populations will it be possible to show broad-spectrum safety and efficacy. Secondly, as studies become more difficult to fill due to the growing number of trials, sponsors will continue to expand their recruiting horizons beyond a handful of nations. Indeed, studies are now ongoing throughout the world.

Table 13 Number of Statement of Investigator FDA Form 1572s Filed

Year	# of 1572s Filed
1990	8,156
1999	28,413

Source: FDA and DataEdge, Inc. Analysis

Methods used to reach enrollment targets vary across the globe, and reflect local interpretations of international clinical trials standards and guidelines, local regulations, character of the people and interest in clinical trials by the local medical establishment. The United States is generally seen as a very open society in terms of recruitment approaches deemed as acceptable and in terms of physician acceptance of industry-based and government sponsored clinical trials. As evidence, there are increasing numbers of physicians involved in clinical studies based on the amount of Form 1572s filed with the FDA. As seen in Table Thirteen, there was a 248% increase in one decade.

Around the world, allowable recruitment initiatives range from multi-media advertising in some countries to a more restrictive approach in others. Perhaps over time, as people become more educated about clinical trials this will serve to change their cultural perceptions about study conduct. In addition, as more people gain Internet access to recruiting sites and clinical trials information, patients may seek access to these studies, possibly resulting in countries facilitating the sharing of information about ongoing trials. Recruitment activities may trend toward less restrictive in some of today's more cautious markets, while still conforming to good clinical practice standards.

* The Common Rule is a succession of policies developed over the years culminating in the current federal regulations for protection of human research subjects. The Department of Health and Human Services has developed the core of these regulations which flow directly from the Nuremberg Code. The Common Rule has been promulgated by seventeen different Federal Department and Independent Agencies.

** Information accurate as this book goes to press in fourth quarter 2000.

*** Direct Mail is known as "Mail Shots" in the U.K.

REFERENCES

[1] "Another Setback for CROs: Strained Relations with Euro Sites," CenterWatch. April 2000, Vol. 7, Issue 4. p. 12.

[2] "No Advertising for Patients in Europe? Not True!" CenterWatch. December 1999, Vol. 6, Issue 12. p. 4.

[3] The Nuremberg Code, 1947. *www.cirp.org/library/ethics/nuremberg.*

[4] The Declaration of Helsinki. *www.faseb.org/arvo/helsinki.htm.*

[5] ICH Harmonised Tripartite Guideline: Guideline for Good Clinical Practice. Introduction, 1996. *www.ifpma.org/pdfifpma/e6.pdf.*

[6] "Council to Develop Direct-to-Consumer Advertising Standards." MedAdNews. August 2000, Vol. 19, No. 8. p. 4.

[7] CenterWatch Survey of 103 Investigative Sites. 1999.

[8] CenterWatch. Boston, Massachusetts. 1997.

[9] *Institutional Review Boards: A Time for Reform*. Office of Inspector General, OEI-01-97-00193. June 1998.

[10] *Recruiting Human Subjects—Pressures in Industry-Sponsored Clinical Research*. Office of Inspector General, OEI-01-97-00195. p. 4. June 2000.

[11] *Recruiting Human Subjects—Sample Guidelines for Practice*. Office of Inspector General, OEI-01-97-00196, p. 2, June 2000.

[12] "Protecting Human Subjects." Department of Health and Human Services, Fact Sheet, May 23, 2000.

[13] Changes in the Relationship Between the NHS and the Private Sector. "The Pharmaceutical and Bio-pharmaceutical Industries." Section 11.11, and 11.12, July 26, 2000. *www.hhs.uknationalplan/npch11.pdf.*

[14] "Early Signs for a Market Shifting Toward For-Profit European Clinical Investigators." CenterWatch. Lisa Henderson. September 2000, p. 3.

[15] "The New System of Review by Multicentre Research Ethics Committees: Prospective Study." British Medical Journal. Joanna Tully, Nelly Ninis, Robert Booy, Russell Viner. April 29, 2000, Volume 320. p. 1179.

[16] Australian Pharmaceutical Manufacturers Association, October 2000.

[17] Therapeutic Goods Administration, Experimental Drugs Section, October 2000.

[18] National Statement on Ethical Conduct in Research Involving Humans, Section 12-Clinical Trials, June 1999, p. 35.

CHAPTER 17

A Patient Recruitment Campaign from Contracting to Completion: A Case Study in Osteoarthritis of the Knee

Melynda Geurts, M.S., Rheumatology Research International

Without study participants there can be no clinical research. Although patient recruitment and enrollment may initially appear simple, in many instances it is only through the employment of a multi-faceted recruitment campaign that enrollment can be accomplished within a reasonable timeframe. However, the use of a multi-faceted campaign is dictated by the study parameters, and therefore, is not always necessary. Yet, given the variables like the number of concurrent osteoarthritis trials being conducted, as in this case study, the use of a multi-faceted approach regardless of the study parameters is growing in popularity among those responsible for speeding clinical trial development.

Over forty percent of all delays occur in the patient enrollment portion of clinical trial process.[1] In addition, Sponsors, Contract Research Organizations (CROs) and Investigator sites identify patient recruitment as their biggest challenge. Moreover, eight out of nine Investigators may overestimate their ability to recruit qualified patients for clinical trials.[2] With the number of clinical research trials rising to an all time high, Sponsors will continue to look for options (i.e., patient recruitment) that will bring their product to the market faster.[3]

Therefore, patient recruitment campaigns must be designed to stimulate immediate response of potential participants to generate required enrollment rates in specific market areas. Employing a comprehensive array of techniques, advertising, public relations, interactive media and grassroots advocacy, are now essential patient recruitment tools for the pharmaceutical and biotechnical companies that are seriously committed to accelerating drug development.[4]

The primary objective of this chapter is to focus on the six-step process in devising a comprehensive patient recruitment campaign from contracting to completion.[5] It is through a case study in osteoarthritis of the knee that the correlation of these steps in the formulation of a comprehensive patient recruitment campaign will be demonstrated.

The steps to be discussed in detail include: (1) evaluating sponsor and trial needs, (2) conducting market research, (3) developing a recruitment proposal, (4) negotiating and securing a separate patient recruitment contract and budget, (5) implementing a patient recruitment campaign, and (6) conducting site management services.

CASE STUDY SYNOPSIS

A case study of osteoarthritis of the knee will be used to explain the six-step process. This example describes a national U.S. study conducted by forty-five research centers. These centers were challenged with enrolling 1200 subjects over a nine-month enrollment period, knowing the screen failure ratio was predicted to be at least 5:1 and possibly as high as 10:1. The predicted high screen failure ratio was largely due to a particular procedure that had to be performed to meet inclusion criteria into the study, in addition to the other laboratory tests that were necessary for study participation.

STEP ONE: EVALUATE SPONSOR AND TRIAL NEEDS

Identifying the sponsor and trial needs accurately is a pertinent step to prove long-term success in a patient recruitment campaign. It is critical to fully understand the sponsor's philosophies, expectations and available resources as well as the impact that patient recruitment has on the study and the bottom line. It is through this awareness that the analysis of enrollment and/or study challenges is possible.

When evaluating the specifics of the trial, it is imperative that these needs are correlated with the Sponsor's expectations (See Table One).

Through correlating the sponsor and trial needs, a patient recruitment campaign can be developed that will accelerate the overall process and decrease the funds necessary for this process. For example, based on the previously mentioned study criteria, the recruitment group may recommend that an advertising campaign with a broad reach be utilized (i.e., television). If the sponsor agrees to implement this campaign initially, it will help ensure that the recruitment group can secure the appropriate programming and take advantage of schedule discounting. In comparison, if such a campaign is held out as a rescue activity, the appropriate scheduling program may be harder to secure or may not be available. Therefore, the overall reach to potential participants and the costs involved in reaching these participants could be impacted.

Table 1

Evaluating Trial Needs	
Number of Subjects	Therapeutic Difficulty
Length of Enrollment	Competition
Inclusion/Exclusion Criteria	Dropout Rates

Finally, before employing Step Two, Market Research, the recruitment team must be identified. Establishing a recruitment team will ensure the continuity of a recruitment plan as well as define the appropriate communication chain between the team (i.e., CRO, SMO, or Recruitment Group serves as the liaison between the sponsor and the sites). Members of this team should include the CRO, SMO, sites, sponsor and the recruitment group (Table Two). The responsibilities that each party will bring to the completion of the trial should be clearly identified prior to study start-up. "The most successful approach involves convening this group regularly throughout the course of the study. Oftentimes, this takes the form of weekly conference calls with representatives of project management from the sponsor and SMO and/or CRO, and the patient recruitment vendor."[5] It is during these conference calls that the recruitment group present site-specific information to the sponsor related to their course of action, potential obstacles, and/or proposed recruitment activities.

Case Study: In this case example, the sponsor contacted the recruitment group and requested that a comprehensive patient recruitment proposal be developed to assist with study enrollment. Through the use of the protocol, historical metrics and discussions with the sponsor, the recruitment group was able to develop a study specific proposal aimed at generating interest among potential participants and assisting the sites with study enrollment. The recruitment vendor was one of several groups that presented their proposals to the sponsor's project management team at their headquarters. After the presentation of the proposal, the project management team and the recruitment group conducted roundtable discussions to accurately ascertain the sponsor's needs as well as their impressions regarding the trial needs. This information was key to the development of the contract and the implementation of the recruitment strategies. Lastly, the recruitment team, as noted in chart two, was identified. The team consisted of the sponsor's project management team, several SMOs, investigator sites, and a recruitment communications group responsible for patient recruitment that was part of one SMO. A CRO was not utilized for this study.

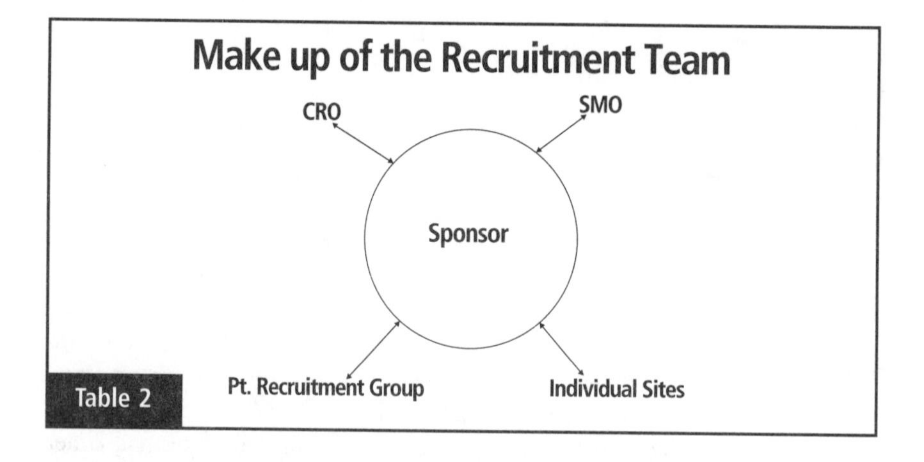

Table 2

STEP TWO: MARKET RESEARCH

Before a successful, cost-effective recruitment campaign can be developed, the target market needs to be identified. This can be accomplished through market research. Oftentimes, this important step in the developmental process is not always allowed. Based on historical metrics and feedback from the participating investigators, many sponsors believe they have a good understanding of the market needs. However, it is imperative the sponsor understands the importance and necessity of conducting market research regardless of how well the sponsor, CRO, SMO or investigator site may think they know their target market. Due to study differences, conducting market research can help identify the target audience, potential recruitment obstacles, and strategies to overcome these obstacles that may otherwise not be recognized and, which may potentially impact recruitment and study completion. Chapter Ten outlines a detailed explanation of the importance of market research.

Case Study: In the case study, the sponsor and recruitment team agreed that initial market research strategies be employed. As mentioned in the case study synopsis, the sponsor was predicting a screen failure ratio to be between 5:1 and 10:1. The sponsor also had concerns about how to effectively reach the ideal study candidate and whether or not compensation should be awarded for time and travel.

Since this was a national study, two market research focus groups were conducted throughout several geographic regions. This allowed for fair geographic representation to be obtained that identified market differences. The primary purpose for conducting these focus groups was to define the most likely target audience for this particular study. In addition, the groups would also help determine: (1) what might motivate people with knee pain to volunteer for a clinical trial (2) to present actual clinical trial and health-related advertising to ascertain appeal of this media, and (3) to explore the effectiveness of various communication venues for disseminating a recruitment message to potential participants in clinical trials for this study.

A total of twenty people with self-reported knee pain participated in these groups. Of the twenty participants, 75% had never participated in a clinical trial, 15% had participated in a clinical trial, and the remaining 10% had taken part in some form of medical testing other than an ongoing clinical trial.

Both groups were asked to give their impressions of five advertisements to gauge their response to headlines, visuals, format, messages regarding clinical trials and to determine if any of the advertising would elicit a response in the form of a telephone call from the respondent. Performing this exercise resulted in identifying barriers and/or motivations to volunteering. The findings and recommendations from these research groups are summarized in Tables Three and Four.

Based on the market research findings, valuable insight was acquired into some aspects of what would and would not influence individuals' participation in this clinical trial. For example, the research findings identified the target audience as being very diverse, meaning they

Table 3 **Market Research Findings**

- The majority of the respondents agreed that stating the study was conducted at a respected, credible organization would predispose participants to believing the study was safe.
- Seventy percent of the respondents reacted positively to a straightforward advertisement headline (i.e., Do You Experience Knee Pain?, Knee Pain?, Fight Pain).
- Information about the investigational medication was imperative to those who indicated they would be interested in learning more about a clinical trial.
- Safety of investigational medication.
- Physician recommendation for participation.
- Projected percentage and/or effects of receiving a placebo.
- Remuneration for time and travel.

Source: Osteoarthritis case study market research findings.

Table 4 **Market Research Recommendations**

- Use a headline in any advertising that speaks simply to the target audience.
- Use a variety of advertising and marketing tactics.
- If possible, provide the name of a credible sponsor and/or site in the ad.
- Offer free information in all advertising (ie. brochures, journal ads).
- Provide as much information about the trial as possible (eliminate skepticism).

Source: Osteoarthritis case study market research findings.

acquired their health information from a wide variety of sources such as healthcare providers, community clinics, Internet, patient associations and media (i.e., journals, brochures). Therefore, it was felt that the use of a multi-faceted campaign would reach a broader number of potential participants, thus yielding a higher response rate. Additionally, it was noted that offering compensation for time and travel was neutral. Although it was important to some of the respondents, there was not a significant difference to justify the expense. Step three in the six-step process, Developing a Proposal, will illustrate how these market research findings play an important role in deciding the overall scope of a patient recruitment campaign.

Once the knowledge related to the target market has been acquired, it is important not to overlook the importance of analyzing historical metrics to further determine effective patient recruitment strategies (See Table Five). It is through a marriage of both market research and historical metrics that a successful campaign will be accomplished.

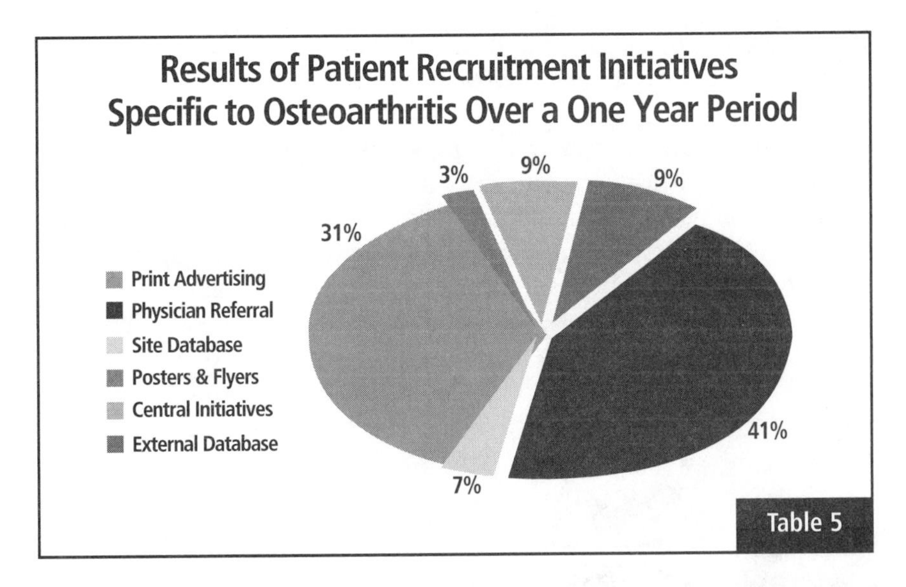

Table 5

Finally, the overall success of a patient recruitment campaign is determined by the sponsor's commitment to the conduct of the campaign. By investing initial resources into the development of the campaign, the sponsor will experience a greater return-on-investments over the length of the study.

STEP THREE: DEVELOPING A PROPOSAL

The third step in the six-step recruitment process is the development of a patient recruitment proposal. The primary objective of a patient recruitment campaign is to achieve an immediate yield of respondents sufficient in volume that will result in the required enrollment.[4] By identifying the needs of the trial and having an awareness of the target market, the recruitment group should be armed with the knowledge to develop a successful, cost-effective patient recruitment proposal.

A patient recruitment proposal is a working document that is drafted on behalf of meeting the sponsor and trial needs. There are many ways to construct a proposal, but one type of proposal that has proven to be well received by the sponsors is one that is presented as a menu of options. Depending on the study criteria, a proposal may include market research, investigator resource materials, both national and local advertising campaigns, Internet advertising, public relations campaign, and screening services. By developing the proposal as a menu of services, it grants the sponsor the flexibility to choose which activities to employ. Table Six is an example of a draft proposal.

Case Study: Based on statistical criteria, forty-five sites were needed to accumulate statistically significant data on 1200 subjects over a nine-month enrollment period. Additionally, the previous market research findings demonstrated the following: (1) print advertisement should speak directly to the target audience, (2) a variety of advertising and marketing tactics should be used, (3) the name of a credible sponsor and/or site should be provided in the advertisement, if possible, and (4) free literature should be offered in all advertising when available. Moreover, data showed that physician referral (41%) and print advertising (31%) yielded the highest response rate among study participants over a one-year period.

Table 6

Patient Recruitment Proposal

Activity	Fees
Market Research: Based on the findings, a patient recruitment campaign would be developed that is tightly directed at the patient with osteoarthritis of the knee per protocol definitions.	$$$ $$$
Investigator Resource Materials: Media kit would be provided to each site to assist with their recruitment needs. A kit might include: posters, fliers, news release, radio script and newspaper ad. All materials would be sponsor and IRB approved prior to distribution.	$$$
Screening Services: Recruitment group would manage screening services through a centralized call center utilizing a toll-free number. Potential patient information would be referred to the appropriate research center for consideration. Recruitment group would gather referral outcome data from the sites and report to the sponsor.	$$$
Local Advertising Campaigns: A protocol specific print advertising campaign would be developed to assist the sites with recruitment efforts. Recruitment group would be responsible for developing the ad and having the ad developed and distributed to the sites. Additionally, the recruitment group would be responsible for assisting the sites with actual placement and coordination. The ad would be sponsor and IRB approved prior to use.	

Given this historical data, an innovative combination of services was planned. The objective of this proposal was to neutralize potential recruitment obstacles that could affect trial enrollment, as noted in the market research findings. The proposal consisted of the following services: (1) develop and design patient recruitment initiatives, (2) ensure sponsor's approval, (3) streamline and coordinate IRB and ethics submission, (4) develop recruitment material, and (5) initiate and manage a central call center. The recruitment vendor was responsible for developing and designing all patient recruitment initiatives and materials. Recruitment initiatives included facilitating the use of direct-to-consumer strategies like targeted direct mailings, Internet based listings and national advertising in trade journals. Recruitment materials also included developing and designing Investigator resource kits that contained a news release, physician-to-patient letter, posters and fliers. All of these initiatives and materials were pre-approved by the sponsor before being submitted to the IRB and/or ethics committee for approval. After IRB and/or ethics approval was obtained, the materials were developed and distributed to the individual Investigator sites for their immediate use. This planning allowed for these initiatives and materials to be in place and/or developed concurrently with study start-up.

STEP FOUR: NEGOTIATING AND SECURING A SEPARATE PATIENT RECRUITMENT CONTRACT AND BUDGET

Step four puts the plan in motion. "It involves negotiating with the sponsor/CRO for an upfront budget that will be specifically earmarked for recruitment strategies. Calculating a meaningful budget results from specifics of the recruitment plan, historic expenditures and revisiting previous metrics for similar studies."[5]

As mentioned earlier, the key to a successful patient recruitment campaign is to secure the sponsor's initial commitment to the proposal. Not only is the recruitment group seeking support regarding the philosophies used to develop the campaign, but financial support as well. Historically, the sponsor would allocate a fixed dollar amount to the sites for advertising. For example, a contract may show the fees associated with different trial procedures (i.e., medical history at screening = $150.00 per patient) and have a line item that reflects advertising monies allocated to each site (i.e., advertising at $2,500.00

per site). In this scenario, centralized patient recruitment campaigns are most likely not utilized. However, sponsors allocating monies to individual sites for recruitment efforts are decreasing. Study staff are not marketing experts, they are health care providers. Many times, they are overburdened with the work of doing the trial, let alone developing and employing a recruitment campaign. Therefore, what is emerging as the norm related to the independent support of recruitment campaigns is the outsourcing of recruitment to vendors or SMOs that specialize in and assume accountability for site enrollment after the proposal has been developed.[5]

New campaign approaches include offering recruitment tactics through a menu of services, which allows the sponsor to choose the venue(s) they wish to support (See Table Seven). A detailed description of each initiative is drafted. A fee for service is then assigned within the budget proposal. The budget will be managed by marketing experts who also have the knowledge and capability of conducting on-going analysis of the strategies employed. The process of matching expenses with the effectiveness of various initiatives will facilitate identification of strategies that are media cost-efficient and cost-inefficient.

Overall, outsourcing patient recruitment may benefit the sponsor and site particularly in difficult to enroll projects. The sponsor should see an increased return-on-investment as well as increased enrollment rates, thus decreasing the length of the trial. The benefit to the site is they are able to focus completely on the conduct of the trial. Allowing a patient recruitment group to manage the recruitment activities decreases the amount of time the research staff must spend to identify

Table 7 **Sample Contract for Services**

Patient Recruitment Services	Fees
• Print Advertisement Development	$$
• IRB/Ethics Coordination & Submission	$$
• Internet Listing & Web Site Management	$$
• Direct Mail	$$
• Site Patient Recruitment Management	$$
• Central, National and International Initiatives	$$
• Central Screening Services	$$
• Patient Retention Program	$$

potential participants. In turn, this approach may actually increase the actual time spent with the study volunteer by the clinical research staff, resulting in a higher quality of participants.

Case Study: As noted in Step Three, Developing a Proposal, an individually priced patient recruitment proposal was presented to the sponsor. Based on the market research findings and the study criteria, the proposal included the following recruitment activities: market research, Investigator resource materials, local advertising, screening services, public relations campaign, Internet advertising, direct mail, and a study specific consumer brochure. The budget for this proposal was $300,000.00. However, due to budgetary constraints, the sponsor elected to implement the following activities: investigator resource materials (which included a print advertisement), direct mail, Internet advertising and screening services. The budget for the selected services was $70,000.00. Each of these services is described in detail in Step Five, Implementing a Patient Recruitment Campaign.

STEP FIVE: IMPLEMENTING A PATIENT RECRUITMENT CAMPAIGN

Once a separate patient recruitment contract and budget has been secured and the sponsor has selected the recruitment activities to be employed from the proposal, then step five focuses on the implementation of the campaign.

Sample Recruitment Timeline — Table 8

Initiatives	Target Date	Status	Party Responsible
Draft recruitment materials to sponsor for approval.	2 weeks	Complete	Recruitment group
Recruitment materials to IRB for approval.	3 weeks	Pending	Recruitment group
Recruitment materials to sites.	4 weeks	Pending	Recruitment group
Coordination of advertisement placement, metrics, site management and screening.		On-going	Recruitment group

Before implementing the recruitment campaign, it is important that a timeline of all the steps involved in launching the campaign is mapped out (See Table Eight). As stated in step one, it is key to include the recruitment team in the timeline process and delineate their responsibilities in the completion of the campaign. This timeline serves as an on-going communication tool for the sponsor, CRO, SMO and investigator site. Finally, an effective timeline should continually be fine-tuned to account for changes in strategy and requirements throughout the clinical trial. After the timeline has been established, then the recruitment materials to launch the campaign can be developed.

MEDIA STRATEGIES

Investigator Resource Kits

With almost forty-percent of all clinical development delays occurring in patient enrollment, it is imperative to provide the sites with effective recruitment tools at study start-up. Ideally, there would be an opportunity to present the prepared recruitment tools at the investigator meeting. Historically, this has generated greater buy-in from the sites, which increases the yield for more successful outcomes.

A tool that can help jump-start the enrollment at the site is the Investigator resource kit. This particular recruitment tool is user friendly and historically has been well received by the sites. The kit presents a multi-faceted approach to subject recruitment. For example, the kit contents may include: posters/fliers, print ad, news release, physician-to-patient letter and educational brochures. (See Table Nine for a sample news release) These materials can be used as internal and/or external marketing tools as well as a referral tool amongst fellow physicians. When developing these materials, it is important to keep in mind that the materials should be designed to be used concurrently to elicit a higher response rate, but may be used independently if elected.

Additionally, surveying the sites at least annually is an effective way of determining what materials are useful to the sites regarding recruitment. From this statistical data, what materials should and should not be included in a resource kit can be deciphered as well as geographic market preferences. In a recent survey of research study coordinators, 84% responded that this type of resource material was helpful in recruiting subjects.[7]

Sample News Release — Table 9

CONTACT: (Insert name of contact person) (Insert Phone Number)

FOR IMMEDIATE RELEASE (Date)

IS KNEE PAIN AFFECTING YOUR EVERY STEP?

City,— It is estimated that 20.7 million Americans are affected by osteoarthritis. A variety of factors such as age and joint injuries may lead to osteoarthritis, which is characterized by a breakdown of cartilage causing the bones to rub against each other creating pain and loss of movement.

(Insert Clinic Name) is currently seeking individuals to participate in a clinical research study to evaluate an investigational medication that may potentially decrease knee pain associated with osteoarthritis.

If you have been diagnosed with osteoarthritis, are between the ages of 30 and 75 and currently experiencing knee pain, you may qualify for this research study. Qualified participants will receive study related physical exams, laboratory tests and study medication.

To learn more about how you may potentially benefit from this research study, call (INSERT CONTACT NUMBER).

Case Study: For this particular study, the resource kits and materials were approved and distributed to all the sites prior to study start-up. The kit contained a news release, radio script, physician-to-patient letter, physician-to-physician letter, fliers, posters, print advertisement and educational brochures. By providing the sites with these materials prior to study start-up, the recruitment group was able to contact each site and help facilitate a recruitment plan with each site. The research staff found the materials to be very helpful in broadening the awareness of the study. Many of the sites used a combination of techniques to generate interest in study participation. For example, one site placed local advertisements in their community paper, mailed the physician-to-patient letter to their database, and provided their local Arthritis Foundation Chapter with study fliers to be included with the distribution of the Chapter's newsletter. (See Table Ten for a sample of an educational brochure)

Direct-to-Consumer Strategies

The public's perception about clinical trials is the greatest hurdle one must overcome when developing direct-to-consumer marketing mate-

Table 10

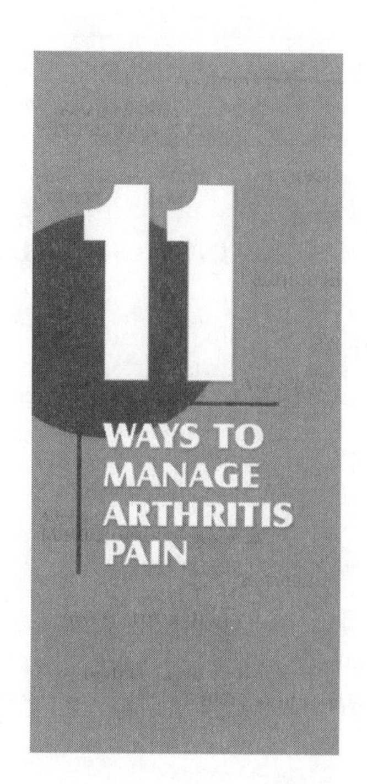

rials. The public's lack of awareness, misunderstanding, and fears about research can be primary deterrents to participation in clinical trials. Successful recruitment in clinical trials is based on how well a message is communicated to the public and how well they understand the purpose of the trial.[8] Some of the newest trends in research subject recruitment are the use of targeted direct mailings and Internet listings.

Direct Mail

The success of a direct mail campaign is dependent upon getting your message into the hands of your target audience. The target audience can be identified through internal database searches (research sites, CRO and SMO) or through external database vendors. By specifically defining the target group, the rate of return can potentially increase. Typically, a general direct mail campaign generates a 1% to 2% return. However, a targeted, direct mail campaign can generate up to a 4% return.

Case Study: In this clinical trial, a national direct mail campaign was implemented within 45 different geographic markets. Potential candidates were identified both through internal and external databases. Through an extensive search, a database vendor was selected who was able to identify individuals with osteoarthritis, met the age requirements, and were located in the desired geographical areas. The mailing went to 16,000 individuals using a toll-free call center number (Table Eleven). This allowed the recruitment vendor to accurately track the results of the campaign and make immediate modifications if necessary. For example, the recruitment team was able to gather responses based on geographic markets and could modify the distribution of the mailing to different zip code areas within a given market that could potentially generate a higher response rate. Although the response rate was approximately 1%, the mailing generated nineteen referrals (37% referral rate), which yielded five randomized patients (26% randomization rate). Overall, this was a cost-effective program. The cost per referral was $86.00.

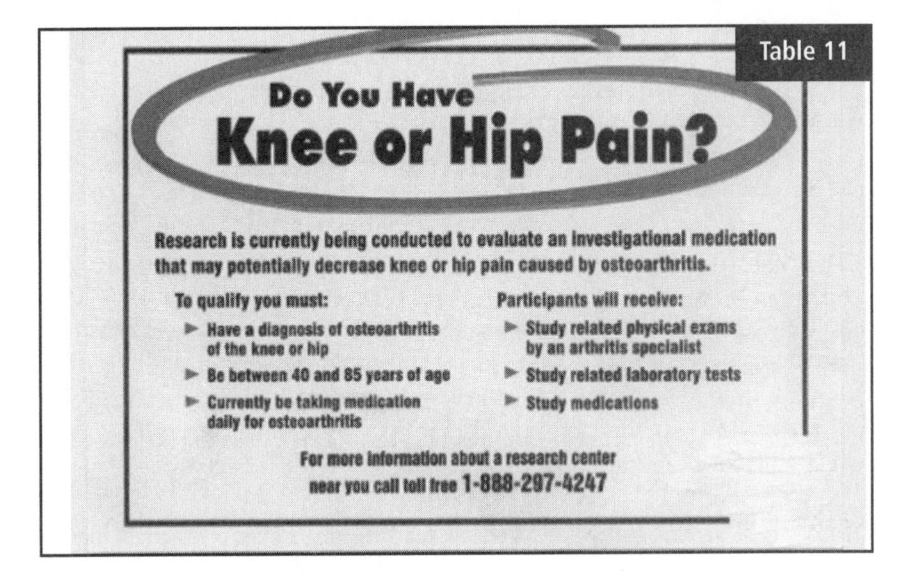

Table 11

Internet Listings

In addition to offering various mediums (TV, radio and newspaper) to reach potential study participants, other options include offering Internet-based patient recruitment solutions (please refer to Chapter Nine—Internet Based Patient Recruitment). Over the past three years, the use of the Internet to recruit subjects has increased by 45%. The success of any web site is to build and maintain high levels of traffic volume.[9] The same holds true for Internet advertising. The more visibility you can garner, the broader your reach, thus potentially increasing your response rate.

Case Study: For this particular study, the recruitment staff listed the trial on several trial listing sites as well as established viable links to credible arthritis web sites. Trial listing sites included the recruitment group's company site, CenterWatch, and the American College of Rheumatology. The recruitment vendor also established a link from the Arthritis National Research Foundation's web site to their web site where the trial was posted. The use of these web sites was chosen due to the therapeutic focus of this study as well as the level of visibility these sites have among the clinical trials industry. Similar to the direct mail campaign, the Internet listings used a toll-free call center number. This venue proved to be a value added supplement to the other recruitment tools employed. These efforts resulted in a 13% response rate and a 33% referral rate.

Call Center

Another important step in the implementation of this recruitment campaign was establishing a call center. Given the broad range of tactics used to recruit subjects for this study, the call center had to be able to receive information from every source.[10] As previously stated, the recruitment group elected to use a call center to handle the calls generated through both the direct mail and Internet campaigns as well as from site's local initiatives. Establishing this service allowed for the following: (1) ensured that the calls were being handled by screening personnel with medical backgrounds, (2) ensured the use of sponsor and IRB approved screening forms, (3) provided unlimited, national phone access, and (4) provided collection and analysis of statistical call screening data.

Not only is it important that the screening staff has a medical background, but it is just as important that they possess a strong understanding of the protocol and related questions that the subject may ask. Additionally, the staff must be able to work a flexible schedule. This allows for appropriate phone coverage to be available based on the campaign's launch as well as the call volume generated. A call center should be operational 24 hours a day, 7 days a week.

Case Study: Probably the most important aspect of utilizing a call center was our ability to concurrently analyze outcomes and make decisions about the campaign's success and next steps. For this particular study, a toll-free line was used to support the recruitment strategies. By establishing the use of a toll-free number, it allowed the recruitment team to accurately determine how well each initiative was working and to recommend which ones to continue, increase, or eliminate from the campaign.

Further, the Sponsor was provided with tracking reports that detailed the total number of calls, the source of the calls, the number of qualified calls and the number of calls referred to the site(s). Tracking the status of the referral(s) to the site is oftentimes the most challenging piece of data to collect. Prior to study start-up, a tracking system was put in place at each participating site to capture the status of each referral. The capturing of this data was handled by a recruitment coordinator; and therefore, did not create any additional burden on the sites. Finally, the use of the call center allowed the call response system to be streamlined. This enables more effective elimination of unqualified subjects, identification of prequalified subjects and provision of management assistance to the sites. Therefore, the recruitment group was able to help the sites process the referrals and ensure the subjects arrival and potential enrollment into the study.

STEP SIX: CONDUCTING SITE MANAGEMENT SERVICES

Once the sites have been armed with a recruitment campaign that provides both local and national support, the recruitment group must establish an action plan to manage these strategies. Step six involves the creation of a system to handle the recruitment funds, track the results, evaluate each site's recruitment needs and assist the sites with the launch of their local initiatives.

Case Study: As stated in the case study synopsis, the SMO was contracted to develop, implement and manage a patient recruitment campaign for 45 sites across the United States. Within the development of the proposal (See Table Six), monies were allocated for each recruitment service. The SMO was responsible for setting up a study budget that captured all study expenses. Capturing this data was key when evaluating which strategies provided cost-effective and successful subject referrals. The following tracking data was collected from the sites and from the recruitment vendor:

- Calculating the number of scheduled patients
- Computing the number of pending appointments
- Determining the number of patients that qualified

- Tallying the number that did not qualify
- Calculating the number that qualified but declined participation
- Determining the number of randomized patients
- Tallying the number that completed the trial

Gathering this data served as to accurately analyze the recruitment team's recommendations to the sponsor regarding the continuation or elimination of particular marketing strategies. One thing to keep in mind is that a recruitment campaign is an on-going work in progress throughout the duration of the study.

Finally, the recruitment team contacted each site after they received their marketing materials to answer any questions the sites may have had at that time as well as evaluate and discuss the site's foreseen recruitment needs. Based on this data, the recruitment coordinator was able to identify with the site which local initiatives proved to be most successful for this particular type of study and in their given geographic area. The contact between the recruitment coordinator and the site is ongoing throughout the study. On a weekly basis, the recruitment team evaluated each site's enrollment performance and weighed it against any recruitment strategies in place. This allowed the team to continually fine-tune the message and media strategy to meet the site's needs, thus achieving maximum results for the overall study. In turn, all of this data was shared with the sponsor on a weekly basis so that they had a first-hand understanding of the campaign results and overall impact on the recruitment budget. For example, the recruitment vendor provided the sponsor with a recruitment report that showed advertising initiatives in place for each site, the responses to these advertisements, and the amount of monies spent on each advertisement. From this data, the recruitment vendor also provided the sponsor with the total cost per randomized subject.

CASE OUTCOMES

The case study selected for demonstration purposes is currently ongoing. However, the recruitment outcomes captured thus far demonstrate the effects these tactics have had on enrollment statistics. First, by providing the sites with user-friendly recruitment materials at the onset of the study, the sites were able to pre-identify potential candidates. Once the study was initiated, the sites already had potential subjects scheduled for screening. Secondly, with the use of the targeted direct mailings and the Internet trial listings, sites were able to receive potential candidates outside their research practice. Thirdly, using the central call center allowed the research staff to focus on the study participants and to conduct detailed chart reviews. The recruitment team was responsible for referring potential subjects to the sites and following up with the sites to determine whether or not the subject was randomized. Finally, conducting site management services was an on-going process throughout the study. In addition to managing the elected recruitment tactics, the recruitment team was able to help the site facilitate grass-roots campaigns in their local communities.

CONCLUSION

With the number of clinical research trials steadily increasing, the need for study subjects continues to grow. Further, the level of difficulty related to study design for these studies is also increasing. This creates additional challenges to identifying potential subjects by narrowing the target audience. Based on the case study, the key to a successful patient recruitment campaign is developing a multi-faceted approach that will reach the target audience through multiple venues. It is through a combination of different mediums that optimal results will be achieved.

This chapter focused on a six-step process that devised a comprehensive patient recruitment campaign from contracting to completion. Through the use of a case study, the correlation of these steps in the formulation of a comprehensive recruitment campaign was demonstrated. Industry trends indicate that sponsors will continue to outsource services, like patient recruitment. Now that resources are flowing into recruitment efforts, the next horizon will be of greater accountability linking those resources to effective recruitment.[5] Ultimately, those coordinating these efforts must be able to establish cost-effective recruitment campaigns that speed the clinical trial process. The tools presented in this chapter should serve as a guide to help create a cost-effective campaign to do just that!

REFERENCES

[1] Chicago Center for Clinical Research, Survey of Sponsors and CROs, 1994.

[2] TheMediciGroup, Inc., 1998.

[3] "Maximizing the Benefits of SMOs." John R. Vogel. Applied Clinical

Trials. November 1999, Volume 8, Number 11. p. 56.

[4] "Patient Recruitment Comes of Age." Medical Marketing & Media. BBK Patient Recruitment. April 1999.

[5] "Planning and Evaluating Patient Recruitment Strategies—The Proof is in the Metrics." European Pharmaceutical Contractor. Diana L. Anderson, Ph.D. February 2000. p. 52-54, 57 & 59.

[6] Osteoarthritis Case Study Market Research Findings, Rheumatology Research International, January–February 1999.

[7] Patient Recruitment Resource Survey, Rheumatology Research International, January 2000.

[8] *Matthews Media Group Report on Patient Involvement in Clinical Trials*. Matthews Media Group, Inc.

[9] "Surfing for Study Subjects." CenterWatch. Lisa Henderson. February 2000, Volume 7, Issue 2. p. 1, 5, & 10.

[10] "Hiring a Call Center." Protocols A Quarterly Patient Recruitment Newsletter. BBK Patient Recruitment, Winter 2000. p. 2-3.

AUTHOR BIOGRAPHY

Melynda Geurts is the Vice President of Communications for Rheumatology Research International (RRI), a comprehensive rheumatology service provider. Ms. Geurts manages the development of new business opportunities for the Communications Division and oversees the scope of services related to patient recruitment, call center, and custom publishing. Additionally, she coordinates the company's image building and branding efforts throughout the pharmaceutical industry.

Previously, Ms. Geurts was a Government Programs Specialist for NYLCare Health Plans of the Southwest, Inc., a nationally known Health Maintenance Organization. She was responsible for expanding the service network for the NYLCare 65 Medicare Risk product. Ms. Geurts' expertise is in healthcare marketing. She holds a M.S. in Healthcare Administration and a B.B.A. in Marketing from Texas Woman's University. She is a member of the Association of Clinical Research Professionals (ACRP), co-chair for the communications committee for the ACRP, and a public education committee member for the North Texas Arthritis Foundation chapter.

CHAPTER 18

Patient Recruitment Campaign From Contracting to Completion: A Therapeutic-Specific Case Study

Leslie Clark Lewis, AmericasDoctor

Patient recruitment—the words strike fear into the hearts of many a pharmaceutical company executive. When enrollment timelines are not met, clinical development programs fall behind, sales opportunities are lost and costs increase. How can a process that seems so straightforward actually present so many opportunities to fail? What are the elements of a successful patient recruitment program? How can we get it right the first time? The following is a case study where planned recruitment initiatives paid off and the sponsor's predetermined enrollment timelines were actually met ahead of schedule.

MARKETING APPROVED DRUGS

To understand how the patient recruitment landscape is changing, it is important to look at what has been happening with the marketing of approved drugs. Traditionally, pharmaceutical companies have marketed directly to physicians through sales representatives who provide educational information and drug samples to stimulate prescribing of the drug.

A newer approach to the marketing of approved drugs is to advertise directly to the consumer. Advertising educates consumers about the pharmaceutical company's therapeutic alternative and drives the patients into physician offices to request the drug. It is expected that the patient will discuss the advertised drug with the physician and, if appropriate, the physician will prescribe the drug to the patient.

Direct-to-consumer advertising by the pharmaceutical industry is the fastest growing segment of DTC advertising. Pharmaceutical companies spent $595 million on direct-to-consumer advertising in 1996. The direct-to-consumer spend is estimated to reach in excess of $1.75 billion in 2000.[1]

THE OLD PATIENT RECRUITMENT FORMULA—WHY IT IS FAILING

Similarly, the "old way" of recruiting patients is to rely exclusively on the investigational sites. The idea is to find the doctors who "have the patients" and avoid sites with competing protocols. Local, site-by-site recruitment advertising might be used, but on a limited basis. If enrollment fails to reach goals, additional sites can be added.

Clinical development programs have become much more competitive. The number of clinical trials per NDA is expected to hit 75 in 2000, up from 36 in 1985.[2] The average number of patients per NDA is expected to grow from 3,233 in 1985 to approximately 4,850 in 2000.[3] The result of this growth is increased competition for patients!

Finally, rescue recruitment is a big part of the old formula. Most sponsors underestimate their need for patient recruitment support. They look at recruitment efforts in terms of money spent, not time saved. Instead of developing proactive plans, they wait until recruitment is in trouble before initiating rescue efforts. So they pay double: once for the expensive rescue program itself, and again for the lost time and opportunity costs.

A CenterWatch poll indicates that 80% of all clinical trials do not meet enrollment timelines.[4]

THE NEW RECRUITMENT FORMULA—TAKING A CUE FROM CURRENT PHARMA MARKETING STRATEGIES

The new way of recruiting patients is to apply the lessons learned in marketing approved drugs: treat the clinical trial as a new product launch. As with marketed drugs, a clinical trial competes with the currently available therapeutic alternatives. So site efforts must be supplemented by a centrally managed, direct-to-consumer advertising program with a well-chosen message targeted to the study patient population.

Of course, not every clinical trial requires or is appropriate for an aggressive recruitment program. But when timelines are critical, and the study is right for a full-service recruitment program, advertising will be the driver of accelerated enrollment.

There are, however, key differences between patient recruitment advertising and post marketing "image advertising." Patient recruitment advertising necessitates a direct response, namely getting people to pick up the phone immediately. This kind of advertising is done in only cities/markets in which a study is being conducted, and under specific time constraints. Therefore, recruitment media must be purchased in sufficient strength to generate significant numbers of calls in each market. The shorter, defined enrollment periods do not allow time for the collateral marketing activities (i.e., detailing, promotions, sponsorships and contests) used to build brand strength and visibility over a sustained period of time.

THE CASE STUDY

This case study involved a Phase III clinical trial of an investigational medication to treat urge urinary incontinence. Urge incontinence is a chronic medical condition that affects nearly 13 million Americans, 11 million of whom are women. The effects of incontinence range from mere inconvenience to near total social isolation because of fear of "wetting accidents" and embarrassment. The financial costs associated with incontinence-related care are high, with over $16 billion spent annually in the U.S.[5]

The sponsor, a mid-size pharmaceutical company, was determined to meet all milestones in its extremely tight drug development timeline. To accomplish this, they contracted with a large contract research organization (CRO) for project management, monitoring, CRF development, drug supply management, laboratory services, report writing and data management.

They also utilized the services of a large site management organization (SMO-A) whose investigators were experienced in conducting urge incontinence trials. SMO-A provided:

- 30 sites
- Site Management Services for site selection assistance, regulatory submission, budgeting and contracting, investigator payments and site communications
- Patient Recruitment Services for development and implementation of a centrally-managed patient recruitment program across all sites

Finally, the sponsor selected six sites from a second SMO (SMO-B), and four independent sites.

Thirty-nine of the forty sites were able to utilize the study's central IRB, which facilitated efficient regulatory approvals, including the recruitment program, and faster study start-up.

PLANNING TO SUCCEED

Approximately four months before study start-up, the sponsor and SMO-A Recruitment Services personnel began discussions about enrollment and recruitment issues. Recruitment Services presented an aggressive proposal that they believed would ensure meeting the sponsor's four-month enrollment goal.

Because SMO-A's sites had conducted forty-four incontinence clinical trials within the past five years, they were uniquely qualified to advise the sponsor about the current challenges in enrolling incontinence studies:

- Two recently approved incontinence drugs were being heavily advertised to patients at that time.
- Investigators advised they could identify fewer patients from within their practices who were not already taking one of the marketed therapies.
- Patients frequently do not care to participate in a trial if they are satisfied with current treatment.
- Competing clinical trials were being conducted concurrently across the U.S.
- Incontinence trial advertising was producing fewer responses post-launch of the two-marketed drugs.

- Similar studies were taking 7–12 months to enroll even with moderate direct-to-consumer recruitment advertising.
- High screen failure rates for urge incontinence studies mandated aggressive outreach for study participants.
- Approved and successful therapies were available to patients without their having to turn to research.
- Patients reported concerns about studies.
- Placebo-control.
- Rx wash-out periods.
- Concomitant medication exclusions.
- Transportation, especially for the elderly.
- Anxieties about a new physician (if identified through advertising or referrals)
- Concern about "accidents" away from home
- The study was scheduled to open for enrollment on December 20. Patient recruitment during the holiday season is significantly slower than at other times of the year.

THE CONTRACT

The sponsor agreed that a proactive program was required and was willing to invest in an aggressive recruitment campaign. They selected SMO-A's Recruitment Services to develop and run the program. The budget was approved, with a "reward/rebate" clause. This provided a bonus to Recruitment Services if enrollment timelines were exceeded, or a rebate from Recruitment Services to the sponsor if enrollment timelines were not met. Recruitment Services contracted directly with the sponsor. The CRO contracted its services separately.

THE SPONSOR'S GOALS

- 480 randomized patients
- 4 month randomization window (including a 1 month run-in)
- 40 sites
- 30 SMO-A
- 6 SMO-B
- 4 independent
- 12 patients per site
- Competitive enrollment
- Estimated 40% screen failure rate

PROGRAM ELEMENTS

Recruitment Services experience shows that a successful patient recruitment program must tackle enrollment challenges on a number of levels. They developed a multi-tiered approach to motivate the sites, maximize opportunities for patient identification and facilitate study leads as efficiently as possible. The plan included the following elements, which will be described below:

- Recruitment Planning
- Site Integration
- Site Buy-in
- Investigator Meeting Presentation
- Site Conference Calls
- Patient Registry
- Media Campaign
- Central Call Screening and Scheduling
- Recruitment Materials
- Management Conference Calls
- Metrics Collection and Reporting

Recruitment Planning—Tapping into Site Expertise

Experienced investigators and coordinators are excellent resources for patient recruitment ideas and planning. Recruitment Services, along with their call center and advertising agency partners, held a conference call with an expert panel of investigators and coordinators from selected study sites. They verified the target patient demographic, and discussed the screening script language and the advertising message. The information provided by site personnel was invaluable to Recruitment Services as they finalized the recruitment program elements.

Pre-study Conference Calls—Getting Site Buy-in

Next in the process was introducing the program study-wide. Recruitment Services held pre-study conference calls with all trial sites to review and reinforce the plan. Getting sites to "buy-in" to the recruitment program would be crucial, as they would be more committed to its implementation. In addition, there were some elements of the program that would be challenging for the sites, such as central call scheduling, that warranted site feedback and input. A newsletter summarizing the discussion was sent to each site.

Investigator Meeting Presentation

The Recruitment Services team, including director, two recruitment managers and call center project manager, reviewed the recruitment program details at the Investigator Meeting and led a feedback discussion. Nearly all of the forty study sites attended. The presentation provided an excellent opportunity to personally introduce Recruitment Services team members to site personnel. Sites were enthusiastic about the recruitment program elements and expressed commitment to the enrollment goals.

During the discussions, special emphasis was placed on central call screening, patient scheduling and the sites' reporting requirements. The sponsor's lead representative reinforced the mandate that sites provide blocks of time for call center personnel to schedule patient screening appointments. This would eliminate the "phone tag" that often occurs between site and patient. The longer a caller must wait for a "close," the less likely the caller will be interested in participating.

A number of sites questioned this requirement. However, because the protocol allowed the screening appointment to be scheduled with the coordinator rather than the investigator, sites more readily agreed to call center scheduling. Study coordinators completed site information forms (site location, directions, parking instructions, after-hours telephone number) for the call center database.

Finally, the television commercial was shown to great enthusiasm.

The sponsor, CRO and Recruitment Services and both SMOs all worked very hard to convey the importance of the study, and there was a sense of excitement among the site investigators and coordinators to participate in a trial with extensive, proactive recruitment support.

Patient Registry Program

Prior to study start-up, sites were asked to prescreen patients from their practices and "register" with Recruitment Services those who were prequalified and interested in taking part. The program ensured that sites got a head start on patient identification and maximized use of their databases. It was also used to keep study staff motivated during the holiday season before the media campaign was implemented.

- Sites forwarded their registry logs to Recruitment Services each Friday for six weeks until study start-up.
- Sites that consented at least three patients from their registry list would receive a thank you gift.
- The goal was to have at least 3 patients per site preregistered and ready to screen at study start-up.

Media Campaign

Past experience shows that significant numbers of leads would be required to fill the trial within the enrollment period. Television advertising, supplemented by limited radio/print in selected markets, was the medium of choice for the study. Because the study's target demographic was women 50 and older, much of the television buy would be during daytime hours, with their more affordable rates.

- The advertising program began on January 3, four weeks after the Investigator Meeting .
- Since direct response advertising is not as effective during the holiday season, Recruitment Services delayed the media campaign until the first of the year.
- Media rates are also less expensive during the first quarter, so the strong media buy required was more affordable.
- Two weeks of advertising were scheduled:
    - One week with ads running
    - One week with no ads running (to allow sites to process patient leads)
    - One week with ads running
- The commercial was filmed, not videotaped, resulting in a higher quality spot.
- All media was researched, placed and billed centrally.
- Call volumes, as expected, were significantly high.

Central Call Screening and Scheduling

Central call screening prescreens volunteers so only those who appear to qualify are referred to the sites. Because a significant number of advertising-generated calls were expected, such screening ensured that calls were answered immediately and screened consistently across all study sites. Initial start-up activities included:

- Call center database programming, including call guide, data entry screens and reports.
- Call center staff training, including script details, frequently asked questions, background information on incontinence, pronunciation guide.
- Additional staff hiring and training due to the anticipated call volume.

The call center leads were facilitated and tracked as follows:

- Callers responding to advertising were screened centrally by call center personnel.
- Qualified leads were scheduled for screening appointments by call center personnel; if available appointment times were not convenient, leads were forwarded directly to the sites for call back.
- Recruitment Services recorded metrics and reported to CRO/sponsor:
    - Number of calls received
    - Number of prequalified volunteers
    - Number of scheduled volunteers
    - Number of volunteers who did not qualify (and reasons for disqualification)

Site personnel completed a telephone "mini-screen" of patients prior to their appointment to confirm eligibility and appointment time, and reported the disposition of referred patients to Recruitment Services.

Recruitment Materials for Site Use

Customized recruitment materials were provided to sites to promote the study within their own practices and communities and included:

- Posters
- Brochures
- Physician to Patient Letters
- Physician to Physician Letters
- Public Service Announcement
- Inclusion/Exclusion Laminated "at a glance" Cards

Periodic site conference calls

During enrollment, conference calls were held with sponsor, CRO, Recruitment Services, SMO and site personnel. They reviewed the on-going program, assessed site recruitment efforts and successes, and secured feedback from sites on the advertising and central call screening efforts. The recruitment program was viewed as a work in progress and open to re-evaluation. When sites had comments, questions, or suggestions for the program, they would share during the calls or one-on-one with Recruitment Services personnel.

Weekly Management Team Conference Calls with Sponsor, CRO, Recruitment Services, SMO-A and SMO-B

To ensure successful communications among the study management personnel, weekly management team conference calls were held. Recruitment and enrollment were included on the call agenda.

Site Metrics Collection

To make a final determination on the recruitment program outcomes, sites reported the source of each patient (i.e., patient registry, advertising, physician referral) on the CRO's screening/enrollment log. Having only one log to complete that was shared by both the CRO and Recruitment Services saved site personnel time and aggravation.

THE OUTCOME

The recruitment program certainly met all expectations. Sites got a great start by screening their preregistered patients, and they immediately began receiving leads from the call center once the media campaign began. Enrollment was completed in 3-1/2 months (including a one month run-in), beating the sponsor's enrollment goal by two weeks.

Combining the Recruitment Services and CRO reports, the outcomes showed:

Calls generated from the media campaign:	8,734
Prequalified leads sent to the sites:	2,806
Patients screened by sites in 2-1/2 months:	1,133
Including 317 preregistered patients	
Patients screen failed:	609
Patients randomized in 3-1/2 months:	522
Including 1 month run-in	

Approximately 70% of the randomized patients came from the advertising program and 30% from practices.

CHALLENGES AS WE WENT ALONG

The screen failure rate turned out to be higher than anticipated. Original projections were 40%; the final rate was calculated at 54%, a 35% increase. Fortunately, the advertising program generated sufficient numbers of volunteers to make up the difference.

Patient scheduling was somewhat problematic. Many patients were unable to make appointments during the blocks of time provided, so their information was forwarded to sites with the understanding that sites would call them back within 24 hours. Some sites were unable to return calls within this timeframe, but nearly all patients were eventually accounted for.

The screening volumes were large. But sites had been chosen on their ability to complete screening and enrollment within four months, and they responded to the challenge.

LESSONS LEARNED

- The squeaky wheel gets the grease! This study was very high profile and had the full attention of site personnel.

- Careful pre-planning, experienced recruitment management personnel and integration of the program with the sites were critical to the program's success.

- The study could never have met its enrollment goal and timeline without the aggressive advertising program coupled with central call screening.

- Even with extensive advertising, study sites can be diligent in accessing their own practice patients for the study. Twenty-one sites received a deluxe cookie assortment as a thank you gift for each screening at least three pre-registered patients. A total of 317 pre-registered patients were screened.

• Studies utilizing central IRBs and SMOs can frequently get off to a faster start. In this trial, all thirty SMO-A sites were IRB approved and ready to screen by January 3 (study start-up was December 20). One budget and one contract covered all SMO-A sites.

CONCLUSION

The study sponsor was extremely pleased that enrollment ended two weeks ahead of plan. The lead sponsor representative noted, "Everyone always underestimates the effort and expense required for a successful recruitment campaign. Even now, only a few months after recruitment ended, it is easy to forget how much effort was put into it. But success is always easier than the strife and expense that failure causes."

REFERENCES

[1] Freeman, Laurie. "Accepting the Risks." Advertising Age. April 3, 2000. p. S-14.

[2] PAREXEL Pharmaceutical R&D Statistical Sourcebook, 1999. p. 56, PAREXEL International Corporation, Waltham, MA.

[3] *Ibid.*, p. 80.

[4] "An Industry in Evolution." Boston, MA: CenterWatch, Inc. 1998: p. 264.

[5] Fantl J, Newman D, Colling J, et al. *Urinary Incontinence in Adults: Acute and Chronic Management*. Clinical Practice Guideline No. 2, 1996 Update. Rockville, Maryland: U.S. Department of Health and Human Services. Public Health Service, Agency for Health Care Policy and Research, 1996.

AUTHOR BIOGRAPHY

Leslie Clark Lewis is the Director of Patient Recruitment at AmericasDoctor. Ms. Lewis oversees the planning and implementation of all study-wide recruitment programs. She joined AmericasDoctor in 1996.

Ms. Lewis has been involved in clinical trials for more than ten years. Immediately prior to joining AmericasDoctor, she directed the Center for Clinical Studies, the clinical research program of the Department of Medicine at Rush-Presbyterian-St. Luke's Medical Center in Chicago. Ms. Lewis began her career in clinical trials at the Chicago Center for Clinical Research where she developed all patient recruitment programs as well as corporate marketing efforts.

Throughout her career, Ms. Lewis has been an enthusiastic advocate for outreach programs that enable the public to access study participation opportunities, and for centrally managed recruitment programs that successfully accelerate study enrollment.

Calls Received 1/15

Cumulative Qualified Count to Date		
Investigator	State	Qualified
101	Los Angeles, CA	122
102	Kansas City, MO	82
103	Washington, DC	121
104	Tucson, AZ	89
105	Los Angeles, CA	131
106	Des Moines, IA	84
107	Austin, TX	79
108	Ft. Lauderdale, FL	118
109	Washington, DC	109
110	Los Angeles, CA	126
Total		1,061

Investigator	Market	Total # Calls	Not Referred -DNQ -No site nearby -Calling for info	Qualified	Appts. Made	Sites to Call
101	Los Angeles, CA	67	39	28	16	12
102	Kansas City, MO	42	19	23	17	6
103	Washington, DC	54	27	27	13	14
104	Tucson, AZ	39	20	19	9	10
105	Los Angeles, CA	62	28	34	18	16
106	Des Moines, IA	41	22	19	10	9
107	Austin, TX	43	24	19	12	7
108	Ft. Lauderdale, FL	66	34	32	17	15
109	Washington, DC	49	23	26	16	10
110	Los Angeles, CA	64	35	29	15	14
site/info only		174	174			
Subtotals		701	445	256	143	113
	Total Qualified Calls			256		

About CenterWatch

ABOUT CENTERWATCH

CenterWatch is a Boston-based publishing company that focuses on the clinical trials industry. We provide a variety of information services used by pharmaceutical and biotechnology companies, CROs, SMOs, and investigative sites involved in the management and conduct of clinical trials. CenterWatch also provides education materials for clinical research professionals, health professionals and for health consumers. Some of our top publications and services are described below. For a comprehensive listing with detailed information about our publications and services, please visit our web site at *www.centerwatch.com.*

PERIODICALS

CENTERWATCH

A monthly newsletter that provides pharmaceutical and biotechnology companies, CROs, SMOs, research centers and the investment community with in-depth business news, feature articles on trends, original research and analysis, as well as grant lead information for investigative sites.

CENTERWATCH EUROPE

A quarterly electronic newsletter dedicated to providing news, information and analyses on the clinical trials industry in the European Union. *CenterWatch Europe* presents in-depth stories, data and analyses on all aspects of the relationship between pharmaceutical companies, CROs and investigator sites.

CWWEEKLY

A weekly fax and electronic newsletter that reports on the top stories in the clinical trials industry. Each weekly newsletter includes business headlines, financial information, market intelligence, drug pipeline and clinical trials results from the prior week.

JOBWATCH

A web-based resource at *www.centerwatch.com* that provides a comprehensive listing of career and educational opportunities in the clinical trials industry. Companies use *JobWatch* regularly to identify qualified clinical research professionals.

Research Practitioner

A peer-reviewed journal published every other month, filled with informative and pertinent articles about clinical research practice and methods. A continuing education component is included with each issue of *Research Practitioner*, so readers can apply for CEUs or CME credits.

Books and Services

An Industry in Evolution

A 300-page source book of charts, data tables and statistics on the clinical trials industry. The material is presented in a well organized and easy-to-reference format. This important and valuable resource is used for developing business strategies and plans, for preparing presentations and for conducting business and market intelligence.

The 2001/2002 Industry Directory

A comprehensive directory with over 1,000 pages of contact information and detailed company profiles for a wide range of organizations and individuals involved in the clinical trials industry. Considered the authoritative reference resource to organizations involved in designing, managing, conducting and supporting clinical trials.

The Investigator's Guide to Clinical Research

A 250-page step-by-step resource filled with tips, instructions and insights for health professionals interested in conducting clinical trials. The *Investigator's Guide* is designed to help the novice clinical investigator get involved in conducting clinical trials. The guide is also a valuable resource for experienced investigative sites looking for ways to improve and increase their involvement and success in clinical research.

Protecting Study Volunteers In Research

Recommended by the National Institutes of Health and the Office of Health and Human Services, *Protecting Study Volunteers in Research* is a 250-page manual designed to assist clinical research professionals in providing the highest standards of safety and ethical treatment for their study volunteers. Written specifically for academic institutions and IRBs actively involved in clinical trials, the manual is also applicable to independent investigative sites. The book has been developed in accordance with the ACCME. Readers can apply for CME credits or Nursing Credit Hours. An exam is provided with each manual.

THE DIRECTORY OF DRUGS IN CLINICAL TRIALS

A comprehensive compilation of new, leading-edge medications currently in research, this directory offers a glimpse at new and upcoming treatment options in phase II–III clinical trials. The Directory provides easy reference information on more than 1,300 drugs in active clinical trials across a variety of clinical conditions. Detailed information is provided on each drug listed.

THE CENTERWATCH CLINICAL TRIALS LISTING SERVICE'

Now in its sixth year of operation, *The CenterWatch Clinical Trials Listing Service*™ provides the largest and most comprehensive listing of industry-sponsored clinical trials on the Internet. In 2001 alone, the CenterWatch web site—along with numerous coordinated online and print affiliations—is expected to reach more than 5 million Americans. *The CenterWatch Clinical Trials Listing Service*™ provides an international listing of nearly 10,000, ongoing and IRB-approved phase I–IV clinical trials.

VOLUNTEERING FOR A CLINICAL TRIAL

An easy-to-read, six-page patient education brochure designed for research centers to provide consistent, professional and unbiased educational information for their potential clinical study subjects. The brochure is IRB approved. Sponsors, CROs and investigative sites use this brochure to inform patients about participating in clinical trials. *Volunteering for a Clinical Trial* can be distributed in a variety of ways including direct mailings to patients, displayed in waiting rooms, or as handouts to guide discussions. The brochure can be customized with company logos and custom information.

Standard Operating Procedures For Good Clinical Practice At The Investigative Site

Designed to be customized for your research facility, this easy-to-use template is based on the ICH/GCP Consolidated Guidelines and the Code of Federal Regulations and is pertinent to the day-to-day conduct of clinical research. The printed template is provided in a 3-ring binder and on 2 diskettes (in Word 95/97) for installation on your computer.

For more information about these and other CenterWatch publications and services, please call us at (617) 856-5940 or visit our web site at *www.centerwatch.com*.